# Key Heterocyclic Cores for Smart Anticancer Drug–Design

## *Part I*

Edited by

**Rajesh Kumar Singh**
*Department of Pharmaceutical Chemistry,*
*Shivalik College of Pharmacy, Nangal*
*IKG Punjab Technical University,*
*Jalandhar, Punjab, 140126,*
*India*

# Key Heterocyclic Cores for Smart Anticancer Drug–Design

*Part I*

Editor: Rajesh Kumar Singh

ISBN (Online): 978-981-5040-07-4

ISBN (Print): 978-981-5040-08-1

ISBN (Paperback): 978-981-5040-09-8

First Published in 2022.

need for a court order if at any point you breach any terms of this License Agreement. In no event will any delay or failure by Bentham Science Publishers in enforcing your compliance with this License Agreement constitute a waiver of any of its rights.

3. You acknowledge that you have read this License Agreement, and agree to be bound by its terms and conditions. To the extent that any other terms and conditions presented on any website of Bentham Science Publishers conflict with, or are inconsistent with, the terms and conditions set out in this License Agreement, you acknowledge that the terms and conditions set out in this License Agreement shall prevail.

**Bentham Science Publishers Pte. Ltd.**
80 Robinson Road #02-00
Singapore 068898
Singapore
Email: subscriptions@benthamscience.net

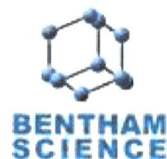

# CONTENTS

# FOREWORD

Cancer is a blemish on the face of humanity in this age of science and technology. While significant progress has been made in the treatment of cancer over the last 50 years, it remains a serious public health concern, necessitating extensive research into new therapeutic approaches. Despite the availability of a number of anticancer medications, problems like multidrug resistance, less therapeutic efficacy, solubility, undesirable side effects, and/or low bioavailability necessitate the creation of novel anticancer treatments. Because of their outstanding pharmacological activity, particularly their anticancer characteristics, heterocyclic compounds have been the primary molecules in organic chemistry for more than a century.

This book entitled **'Key Heterocyclic Cores for Smart Anticancer Drug-Design'** is a detailed assessment of some of the most intriguing hot topics for developing novel anticancer chemotherapeutics. This book aims to help readers quickly grasp the biological targets, structure-activity relationship (SAR), existing problems, and future prospects of heterocyclic-based anticancer medicines.

I'm really enthusiastic about this book and looking forward to its publication at the earliest possible. This book serves as a resource for health care providers, researchers, academicians, and medicinal chemists. The authors and Bentham publishers deserve praise for delivering timely and relevant information.

**Raj Kumar, Ph.D., FRSC**
Department of Pharmaceutical Sciences and Natural Products
Central University of Punjab
Bathinda 151 401,
Punjab, India

# PREFACE

Cancer, which is spreading worldwide, is becoming the leading cause of significant deaths. Today's most daunting task for global researchers is to develop anticancer leads with minimal side effects. Heterocyclic chemistry is an important and unique class of medicinal chemistry as many drugs being used in chemotherapy have a heterocyclic ring as their basic structure, despite various side effects.

The first part of this book **"Key Heterocyclic Cores for Smart Anticancer Drug-Design"** is focused on various green methodologies for the synthesis of these heterocyclic cores. Furthermore, different chapters provide insight into the structure-activity relationship (SAR) of heterocyclic cores to reveal different pharmacophores accountable for anticancer activity. The Part I comprises 6 scholarly-written review articles by leading researchers in the field, covering a broad range of topics.

The variety of natural compounds is indispensable for their anticancer action. For many years, these natural compounds have provided the basis for the development of diverse new classes of synthetic chemotherapeutic agents. In the first chapter of this book, Bachar *et al.* concentrate on recent research on various classes of natural scaffolds and their analogues that possess potent antitumour activity. Analysis of preclinical and/or clinically investigated natural compounds along with structural modification, structure-activity relationship, and molecular mechanisms of anticancer activity has also been discussed.

Recent efforts in the research and development of anticancer drugs derived from natural products have led to the identification of numerous heterocyclic terpenes that inhibit cell proliferation, metastasis, apoptosis, and other mechanisms. Chapter 2 by Chopra *et al.* explores the anticancer terpenoidal components that may promise and potentially open new opportunities for cancer therapy.

Among various heterocyclic scaffolds, benzothiazole (BT) is one of the most privileged moieties that exhibit a broad spectrum of biological activities such as anticancer, antidiabetic, anti-inflammatory, antiviral, antifungal, *etc*. The third chapter by Kumar *et al.* discusses the recent research done on benzothiazole scaffolds against the various biological targets for their anticancer activity. The chapter furnishes advancements on benzothiazole-containing drugs under clinical trials and those drugs that have been granted patents recently.

Nowadays, hybrid molecule drug designs attract a great deal of attention among organic and medicinal chemists. Among the different natural sources, quinoline, quinolone, and their hybrid derivatives are the most privileged ones. In Chapter 4, Panda *et al.* reviews the SAR study of recent literature (2017–2020) of hybrid quinoline and quinolone derivatives that act as anticancer agents through various mechanisms such as Bcl-2 inhibition, ALDH inhibition, kinase inhibition, topo-II, and EGFR-TK inhibition, *etc*.

Among all heterocycles, tetrazoles have gained attention in recent years due to their vast biological activity spectrum. The tetrazole ring has a structural similarity to carboxylic acids and hence serves as a bio isostere analogue. Chapter 5 by Unnamatala *et al.* explores the synthetic chemistry of the tetrazole nucleus and SAR studies of various tetrazole derivatives with promising activity, bioavailability against both drug-resistant and sensitive cancers, and reduced toxicity with numerous mechanisms of action.

Researchers and scientists have paid much attention to the drug design and drug discovery of nitrogen (N) and oxygen (O) based heterocyclic compounds in the last decade. Chapter 6 by Choudhary *et al.* compiles a dataset of advances (2017-2020) in various nitrogen and oxygen-containing heterocyclic rings with anticancer activities along with their structure-activity relationship (SAR) studies.

The editors would like to convey their gratitude to all contributors s for their hard and scholarly work.We are also grateful to Mr. Mahmood Alam (Director of Publication) and Ms. Humaira Hashmi (Manager Publication) of Bentham Science Publisher, who took over the management of the production of this book under the challenging circumstances of the COVID pandemic and whose contribution is much appreciated. We are confident that this book will help researchers, pharmacologists, and medicinal chemists learn about designing new and valuable novel heterocyclic anticancer drugs from synthetic and natural sources based on structure-activity-relationship studies.

**Rajesh Kumar Singh**
Department of Pharmaceutical Chemistry
Shivalik College of Pharmacy, Nangal,
IKG, Punjab Technical University
Jalandhar, Punjab, 140126,
India

# List of Contributors

| | |
|---|---|
| **Abdullah Al Hasan** | Department of Pharmacy, Southeast University, Dhaka, Bangladesh |
| **A.K.M. Shafiul Kadir** | Institute of Biological Sciences (IBSc), University of Rajshahi, Bangladesh |
| **Archana Kumari** | School of Pharmaceutical Sciences, Lovely Professional University, Phagwara - 144411, Punjab, India |
| **Ashwani Dhingra** | Guru Gobind Singh College of Pharmacy, Yamuna Nagar-135001, Haryana, India |
| **Bhawna Chopra** | Guru Gobind Singh College of Pharmacy, Yamuna Nagar-135001, Haryana, India |
| **Deo Nandan Prasad** | Shivalik College of Pharmacy, Nangal-140124, Punjab, India |
| **Erick Cuevas Yañez** | Facultad de Química, Universidad Autónoma del Estado de México, Carretera Toluca-Atlacomulco Km 14.5, Unidad San Cayetano, Toluca, Estado de México, C. P. 50200 México<br>Universidad autonoma del estado de Mexico, Toluca de Lerdo, Mexico |
| **Fazlur-Rahman Nawaz Khan** | Organic and Medicinal Chemistry Research Laboratory, School of Advanced Sciences, Vellore Institute of Technology, Vellore-632 014, Tamil Nadu, India |
| **Kanaya Lal Dhar** | Emeritus Scientist, Indian Institute of Integrative Medicine, CSIR, Jammu-180016, India |
| **Kunal Nepali** | Taipei Medical University, Taiwan |
| **Monika Sharma** | Department of Pharmaceutical Chemistry, Shivalik College of Pharmacy, Nangal Distt. Rupnagar, 140126, Punjab, India |
| **M.V. B. Unnamatla** | Universidad autonoma del estado de Mexico, Toluca de Lerdo, Mexico |
| **Pravati Panda** | Department of Chemistry, Ravenshaw University, Cuttack, Odisha 753 003, India |
| **Rajesh Kumar** | Department of Pharmaceutical Chemistry, Shivalik College of Pharmacy, Nangal Distt. Rupnagar, 140126, Punjab, India |
| **Rajesh K. Singh** | Department of Pharmaceutical Chemistry, Shivalik College of Pharmacy, Nangal Distt. Rupnagar, 140126, Punjab, India |
| **S.M. Riajul Wahab** | School of Pharmacy, The University of Texas at El Paso, Texas, USA |
| **Sahil Kumar** | Department of Pharmaceutical Chemistry, Delhi Institute of Pharmaceutical Sciences and Research (DIPSAR)-Delhi Pharmaceutical Sciences and Research University (DPSRU), New Delhi, 110017, India |
| **Sakshi Choudhary** | Department of Pharmaceutical Chemistry, Shivalik College of Pharmacy, Nangal, Dist. Rupnagar, 140126, Punjab, India |
| **Sarita Sharma** | Mount Carmel Sr.Sec. School, Rakkar Colony Distt. Una, 174303, Himachal Pradesh, India |
| **Sitesh C. Bachar** | Department of Pharmacy, Faculty of Pharmacy, University of Dhaka, Dhaka-1000, Bangladesh |
| **Subhendu Chakroborty** | IES University, Bhopal, Madhya Pradesh, 462044, India |

# CHAPTER 1

# Heterocyclic Anti-cancer Compounds Derived from Natural Sources with their Mechanism of Action

**Sitesh C. Bachar**[1,*], **A.K.M. Shafiul Kadir**[2], **S.M. Riajul Wahab**[3] **and Abdullah Al Hasan**[4]

[1] *Department of Pharmacy, Faculty of Pharmacy, University of Dhaka, Dhaka-1000, Bangladesh*

[2] *Institute of Biological Sciences (IBSc), University of Rajshahi, Bangladesh*

[3] *School of Pharmacy, The University of Texas at El Paso, Texas, USA*

[4] *Department of Pharmacy, Southeast University, Dhaka, Bangladesh*

**Abstract:** The variety of natural compounds is indispensable due to their mechanism of action. For many years, natural compounds have been used to develop new classes of chemotherapeutic agents. Chemotherapeutic agents derived and synthesised from natural sources could be the best possible alternatives to minimise the harmful after-effects of conventionally used agents against cancer, especially oral and maxillofacial carcinoma and tumors. The proposed chapter concentrates on recent research on various classes of natural scaffolds and their analogues that possess potent antitumor activity. Moreover, we would like to provide an analysis of preclinical and/or clinically investigated natural compounds. These compounds and their synthetic heterocyclic analogues were found to be obtained through bioactivity and mechanism of action-directed isolation and characterization, conjoined with modification using rational drug design-based approaches and analogue synthesis. Structure-activity relationships, structural change, and molecular mechanisms of action will all be examined.

**Keywords:** Anti-cancer, Drug-design, Heterocycles, Natural compounds, Natural scaffolds, Oral and maxillofacial carcinoma.

## INTRODUCTION

The anti-cancer drugs are accustomed to demonstrating considerably excessive lethal effects on the cancer cells and the body's normal cells. All over the world, for health benefits or to treat diseases, a large number of plants and herbs in different forms are consumed as traditional or folk medicine. The increased preva-

\* **Corresponding author Sitesh C. Bachar:** Department of Pharmacy, Faculty of Pharmacy, University of Dhaka, Dhaka-1000, Bangladesh; E-mails: bacharsc@du.ac.bd, bacharsc63@gmail.com

lence rate of different cancer types is creating a necessity for novel anti-cancer drugs. Plants that have long been used in conventional medicaments are now being used as the origin of biologically active remedies [1]. Extracting these compounds from plant materials is one process. Another alternative is to use biotechnology to develop plant-derived anti-cancer compounds. The anti-cancer attributes of natural substances can be found in a variety of chemical groups of compounds, such as alkaloids, diterpenes, diterpenoquinone, purine-based compounds, lactonic sesquiterpene, peptides, cyclic depsipeptides, proteins, macrocyclic polyethers, *etc*. The expense of extracting these compounds from natural sources is sometimes much less than synthesising them chemically or vice versa, such as one ton of *Catharanthus roseus* leaves yields 50 g of raw vincristine, a heterocyclic alkaloidal anti-cancer drug. Vinblastine, however, which is found in this plant, occurs at a 1000-fold higher drug level than vincristine and costs one-third less [2]. The prodrug vincristine (Fig. **1**) can be made from its parent drug, vinblastine, by modifying its structure using various synthetic and biotechnological methods [3].

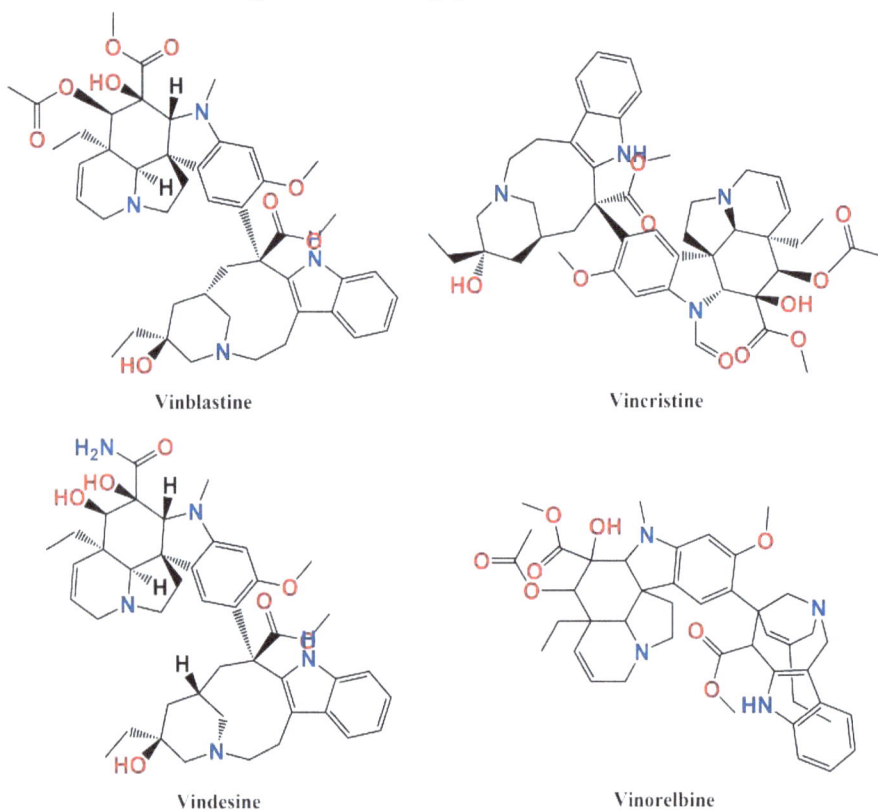

Vinblastine

Vincristine

Vindesine

Vinorelbine

**Fig. (1).** Structures of vinca alkaloids.

Paclitaxel is obtained from *Taxus brevifolia*. It can also be prepared by semi-synthesizing its precursors, which include paclitaxel C, 7-epipaclitaxel baccatin III, and 10-deacetyl baccatin III [4]. However, extracting this active diterpene heterocyclic anti-cancer compound from the bark of trees contributes to a decline in the raw materials of these trees. Furthermore, the compound used as a drug when isolated from the Pacific yew tree is supplied in a small amount, *i.e.*, only 100 mg of Taxol per kg of bark [5]. However, the leaves of the European yew tree can be used to isolate this bioactive compound too. So, various synthesis methods have been developed for obtaining taxanes, such as paclitaxel, docetaxel, and cabazitaxel (Fig. **2**), to protect the *Taxus* plant [6 - 9]. These taxanes are commonly used as a single therapeutic agent and/or in conjunction with other anti-cancer medications to treat breast cancer [10 - 12]. Vincristine, vinblastine, and paclitaxel isolated from plants have become blockbuster molecules and attracted the interest of world-leading pharmaceutical companies.

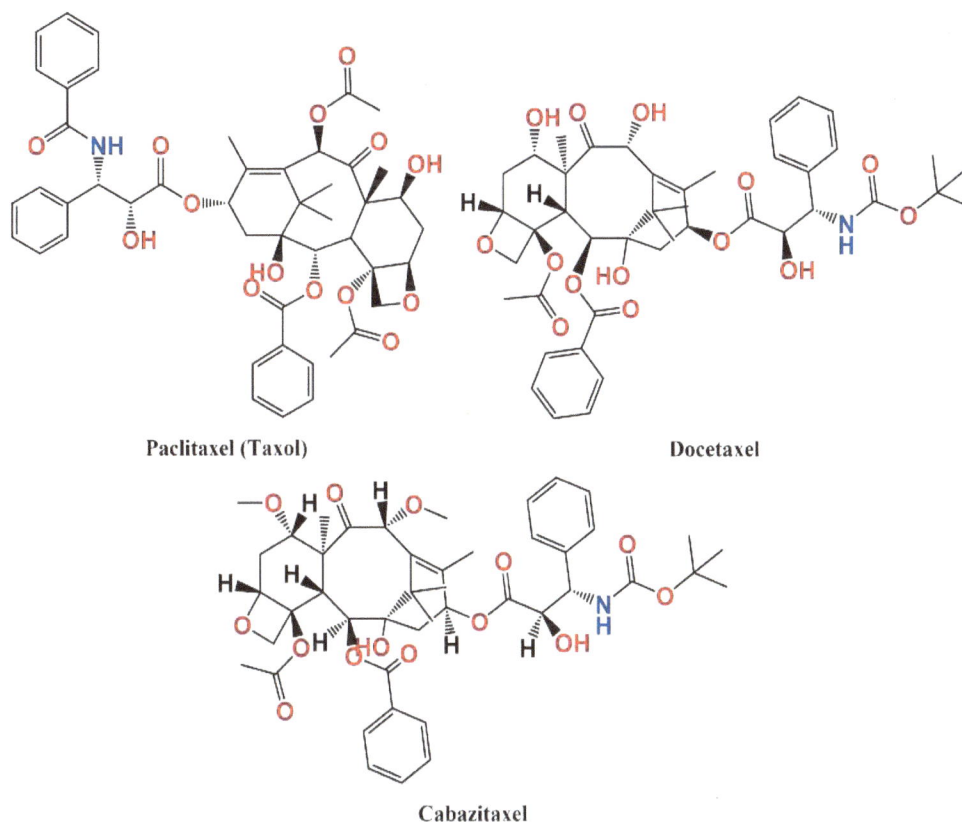

Paclitaxel (Taxol)                                   Docetaxel

Cabazitaxel

**Fig. (2).** Structures of taxanes.

Camptothecin is a heterocyclic compound, and its derivatives, irinotecan and topotecan (Fig. **3**), are a pentacyclic group of quinoline alkaloids extracted from *Camptotheca acuminata* and have anti-cancer effects [13]. Camptothecin and its by-products have also been synthesised using various techniques [14 - 18]. Another derivative, exatecan, is a comparatively more potent anti-cancer drug than topotecan [19].

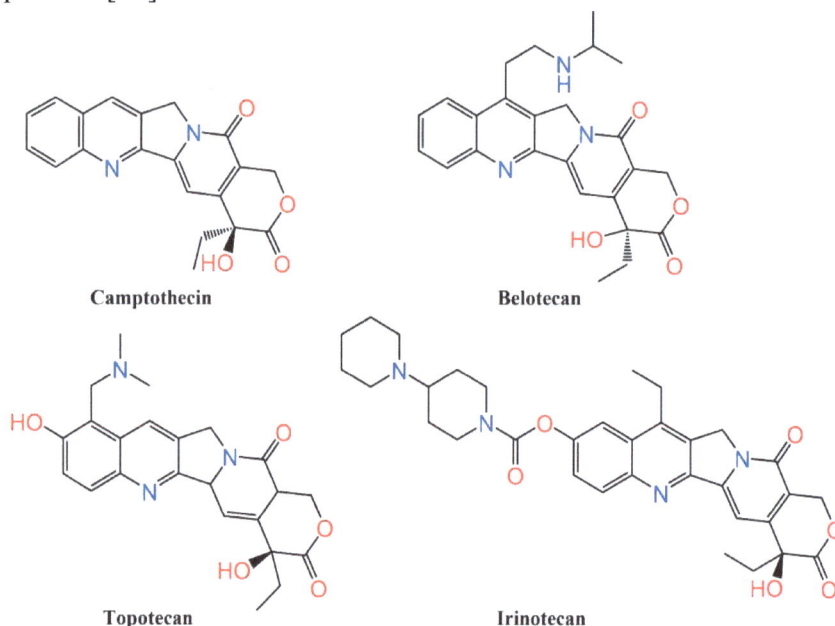

**Fig. (3).** Structures of camptothecins.

Podophyllotoxin is a lignan derived from Podophyllum [20]. Its semi-synthetic derivatives are etoposide and teniposide, which exhibit cytostatic activity [21]. For a long time, geniposide, derived from the *Gardenia jasminoides* Ellis (Rubiaceae) fruits, has been used in the medicaments of China. Its iridoid glycoside derivative was considered for critical review due to its prominent antitumor activity [22, 23]. The homoharrigtonine, which was isolated from several *Cephalotaxaceae* species, was synthesised for the first time in 1982 [24] with the intention of treating chronic myeloid leukemia, with 92% of patients achieving remission [25]. Woodward *et al.* synthesised ellipticine (5,11-dimethy--6*H*-pyrido-(4,3-b)-carbazole), an alkaloid found in *Apocyanaceae* species, and found it to have significant antitumor activity when combined with its more dispersible derivatives [26]. The following is a purine-based, semi-synthetic R-roscovitine by-product, which Meijer and co-workers later purified as distinct, more viable constituents of the cyclin-dependent kinase (CDK)-inhibitor, insulated from the *Raphanus sativus* L. (Brassicaceae) cotyledons [27]. Corey and co-workers processed maytansine, a cytotoxic agent derived from the *Maytenus serrata* (Celastraceae), a plant found in Ethiopia [28]. Maytansine and its derivatives have antimitotic properties due to their ability to bind to tubulin near the vinblastine binding site and prevent microtubule aggregation [29].

Thapsigargin, which is a lactonic sesquiterpene, is derived from *Thapsia garganica* L. (Apiaceae) roots. Ball *et al.* developed thapsigargin and its derivatives as anti-neoplastic drugs that inhibit the sarcoplasmic/endoplasmic reticulum calcium adenosine triphosphatase (SERCA) enzyme in the sarcoplasmic/endoplasmic reticulum [30]. Bruceantin was synthesised by Sasaki and Murae (1989) from a tree named *Brucea antidysenterica* (Simaroubaceae) found in Ethiopia and is utilised by the natives to treat "cancer" [31, 32]. In the treatment of different cancers in mice, bruceantin has been shown to have an anti-cancer effect. However, after the phase I and phase II trials on patients, its usage was terminated when no objective tumour retrogressions were observed. Alternatively, in independent research, bruceantin demonstrated significant pursuit against leukemia, lymphoma, and myeloma cell lines in animal models [33].

Another anti-cancer compound is Psammaplin A, extracted from *Poecillastra* species and *Jaspis* species from *Psammaplin aplysilla*, a marine sponge and microalgae (cyanobacteria) associated with these sponges, tunicates, and soft corals [34]. Later, Hoshino and co-workers (1992) synthesised it [35]. Psammaplin A and its derivatives, psammaplin F, psammaplin G, and biprasin, have potential tumorigenesis and angiogenesis activity by inhibiting histone deacetylase. NVP-LAQ824, a formidable histone deacetylase inhibitor, is a synthetic indole derivative that has been tested in patients with solid tumours or leukaemia [36, 37]. Didemnin B, for example, is a cyclic depsipeptide discovered in the marine tunicate *Trididemnum solidum* and synthesised by Ramanjulu and co-workers (1997) [38]. Dolastatin 10 is a pentapeptide that was extracted with increased supply from the marine cyanobacteria *Symploca hydnoides* and *Lyngbya majuscule*, both of which were synthesised earlier [39]. Auristatin, soblidotin, synthadotin, and cematadin, the synthetic and semi-synthetic derivatives of dolastatin 10, possess improved antitumor activity [40, 41]. Trabectedin is a tetrahydroisoquinoline alkaloid derived synthetically or semi-synthetically from the Caribbean marine tunicate *Ecteinascidia turbinate* [42]. Changes in the tumour microenvironment can be related to trabectedin's anti-cancer activity against advanced ovarian, breast, and mesenchymal tumours [43]. A complex type of compound is halichondrin B, which is a polyether and is sequestered from marine sources such as sponges and tunicates [44]. In addition, the other compounds of homohalichondrin B, including halichondrin B, confirmed their inhibitory activities against murine cancer cells in *in-vitro* and *in-*

*vivo* studies [45]. The quest for various scaffolds is enticing in medicinal chemistry as diverse structures can be discovered in terms of possibilities for lead optimization [46 - 48]. The present chapter deals with known heterocyclic anti-cancer drugs primarily derived from natural plant, marine, and microbiological sources. Some of them have already been approved for use, including potential novel synthetic or semi-synthetic anti-cancer analogues.

## DEATHS FROM CANCER ARE A GLOBAL THREAT

Globally, cancer is the most common cause of death after cardiovascular diseases. According to the World Health Organization, cancer is the leading cause of one in six deaths [49]. The worldwide incidence of cancer is estimated to have gone up to new cases of 19.3 million and deaths of 10.0 million in the year 2020 [50]. Cancer affects one out of every five people in the world at some point in their lives, and one out of every eight men and one out of every eleven women dies from it.There are many types of cancer listed worldwide. In a current report, female breast cancer is reported as the type of cancer that is the most common worldwide. Leukemia and pancreatic cancer are two other types of cancer that have been reported [51]. Cancers of the lip and oral cavity account for the 16th most common form of cancer in the world. In South Asia, Pakistan had the highest incidence of cancer of the lip and oral cavity at 12.2 individuals per 100,000 people, followed by Bangladesh at 9.5 individuals per 100,000 people, and India at 9.1 individuals per 100,000 people [52]. Statistically, across the globe, middle-income and high-income countries have been suffering from cancer of the respiratory tract, which includes tracheal, bronchial, and lung cancer, which raises death tolls there. It varies in the countries with lower-income status, from colon and rectal cancer, liver cancer, cervical cancer, stomach cancer, breast and prostate cancer, and it shuffles the list [53]. According to the World Health Organization (WHO), cancer's deadly strike will affect one in five men and one in six women before they reach the age of 75. Again, one in eight men and one in twelve women will die from the disease. Around 27 million people have a chance of being affected by cancer within 2040 [54].

## THE ANTI-CANCER NATURAL COMPOUNDS' RATIONALE

Mother Nature is the birthplace of varieties of medicinal drugs. According to history, shamans and medicine men used a diverse variety of natural compounds for the remediation of ailments. The first potent bioactive compounds were isolated at the start of the nineteenth century. In developing modern drugs, such pure compounds are accepted as pharmaceutical agents, allowing effective dosage of treatment and drug delivery control in the human body. Medicine based on raw natural supplements still reigns supreme in many parts of the world.

New and modern biotechnologies have made it possible to synthesize many bioactive compounds nowadays. Nonetheless, it could not eliminate the need for a premier new drug's natural sources [55]. This organic diversity comes from earthbound and aquatic life-forms and various organisms, which provide diversified biologically active molecules [56, 57]. Plant species, livestock, and microorganisms manufacture a range of compounds that could be used to research drug discovery to identify molecular structures with useful therapeutic actions [56, 58].

## MECHANISMS OF ACTION OF ANTI-CANCER COMPOUNDS

Carcinogenesis consists of three phases, such as initiation, promotion, and tumour development. The initiation of cancer is an irreversible and rapid procedure that takes place following damage to DNA, RNA, proteins, and other macromolecules. Tumor promotion involves the formation of benign tumours from transformed cells, and this is a reversible phase. The cancer cells enter into the progression phase once the cells in the benign tumour gain the ability to be invasive and have metastatic potential. Phytochemicals can inhibit the cancer initiation phase by inactivating metabolic carcinogens and protecting the DNA from oxidative damage and covalent modification *via* modulation of cellular detoxification pathways. The anti-cancer effects of most of the phytochemicals are largely attributed to their ability to inhibit cell proliferation, angiogenesis, inflammation, invasion, migration, altering cell cycle kinetics, targeting cancer stem cells (Fig. **4**), and so on.

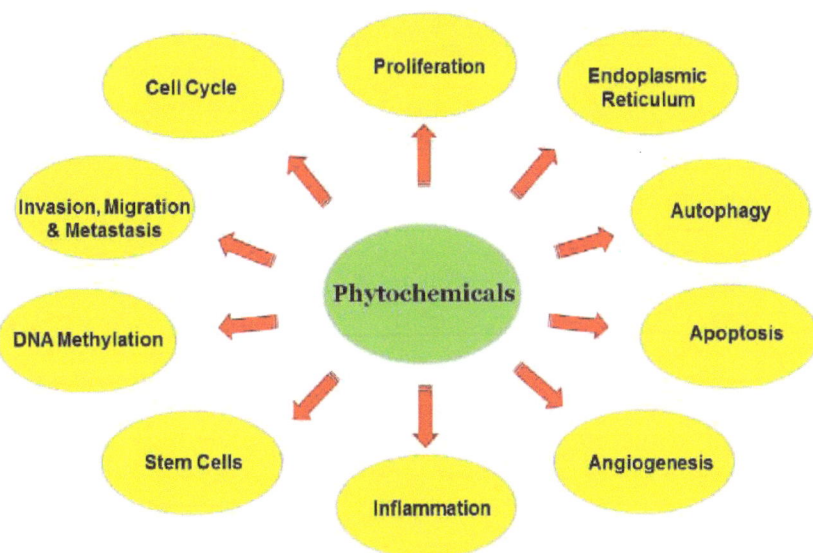

**Fig. (4).** Phytochemicals targeting different steps to exert antineoplastic effect.

**Inhibition of Angiogenesis**

Angiogenesis is known as the development of blood vessels or the formation of new blood vessels. The study suggested that angiogenesis develops blood vessels anew from the pre-existing vessels [59]. It is regulated by some factors like angiogenin, angiopoietins, interleukin-8, fibroblast growth factors (FGFa and FGFb), hepatocyte growth factors (HGF), tumour necrosis factor (TNF-α), transforming growth factor (TGF-α and TGF-β). The most critical factor among all of these is the vascular endothelial growth factor (VEGF), which vastly contributes to the development of new blood vessels. *In vitro*, VEGF triggers endothelial cells to predominantly emanate from nerves, lungs, and lymphatic drainage vessels. In fact, it is one of the most important survival mechanisms for endothelial cells in both *in vitro* and *in vivo* environments [60].

Thymoquinone significantly reduces angiogenesis by regulating VEGF signalling *via* the Akt and extracellular receptor kinase pathways [61, 62]. The development of new blood vessels in osteosarcoma (SaOS-2) and human prostate cancer cells (PC3)[53] decreases with thymoquinone administration in a xenograft model in nude mice. Specifically, the angiogenesis markers CD34 and VEGF are suppressed in osteosarcoma cells. Moreover, thymoquinone treatment in combination with resveratrol demonstrated that they suppressed angiogenesis by inhibiting VEGF directly. Also, they might stimulate the necrosis in that specific area of cancer expansion. Following this pathway, it can obstruct the emergence of new blood vessels [63].

In colon carcinoma cells (HCT116), management with formononetin (Fig. **5**), a phytochemical, suppressed the gene and protein expression of VEGF [64]. Besides this, formononetin demonstrated its significant inhibitory activity on fibroblast growth factor receptor 2 (FGFR2). In an *in vitro* model, it suppressed the stimulation of FGF2 on FGFR2, which results in down-regulation of the signalling pathway of FGFR2, such as PI3K and Akt phosphorylation. Formononetin reduced angiogenesis progression in the human breast cancer xenograft mouse model by inhibiting microvessel density and decreasing the number of phosphorylated FGFR2-positive cells in tumours [65].

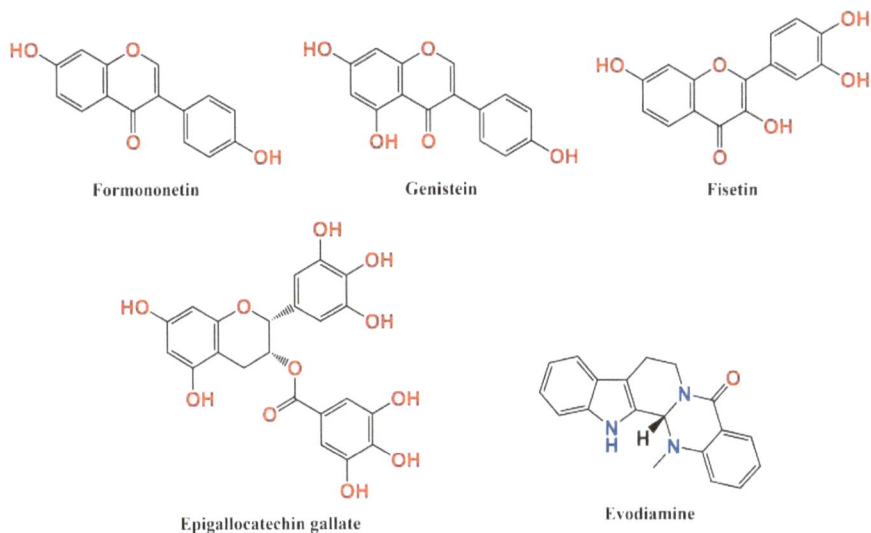

Fig. (5). Structures of formononetin, genistein, fisetin, epigallocatechin gallate and evodiamine.

## Induction of Apoptosis

Apoptosis is a planned cell death that plays several vital roles, such as the embryo's growth to maintain the normal cell turnover and cell population [66]. It can occur in both intrinsic and extrinsic pathways, where internal signals trigger the intrinsic pathway. The intrinsic process of apoptosis is regulated by Bcl-2, Bax, cytochrome C, and caspase-9. Bax-mediated inhibition of apoptosis may occur through the inhibition of BCL-2 protein. In the case of intrinsic pathway, Bax protein becomes stimulated and transferred to the outer membrane of the mitochondria, forming a channel on the membrane of the mitochondria that allows cytochrome C to travel to the cytoplasm and stimulate the formation of apoptosomes that trigger caspase-9 and gradually lead to cell death [66, 67]. On the other hand, death domains, complement ligands, caspase-8, and death receptors are implicated in the extrinsic apoptotic pathway. In a nutshell, in the extrinsic pathway, apoptotic signals interact with the death receptor and activate the death domains by converting procaspase-8 to caspase-8. It ultimately results in the death of cells [66].

Many studies have suggested the apoptosis-inducing effect of formononetin on various cancer cells. A study showed that formononetin administration in ovarian cancer cells augmented the manifestation of cleaved caspase-3 and-9 in a dose-dependent manner [68]. In human nasopharyngeal cancer cells and human multiple myeloma, formononetin induces apoptosis by stimulating caspase-3, which leads to the formation of cleaved PARP, which inhibits the repair of DNA damage [69, 70]. Some other investigations confirmed that formononetin considerably increased the level of caspase-3 expression in human non-small cell lung carcinoma and human osteosarcoma in a dose-dependent fashion [71, 72].

Bcl-2 and Bax proteins are significant controllers in the intrinsic pathway of apoptosis. Several studies have suggested that formononetin directly regulates the expression of anti-apoptotic and pro-apoptotic members of the Bcl-2 family in different cancer cells such as breast cancer cells [73], nasopharyngeal [69], prostate [71, 74], and colon [75]. Numerous studies reported that upon treatment with formononetin, Bax protein expression surged, whereas the level of Bcl-2 protein was reduced [71, 74 - 76]. An increased pro-apoptotic to anti-apoptotic Bcl-2 family protein ratio stimulates the release of cytochrome C and other apoptogenic factors into the cytoplasm from the mitochondria, resulting in caspase cascade activation and programmed cell death [77].

Another phytochemical, honokiol, demonstrated caspase-dependent apoptosis in various kinds of carcinomas. Administration of honokiol in chondrosarcoma cells results in the loss of the mitochondria's membrane potential and leads to programmed cell death. It also significantly interrupted the Bax/Bcl-2 ratio's stability in different cancer cells [78 - 80]. Besides, honokiol markedly reduced the expression of anti-apoptosis mRNA and proteins such as Bcl-xL [78], MCL-1 [78], and escalation of the expression of pro-apoptotic proteins like Bak, Bad, and Bax [78, 81].

In p53-deficient cancer cell lines such as MDA-MB-231 breast carcinoma cells, lung carcinoma cells, and bladder carcinoma cell lines, honokiol significantly induced cell death by preventing Ras' initiation phospholipase D [82 - 84]. Moreover, honokiol also increases the expression of cancer suppressor genes like p21$^{wafl}$ [85], p62 [86, 87], p21 [88], and p38 MAPK [89, 90].

Several other reports suggested that honokiol could target the death receptors, TNF-related apoptosis-inducing ligand (TRAIL) receptors as well as tumour necrosis factor receptors (TNFR). It leads to the orchestrated activation of caspase-8 and-3, resulting in the breakdown of the target protein and eventually apoptosis [91, 92].

Capsaicin can trigger selective programmed cell death in human pancreatic cancer cells (BxPC-3 and AsPC-3) without obstructing the growth of normal pancreatic acinar cells through decreasing the survival factor, Bcl-2, and increasing Bax expression, thus promoting the discharge of apoptosis-inducing factor (AIF) and cytochrome C from mitochondria into the cytosol [93]. It can also cause the death of human liver cancer cells (SK-Hep-1) by activating caspase-3 and partly reducing the Bcl-2/Bax ratio [94]. Moreover, besides the initiation of caspase and inhibition of Bcl-2 expression, capsaicin can also reduce the expression of carcinogenic genes like BRAF, PTPN1, MAPK7, and K-ras Akt in severe lymphoblastic leukaemia cell lines [95].

In human oesophageal epidermoid cancer (CE 81T/VGH) cells [96] and human prostate neoplasm (DU-145, LNCaP, and PC3) cells [97], cell death is induced *via* induction of p53 and its target proteins such as Bax and p21. Capsaicin caused apoptosis in human leukaemia cells and SNU-1 cells by increasing phosphorylated p53 at serine 15 residues and increasing p53 overexpression [98].

## Induction of Autophagy

Autophagy is a natural catabolic evolutionary conservative method for removing unnecessary, dysfunctional cellular components for lysosomal degradation [99, 100]. During stressful and harsh conditions, autophagy supports cell survival and continues cell growth by reducing the cell's energy requirements by breaking down unnecessary components [100, 101]. In cancer cells, it plays a dual role by facilitating both tumour dominance and tumorigenesis through the stimulation of cell death and elevating cancer cell growth rate [102].

Honokiol is a potent bioactive compound commonly found in Magnolia species. Numerous studies have described how honokiol induces cell death *via* autophagy in human thyroid cancer [103], human glioma cells [104], and human prostate tumour cells [105]. Chang *et al.* have reported that two crucial autophagic proteins, LC3 and Beclin-1, were detected to be increased after honokiol treatment in glioblastoma multiforme cells [106]. Honokiol treatment in osteosarcoma HOS and U2OS cells results in the build-up of autophagic vacuoles by instigating the atg5/atg7-dependent pathway *via* the overexpression of Atg5, Atg7, and LC3B-II levels [107].

The human high-mobility group box 1 protein (HMGB1) is required for stress signalling as well as autophagy stimulation *via* extracellular, cytoplasmic, and nuclear function [108 - 111]. Lycorine, a phytochemical compound, diminishes the expression of HMGB1 protein and consequently inhibits it. Lycorine-mediated proteasomal degradation of HMGB1 suppresses the initiation of the MEK-ERK signalling pathway, thus reducing Bcl-2 phosphorylation, which leads to the constructive association of Bcl-2 with Beclin-1, resulting in inhibition of autophagy [112].

Another plant-derived compound, bardoxolone methyl, can prompt lysosomal degradation in prolonged myeloid leukaemia cells where the toxic effects on mitochondria lead to the engulfment in autophagosomes of dysfunctional organelles [113]. Stimulation of autophagy in K562 cells by bardoxolone methyl happens *via* subduing the PI3K/Akt/mTOR signalling pathway [114]. A similar mechanism has been found in the oesophageal squamous cell lines Ec109 and KYSE70 [115].

## Arresting Cell Cycle Kinetics

There are four phases in eukaryotic cell cycles: G1, S, G2, and M. The G1 phase controls cell proliferation. When the cell cycle continues from the G1 phase to the S phase, it is not reversible, and the cell is dedicated to undergoing cell division if there is no stress, such as DNA damage. According to research, cyclin-dependent kinases (CDKs) phosphorylate a group of retinoblastoma (Rb) proteins, allowing the cell cycle to enter the S phase [116]. Therefore, CDKs play a pivotal role in the modulation of cell proliferation. Deregulation of the cell cycle results in uncontrolled cell proliferation, leading to cancer development. So, targeting cell cycle arrest demonstrates an operational approach to inhibiting cancer.

Numerous studies have demonstrated that formononetin induces cell cycle arrest in a number of cancers, like ovarian cancer [117], prostate cancer [118], breast cancer [119], and lung cancer cells [72]. Formononetin treatment in ovarian cancer cells (OV90 and ES2) prompted significant cell populations at the sub-G0/G1 phase with reduced cell populations at the G2/M phase [117]. Li *et al.* also reported the similarly increased accumulation of prostate carcinoma cells (PC-3) at the G0/G1 phase and the down-regulation of cyclin D1 and CDK-4 [118]. In another study, formononetin administration in human non-small lung carcinoma cells induced cell cycle arrest at the G1 phase with reduced cell accumulation at the S phase [72]. The majority of formononetin studies showed cell cycle arrest at the sub G0/G1 and G1 phases *via* modulation of cyclin expression regulating proteins like CDK-2, CDK-4, cyclin D1, and cyclin E [70, 72, 117].

Honokiol can cause cell cycle arrest at G0/G1 and G2/M in several types of cancers, including oral squamous cancer [120], prostate cancer cells [121, 122], lung squamous cell carcinoma [123], and oral squamous cell carcinoma [120]. In most cancers, honokiol-induced cell cycle arrest is associated with decreased expression of cyclin-dependent kinase CDK-2 and CDK-4 and increased expression of cell cycle suppressor proteins p21 and p27 in human oral squamous cell carcinoma cells [86, 124], and decreased expression of cyclin-B1, CDC2, and Cdc25C in human gastrointestinal cancer and human neuroglioma cancer cells [124 - 126].

## Modulation of DNA Methylation

Methylation of DNA is one of the best-known mechanisms for silencing genes *via* transcriptional repression. DNA methylation is a prominent event in the cell related to definite progressions, including suppressing recurrent elements or genomic imprinting and X-chromosome inactivation [127]. Cancer initiation, promotion, and progression are controlled by both epigenetic and genetic events [128]. Gene expression is controlled by epigenetic alterations such as histone chemical modification, RNA mechanisms (microRNA and non-coding RNA), and DNA methylation, which are crucial for gene expression by controlling transcription [129]. Cellular DNA methyltransferases (DNMTs) catalyse DNA methylation, which denotes critical physiological stages that endorse cellular and tissue homeostasis, which plays a unique role in cells' various functions [130, 131]. Aberrant DNA methylation is responsible for the carcinogenic transformation of eukaryotic cells, including changes in proliferation, apoptosis, cell cycles, invasion, migration, and differentiation [132].

A number of preclinical investigations using cancer cell lines have reported DNA methylation variation following treatment with phytochemical compounds. Treatment with the combination of proanthocyanidines from grape seeds with trans-resveratrol reduced DNA methyltransferase activity (DNMT) in MDA-M--231 and MCF-7 cells [133]. Additionally, this combination therapy synergistically reduced post-treatment cell proliferation and cell viability in both cell lines and increased apoptosis in MDA-MB-231 cells with a remarkable upsurge in the ratio of Bax to Bcl-2 expression. In a different study, indicaxanthin, a phytochemical derived from beets, demonstrated anti-proliferative activity by inducing demethylation in the promoters of specific methylation-silenced tumor-suppressor genes in colorectal cancer cell lines (HT29) [134]. Moreover, indicaxanthin upregulated the levels of specific genes accountable for DNA methylation.

Numerous reports also confirmed that treatment with phytochemicals increased the responsiveness of specific cancers by modulating DNA methylation. A study reported that withaferin A (WA) reduced HER2/PR/ESR-dependent gene expression interactions and suppressed the triple-negative MDA-MB-231 breast cancer cells with a precise hypomethylation profile [135]. Unlike the DNA methylating agent 5-aza-20-deoxycytidine, treatment with WA in MDA-MB-231 breast cancer cells modulated the epigenetic signalling network *via* gene-specific DNA hypermethylation of oncogenes containing ADAM metallopeptidase domain 8, urokinase-type plasminogen activator, tumour necrosis factor superfamily member 12, and cell detoxification enzymes like glutathione S transferase mu1. Another study suggested that dietary phytochemicals like EGCG, DIM, curcumin, genistein (Fig. **5**), and indole-3-carbinol (I3C) altered the expression of genes such as p21$^{Cip1}$, Cadherin-11, interleukin-6, and urokinase-type plasminogen activator through the modulation of DNA methylation. As a result, MDA-MB-231 breast cancer cells were induced to apoptosis [136].

The role of different plant-based components in DNA methylation variation has been helped by several study models involving animals. Several studies have demonstrated the role of curcumin in the regulation of epigenetic events that comprise this mechanism. A study using MCF-7 cell lines reported that curcumin decreased tumour size with the correlation of specific CpG site hypomethylation of the RASSF1 promoter [137]. Likewise, in a lung cancer experimental model using female BALB/c nude mice, curcumin reduced the condition of the methylated RARβ promoter zone, which led to the revival of the gene [138]. Treatment using curcumin also suppressed the level of DNMT1 in a xenograft model of severe myeloid leukaemia in female athymic nu/nu mice [139]. Trans-resveratrol is a nourishing element related to several meditative outcomes that validated significant anti-cancer features in observational mammary carcinogenesis by reducing DNMT3 levels in ACI rats [140]. Genistein is an epigenetic modifier that suppresses tumour growth and reduces the degree of methylated CDH5 promoter zone by reducing the DNMT3 activity in the neuroblastoma animal model [141]. Furthermore, in a mammary cancer experimental model using virgin female immunodeficient nu/nu mice, genistein was linked to the revival of oestrogen receptor (ER) as a result of a lower level of DNMT1 [142].

## Modulation of Endoplasmic Reticulum Stress

The endoplasmic reticulum (ER) is a component of eukaryotic cells that was discovered by Porter *et al*. in 1945 [143] after analysing chicken fibroblasts under electron microscopy. ER can be classified as rough and smooth ER, which can exist either as separate compartments or interconnected [144]. It is physically connected with mitochondria-associated membranes and plays a crucial part in $Ca^{2+}$ homeostasis [145]. The functions of ER include folding and post-translational dispensation of secreted and membrane-bound proteins, glycogen degradation, lipid synthesis detoxification, and release and storage of $Ca^{2+}$ [146]. Stress factors like starvation, hypoxia, change in pH, oxidative insults, depletion of $Ca^{2+}$, hypoglycaemia, depletion of ATP, and infections can alter ER homeostasis. All these factors can disrupt the appropriate protein folding, resulting in the build-up of unfolded or misfolded proteins, leading to a state known as ER stress [147]. Under these kinds of stress states, cells can adopt an evolutionary signalling pathway referred to as "unfolded protein response" (UPR), which acts to repair the ER homeostasis [148]. In unresolved stress and toxic conditions, UPR converts the cell destiny from existence to death [149].

Natural compounds derived from plants are categorised by their anti-carcinogenic, antioxidant, antimutagenic, and detoxifying properties, which could be used to develop new effective antineoplastic drugs [150]. Numerous studies have reported that different phytochemicals induce ER stress-related apoptosis in cancer cells [151 - 153].

Turmeric, a yellow spice used widely in cooking and ancient Ayurvedic remedies, contains curcumin, a polyphenol compound derived from this spice [153]. Recently, a study established that curcumin has the ability to induce cell death through the paraptosis pathway encompassing the ER in the A172 human glioblastoma cell line. They also noticed the alteration in expression of ATF6 and IRE1α genes, miR-222, miR27a, and miR-449, after treatment with curcumin [154]. In colorectal cancer, cell lines such as HT-20 and LoVo demonstrated the improved anti-cancer activity of irinotecan by activating the ER stress pathway and increasing ROS production [155]. In the SW620 colon carcinoma cell line, a mono carbonyl analogue (B63) of curcumin showed significant pro-apoptotic and anti-proliferative effects by increasing Bad and Bim proteins with enhanced release of cytochrome C from mitochondria. Additionally, its anti-neoplastic function was ER stress activation-dependent [156]. The curcumin analogue B19 caused ER stress activation and ROS production at an apoptosis-stimulating concentration [157].

Several studies have reported that resveratrol suppresses cancer development by aiming molecules and signalling pathways at cancer advancement [158]. Some studies suggest its capacity to invoke apoptosis related to ER stress initiation in diverse cancer cell types. Resveratrol induces ER-stress-related apoptosis in human multiple myeloma cell lines *via* hindering the pro-survival XBP1's activity and stimulating the enhancement of its molecular target sirtuin1 [159]. In another investigation, resveratrol treatment in a malignant melanoma cell line (A375SM) induced apoptosis and cell cycle arrest by promoting ROS production and ER stress concurrently [160].

Green tea extract (GTE) has anti-neoplastic properties due to the existence of flavan-3-ols, particularly epigallocatechin gallate (EGCG) (Fig. **5**). Flavan-3-ols derived from GTE, according to research, primarily target the ER function [161]. A GTE extract, Polyphenon E®, induced prolonged and severe ER stress in the human prostate cancer cell line PC3 by stimulating the PERK pathway, which is characterised by prolonged expression of ATF4 and p-eIF2α [162]. Substantial activation of XBP1 mRNA splicing in these cell lines also indicated the involvement of ATF6 and IRE1α signalling arms of ER stress in the cellular response to Polyphenon E®. The generation of XBP1s by braiding after the disruption of ER homeostasis indicates ER stress activation. It contributes to the over-expression of the pro-death protein CHOP [163].

## Regulation of Inflammation

Homeostasis and pathogenesis are part of inflammation. Any physical injury and/or microbial attack initiates an inflammatory response to improve homeostatic tissue stability between physiological function and its composition. Chronic inflammation may lead to tissue damage and that may result in non-functioning organs [164]. The complex mechanism of inflammation is linked to the progression of various diseases like malignancy, cardiovascular and neurodegenerative diseases [165]. In 1863, Rudolf and Virchow first proposed the relationship between inflammation and carcinoma. Numerous studies have recently reported that acute inflammation with concurrent cytokine activity and reactive oxygen species production is associated with cancer-promoting diseases [166, 167].

The nuclear factor kappa B (NFκB) family proteins can modulate the transcription of genes responsible for numerous cellular activities like inflammation, invasion, migration, proliferation, angiogenesis, and apoptosis [168, 169]. Persistent stimulation of NFκB has been observed in various categories of cancers. Honokiol interferes with the indigenous activation of NFκB and the level of NFκB-regulated genes involved in inflammation (COX-1, COX-2) [170]. Several studies have confirmed honokiol's NFκB-mediated inhibitory activity in a variety of tumour cells, including pancreatic cancer cells [171], breast cancer cells [172, 173], colon cancer cells [174], and human leukemic cells [175].

Another phytochemical, curcumin, has been reported to have therapeutic efficacy and preventive perspective for cancer patients *in vitro* and *in vivo* human and animal clinical studies for various types of cancers [176 - 178]. Curcumin plays a pivotal role in modulating various intracellular signalling pathways on multiple targets that regulate inflammation [179]. Most carcinogenic agents activate the NFκB pathways, leading to the expression of inflammatory mediators such as LOX-2, COX-2, inflammatory cytokines, TNF-α, and several chemokines [180].

## Reduction of Invasion, Migration, and Metastasis

Through metastasis, a multifaceted, multistep procedure, cancer cells can spread to a distant region through the blood and lymphatic system. The steps in metastasis include detachment, relocation, and invasion. One of the crucial steps in managing cancer in the early detection stage is controlling metastasis to other organs.

Several studies demonstrated that formononetin could reduce the metastasis of various types of carcinomas, such as bladder cancer [65], colon cancer [64, 181], ovarian cancer, and breast cancer [182]. Several studies have shown that formononetin exerts anti-metastatic effects by inhibiting the expression of matrix metalloproteinases (MMPs) like MMP-2 and MMP-9 proteins that maintain cell survivability *via* induction of angiogenesis and metastasis [64, 68, 181 - 183]. Zhou *et al.* also demonstrated that formononetin inhibits invasion by increasing the levels of MMPs negative controllers such as tissue inhibitors of metalloproteinase (TIMPs) TIMP-1 and TIMP-2 in breast carcinoma cells [182].

Evaluation of thymoquinone in CaSki and SiHa cervical tumour cell lines demonstrated that it could modulate the expression of EMT-regulated (epithelial to mesenchymal transition) proteins and metastasis. Thymoquinone treatment on cervical tumour cells reduced migration and invasion in a dose-dependent and time-dependent manner through the upregulation of E-cadherin and suppressed expression of Zeb1 and Twist1. These findings support the notion that thymoquinone targets Zeb1 and Twist1. Thus, it can be concluded that thymoquinone-mediated inhibition of metastasis of cervical cancer cells is mainly caused *via* the signalling pathway of Zeb1/E-cadherin/EMT and Twist1/E-cadherin/EMT [62].

## Reduction of Proliferation of Cancer Cells

Cancer cells possess unique characteristics that allow them to survive longer than their normal life length and to undergo proliferation aberrantly. Standard cancer therapy should ideally kill the highly proliferative and regenerative cells. However, these kinds of anti-neoplastic drugs target tumour cells and kill the normal proliferating cells of the hair, skin, and epithelium of the gastrointestinal tract. This type of toxicity is one of the major disadvantages of currently available anti-cancer drugs. Phytochemicals that are well known for their low or no side effects could play a vital role in overcoming the disadvantages of conventional anti-cancer therapy.

Capsaicin exerts its anti-cancer effect by preventing cancer cell proliferation. In human oesophageal epidermoid tumour cells, capsaicin inhibits proliferation by cell cycle arrest at G1 followed by the down-regulation of transcription factor E2F, cyclin E, CDK-4, and CDK-6 up-regulation of CDK inhibitor p21 [96]. The proliferation of human multiple myeloma cells was inhibited at the G1 phase by arresting the cell at the G1 phase after treatment with capsaicin [184]. Furthermore, capsaicin also inhibited the proliferation of immortalised human endometriotic cells [185].

Evodiamine (Fig. **5**) inhibits the proliferation of A549 cells. This was associated with the capacity of evodiamine to up-regulate the level of oncoprotein metadherin, oxidative injury, and regulation of cancer-causing gene expression by governing protein kinase B/NFκB and sonic hedgehog/GLI family zinc finger 1 pathways [186, 187]. Through the inactivation of topoisomerase I and II, evodiamine demonstrated its anti-proliferative activity in human leukaemia cells K562, CCRF-CEM, THP-1, and camptothecin-resistant CCFR-CEM/C1. Furthermore, the cleavage complex formation of topoisomerase with DNA was not affected by evodiamine [188].

Fisetin (Fig. **5**) is a flavonoid compound extensively found in edible and medicinal plants. A study revealed that fisetin repressed the proliferation of Mcf-7, MDA-MB-231, and MDA-MB-468 cells [189, 190]. Xu *et al.* reported that fisetin considerably subdued the proliferation of breast carcinoma cells 4T1 [191].

## Targeting Cancer Stem Cells

Cancer stem cells (CSC) in a tumour have the dual capability to self-renew and build up the heterogeneous families of cancer cells that involve the carcinoma [192]. Generally, the current standard of chemotherapy, like paclitaxel for different cancer categories and imatinib for chronic myelogenous leukemia, mainly targets proliferating cells. Nonetheless, CSCs are resistant to a wide range of conventional therapies, including these two drugs [193]. A standard curative anti-cancer drug should acknowledge CSC plasticity and its elimination.

Curcumin, a diferuloylmethane, is present abundantly in the Indian spice turmeric, which gives it a yellow colour. Curcumin has been shown in studies to have anti-cancer properties by targeting CSC [194 - 197]. Standard anti-cancer drug-resistant CSC is vulnerable to curcumin. Stem cell signalling pathways are connected in the process of carcinogeneses like Notch, Wnt, Hedgehog, and STAT. Tsai *et al.* reported that in liver cell carcinoma CSCs, curcumin reduced tumour size, lung metastasis, inhibited SP, invasion, and EMT in a nude mouse xenograft model. In the same study, they found that the sphingosine-1-phosphate receptor signalling pathway was inhibited [198]. Another study showed that curcumin reduced oesophageal CSC spheroid size and number. The molecular machinery was inhibition of the Notch pathway, proved by the reduction in RNA and protein manifestation of $\gamma$ secretase, Notch-1 protein, and its related ligand Jaggard-1 [199]. In colorectal cancer, curcumin induced epigenetic modification, including expression of microRNA oncomirs related to metastasis, methylation of the epidermal growth factor receptor (EGFR) promoter, and suppression of CSC markers (ALDH+, CD133) [197]. Using co-culture and immunoblotting to assess EMT markers, Buhrmann *et al.* discovered that curcumin sensitised colorectal CSCs to fluorouracil (5-FU). It suppressed cross-talk between stromal fibroblasts and CSCs in the tumour niche [200].

Soybeans contain the isoflavone genistein (4',5,7-trihydroxyisoflavone). It is classified as a phytoestrogen because it binds to oestrogen receptors. It targets

CSCs in many solid tumours. A study showed that genistein repressed spheroids' "stemness" (Oct4 and Nanog gene expression) and decreased the xenograft tumour volume of gastric CSCs [201]. It also inhibited the extracellular signal-associated kinase (ERK) pathway and drug transporters in these CSCs. Genistein suppressed spheroid formation and tumour formation in the xenograft model. It also down-regulated the hedgehog pathway (reducing Gli1 gene expression) in both breast and prostate CSCs [202, 203].

Genistein can show a synergistic anti-cancer effect with standard anti-cancer drugs, and it also targets the CSC microenvironment. It overcomes the docetaxel resistance in prostate CSCs and decreases the size of tumours more than either compound administered separately [203]. It is well known that breast adipose tissue has contributed to the development of breast cancer. The study found that genistein inhibited the differentiation of mammary stromal fibroblast-like cells into adipocytes by inhibiting PPARγ and fatty acid synthase gene expression [204].

Resveratrol is a stilbene found primarily in red grape skin (3,4',5-tri-hydro-y-trans-stilbene). Studies have suggested that resveratrol can significantly target CSCs. Fu and colleagues have reported the cytotoxic effect of resveratrol on the breast CSCs *in vitro* [205]. A mechanistic study of microtubule-linked protein light chain 3 (LC3) and β-catenin protein revealed that it induced autophagy and suppressed the Wnt signalling pathway. Moreover, resveratrol decreased ALDH+ cells, inhibited tumour formation, and reduced tumour size in murine xenografts. Another study found that resveratrol suppressed pancreatic CSC spheroid development *via* the induction of apoptosis, suppression of mRNA expression responsible for pluripotency maintenance transcription factors such as Nanog and Oct4, and interfering with EMT [206]. Yang and colleagues discovered that CSCs pre-treated with resveratrol *in vitro* were not carcinogenic in glioblastoma multiforme, as the xenografted SCID mice survived longer than their untreated counterparts [207].

Resveratrol can spare the normal stem cells and attack only CSCs. The study revealed that resveratrol suppressed the expression of the fatty acid synthase gene and repressed breast CSC growth. However, the enzymes produced by the normal mammary epithelial cells were not affected [208]. In different studies, resveratrol showed cytotoxicity to breast CSCs but not to normal breast epithelial cells [205]. In another study, the CSC specificity of resveratrol was also reported. It blocked the enzymatic stimulation of sirtuin activity and suppressed the growth of glioma CSCs without any effect on normal neural stem cells (from fetal brains) [209].

Epigallocatechin gallate (EGCG), the main component in green tea, is a polyphenol (flavon-3-ol) found in the *Camellia sinensis* plant. EGCG can target CSCs in different types of cancer. The study reported that EGCG in human neuroblastoma CSCs inhibited ALDH, the formation of a spheroid, and down-regulated the stemness-related genes called Oct4 and Nanog [210]. Treatment with EGCG significantly decreased the number of ALDH+ cells, decreased the expression of Nanog, and reduced the tumor volume in mouse xenografts [211].

EGCG, in combination with other conventional drugs and phytochemicals, enhances the anti-cancer effects, mainly targeting the CSCs and bulk cancer cells [212]. EGCG, when used with quercetin, exhibits synergistic effects in inhibiting the activation of EMT, increasing apoptosis, and reducing the spheroid formation in prostate CSCs [213]. Another study revealed that EGCG enhanced the sensitivity of nasopharyngeal CSCs to cisplatin by inhibiting phosphorylation of STAT3 and increasing apoptosis [214].

## ANTI-CANCER NATURAL COMPOUNDS

More than 60% of synthetic drugs are obtained from natural sources [215]. Natural anti-cancer heterocyclic molecules serve as models for the development of more potent analogues and prodrugs by metabolomics, total or combinatorial manufacturing, or biosynthetic pathway alteration.

### Potential Anti-Cancer Compounds from Plant Sources

### *DNA Topoisomerase Inhibitors*

Topoisomerase inhibitors associate with topoisomerase-DNA complexes and inhibit the re-ligation step of the topoisomerase mechanism, leading to apoptosis and cell death [216]. Because of this capability to induce apoptosis, topoisomerase inhibitors have earned an interest as therapeutics against infectious and cancerous cells. Studies searching for antibiotics and anti-cancer agents have resulted in the discovery of camptothecins, anthracyclines, and epipodophyllotoxins.

The discovery of camptothecin from the *Camptotheca acuminata* tree contributed to the synthesis of three currently FDA-approved derivatives: topotecan, irinotecan, and belotecan (Fig. **3**) [217]. Camptothecins bind to the topoisomerase I and DNA complex, thereby stabilising it (Fig. **7**) resulting in the prevention of DNA re-ligation and therefore causing DNA damage which results in apoptosis. Topotecan is normally used in the treatment of ovarian and small-cell lung cancer (SCLC) and irinotecan is known to ameliorate colon cancer [217, 218]. Usually, topotecan is utilised in conjunction with a combination of drugs such as cyclophosphamide, doxorubicin, and vincristine [218]. Belotecan is a recent camptothecin derivative found to be effective in the treatment of SCLC [219]. Other camptothecin compounds, such as gimatecan, are still undergoing research and clinical studies [219, 220].

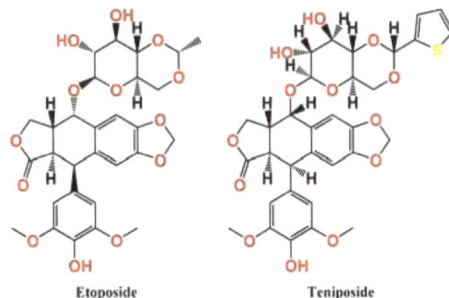

**Etoposide**          **Teniposide**

**Fig. (6).** Structures of epipodophyllotoxins.

Epipodophyllotoxins are natural products commonly found in the root of American Mayapple plant (*Podophyllum peltatum*) [221]. The discovery of podophyllotoxin has contributed to the synthesis of some derivatives that are currently used in the treatment of cancer including etoposide (Fig. **6**) and teniposide which exert the anti-cancer effect by inhibiting topoisomerase II (Fig. **7**) [222, 223].

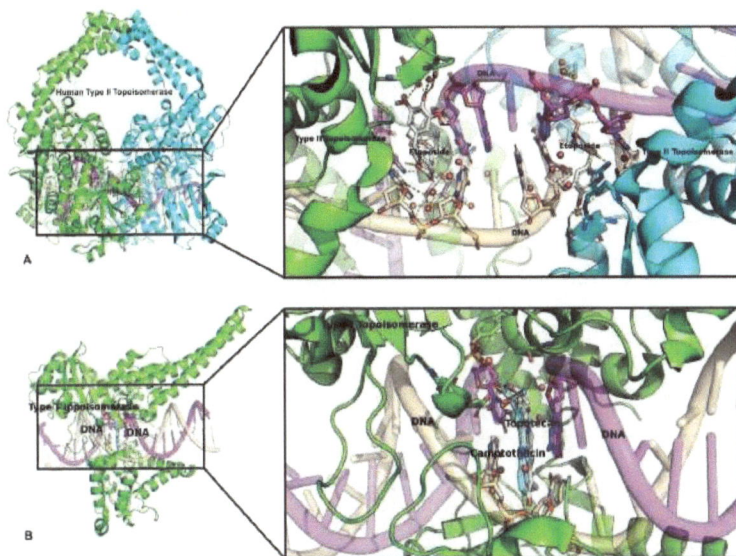

**Fig. (7). (A)** Human type II topoisomerase (green and cyan) inhibition by the anti-cancer drug etoposide (white); based on PDB ID 3QX3 [224]. **(B)** Overlay of the anti-cancer molecules camptothecin (cyan) and topotecan (white) bound to the human type I topoisomerase (green); based on PDB IDs 1T8I [225] and 1K4T [226].

## Mitotic Inhibitors

Mitotic inhibitors disrupt microtubules and are used in cancer treatment. Cancer cells are able to grow and eventually metastasize by continuous mitotic division. As a result, mitotic inhibitors like taxanes (Fig. **2**), such as paclitaxel, docetaxel, and cabazitaxel, and vinca alkaloids (Fig. **1**), such as vinblastine, vincristine, and vinorelbine, are particularly effective against cancer cells.

Taxanes, a class of diterpenes, were in the beginning identified as being from plants of the genus *Taxus* (yews) and have a taxadiene core. Paclitaxel (Taxol) and docetaxel (Taxotere) are widely used to treat many forms of cancer [227], and cabazitaxel is used to treat metastatic castration-resistant prostate cancer [228]. The primary mechanism of action of the taxanes is the perturbation of microtubule function. Microtubules are essential for cell division, and taxanes hyperstabilize GDP-bound tubulin in the microtubule (Fig. **8**), preventing cell division by inhibiting depolymerization [229].

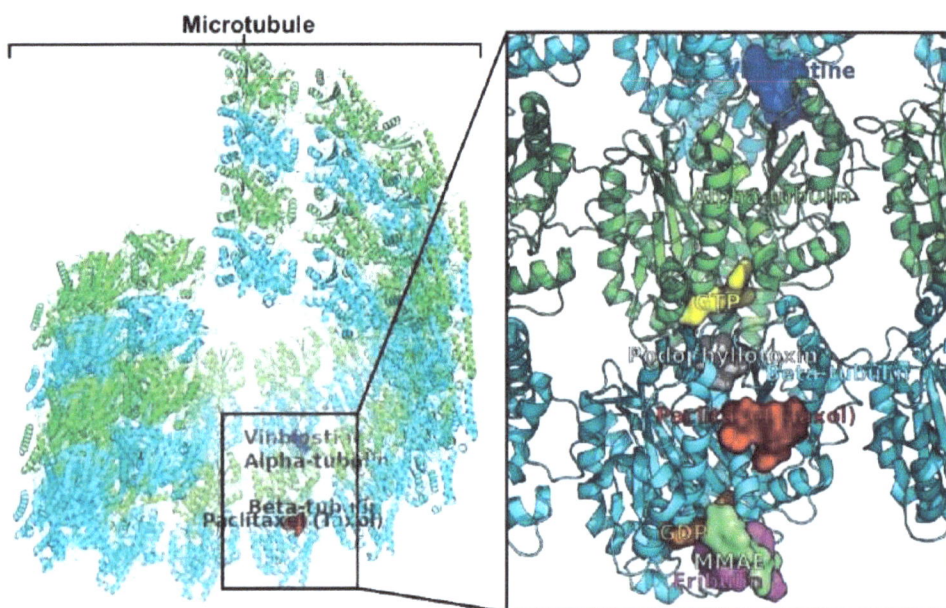

**Fig. (8).** Overview and enlargement of tubulin inhibitor binding sites, including paclitaxel (PDB ID 5SYF) [230], vinblastine (PDB ID 5J2T) [231], podophyllotoxin (PDB ID 1SA1) [232], eribulin (PDB ID 5JH7) [233], and monomethyl auristatin E (MMAE) (PDB ID 5IYZ) [231].

Vinca alkaloids are anti-mitotic agents originally obtained from the periwinkle plant, *Catharanthus roseus*, and other Vinca plants [234]. Vinca alkaloids are now produced synthetically and used as anti-cancer as well as immunosuppressive drugs. Examples of vinca alkaloids are vinblastine, vincristine, vindesine, vinorelbine, and so on (Fig. **1**) [235]. In contrast to the taxanes, the vinca alkaloids inhibit mitotic spindle formation by preventing tubulin polymerization (Fig. **8**) [229]. Both taxanes and vinca alkaloids are, therefore, regarded as spindle poisons or mitosis poisons, but their actions are different. Interestingly, podophyllotoxin also destabilises microtubules by binding to tubulin and therefore preventing cell division [232].

## Potential Anti-Cancer Compounds from Microbial Sources

### DNA Intercalating Agents

Bleomycin (Fig. **9**) belongs to a subfamily of glycopeptide antibiotics produced from the fermentation of *Streptomyces verticillus* and is used in the treatment of various malignancies [236, 237], including squamous cell carcinoma, metastatic germ cell cancer, and non-Hodgkin's lymphoma [238], generally in combination with radiation or other chemotherapeutic agents.

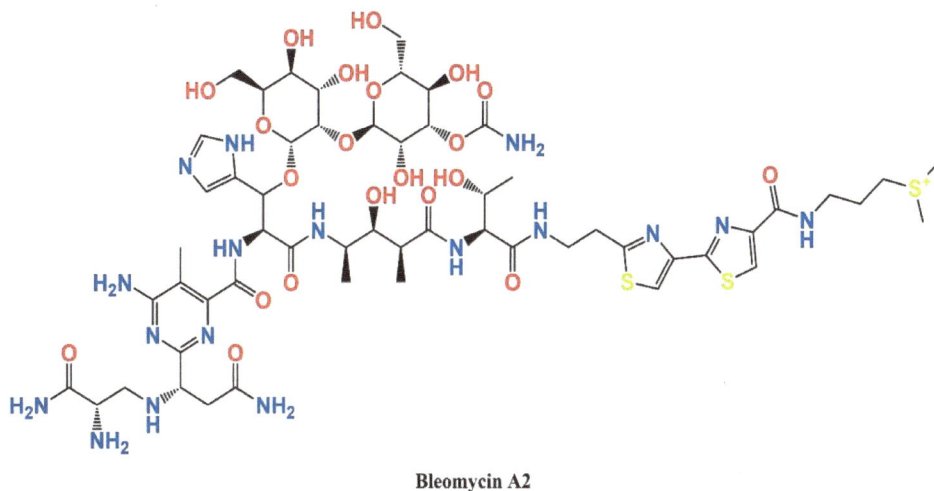

Bleomycin A2

**Fig. (9).** Structure of bleomycin.

It acts by inducing iron-dependent degradation of DNA (Fig. **10**) [239, 240]. However, the therapeutic applications of bleomycin are limited by the accompanying potential of lung toxicity. Many attempts have been made to develop novel bleomycin analogues for the search for drug leads with improved antitumor activity and/or reduced toxicity [241].

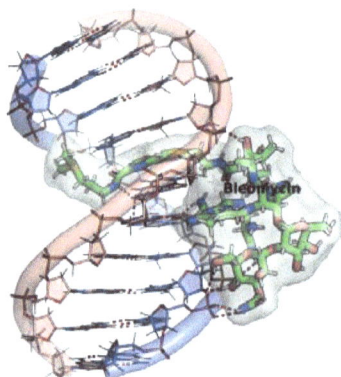

**Fig. (10).** Bleomycin (green) (PDB ID 1MXK) as an intercalating agent [242].

Dactinomycin, also known as actinomycin D (Fig. **11**), is used to treat various types of cancer, including Wilms' tumour [243], rhabdomyosarcoma [244], Ewing's sarcoma [245], trophoblastic neoplasm [246], and so on. It was the first antibiotic shown to have anti-cancer activity.

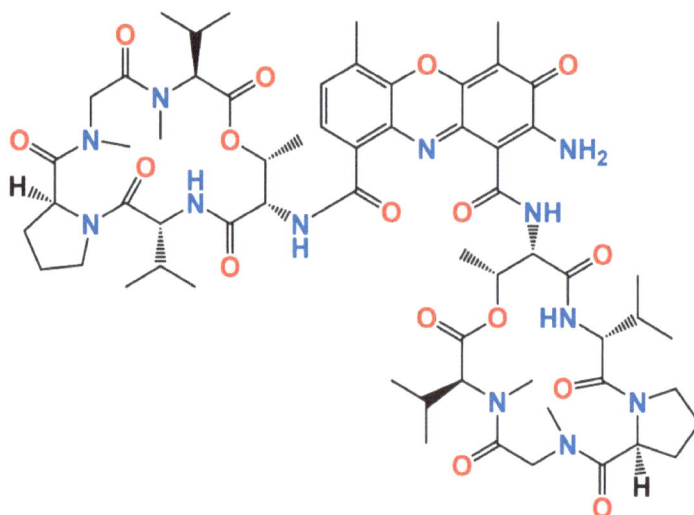

**Dactinomycin**

**Fig. (11).** Structure of dactinomycin.

Dactinomycin inhibits transcription by binding DNA (Fig. **12**) at the transcription initiation complex and preventing elongation of the RNA chain by RNA polymerase [247]. It was first isolated in 1940 by Selman Waksman and his co-worker H. Boyd Woodruff [248].

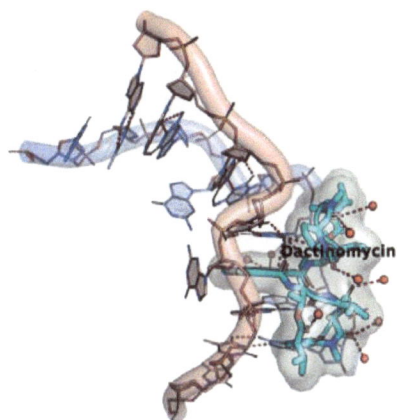

**Fig. (12).** Dactinomycin (cyan) (PDB ID 6J0H) as an intercalating agent [249].

Anthracyclines are utilised in cancer chemotherapy and are mainly obtained from the *Streptomyces* bacterium [250]. The first anthracycline found was daunorubicin, also known as daunomycin, which is produced by *Streptomyces peucetius* actinobacteria. Anthracyclines are among the most effective anti-cancer therapies ever developed and are effective against more types of cancer than any other class of anti-cancer drugs, including leukemias, lymphomas, breast, stomach, uterine, ovarian, bladder, and lung cancers [251, 252]. Clinically, the most significant anthracyclines are doxorubicin, daunorubicin, epirubicin, and idarubicin (Fig. **13**) [253].

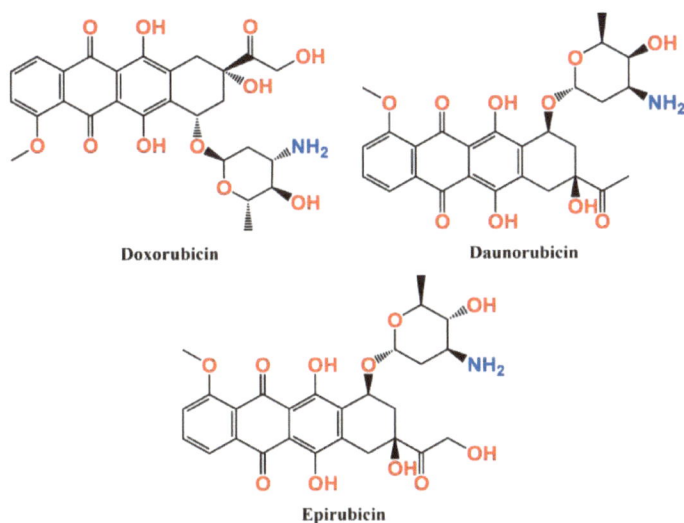

**Doxorubicin**                    **Daunorubicin**

**Epirubicin**

**Fig. (13).** Structures of anthracyclines.

These drugs act primarily by intercalating with DNA (Fig. **14**) and interfering with DNA metabolism and RNA production [254]. However, two considerable dose-limiting toxicities of anthracyclines include myelosuppression and cardiotoxicity [255].

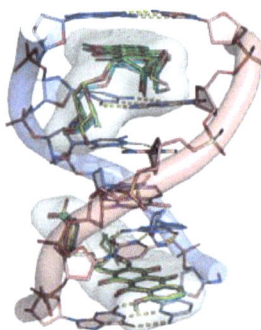

**Fig. (14).** Overlay of doxorubicin (cyan; PDB ID 1P20) [254], daunorubicin (green; PDB ID 1JO2) [256], and epirubicin (yellow; PDB ID 1D58) [257] molecules intercalated within DNA.

## Histone Deacetylase Inhibitors

Histone deacetylase (HDAC) inhibitors (HDIs), such as romidepsin (Fig. **15**), are being investigated as possible treatments for cancers. *In vitro* and *in vivo* studies on pancreatic, esophageal squamous cell carcinoma, multiple myeloma, prostate carcinoma, gastric cancer, breast cancer, ovarian cancer, non-Hodgkin's lymphoma, and other cancers revealed anti-cancer activity of Pan-HDAC inhibitors [258].

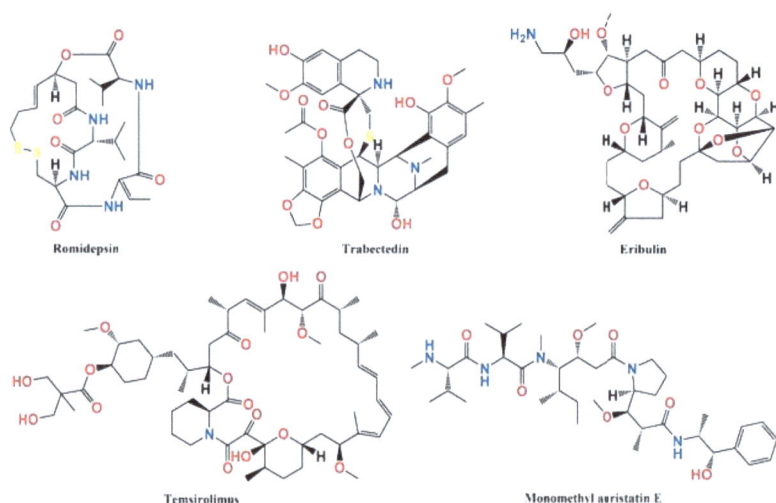

**Fig. (15).** Structures of romidepsin, trabectedin, eribulin, temsirolimus, and monomethyl auristatin E.

Romidepsin, also known as Istodax, is an anti-cancer drug utilised in the treatment of cutaneous T-cell lymphoma and other peripheral T-cell lymphomas. It was obtained from the bacterium *Chromobacterium violaceum*, and it works by blocking histone deacetylases, thus inducing apoptosis [259, 260].

## mTOR Inhibitors

A mammalian target of rapamycin (mTOR) is a serine/threonine-specific protein kinase enzyme inside the cell that collects and interprets the numerous and varied growth and survival signals received by cancer cells. Many mTOR inhibitors, also called rapalogs (rapamycin and its analogues), have shown tumour responses in clinical trials against several tumour types [261].

Temsirolimus (Fig. **15**), sold under the brand name Torisel, is an intravenous drug for the treatment of renal cell carcinoma. It is a prodrug of rapamycin and is a specific inhibitor of mTOR. It interferes with the synthesis of proteins that regulate the proliferation, growth, and survival of tumour cells. However, temsirolimus is associated with lung toxicity, and the risk of developing this complication may be increased among patients with a history of lung disease [262].

## Potential Anti-Cancer Compounds from Marine Sources

### *Mitotic Inhibitors*

Monomethyl auristatin E (MMAE) (Fig. **15**) is a highly toxic mitotic inhibitor, *i.e.*, it inhibits cell division by blocking the polymerization of tubulin (Fig. **8**) and is linked to a monoclonal antibody which directs it to the cancer cells. It was derived from peptides present in the marine sea hare *Dolabella auricularia* called dolastatins, which display potent activity both *in vitro* and *in vivo* against a range of lymphomas, leukemia, and solid tumors. These drugs display a potency of up to 200 times that of vinca alkaloids [263].

Eribulin (Fig. **15**) is a fully synthetic macrocyclic ketone analogue of the marine natural product halichondrin B [264], which is a potent, naturally occurring mitotic inhibitor found in *Halichondria* sponges [45]. It is a mechanistically unique inhibitor of microtubule dynamics [265], binding mostly at the plus ends of existing microtubules (Fig. **8**).

### *DNA Minor-Groove Alkylators*

Alkylating agents bind to DNA, cross-linking two strands, thereby preventing DNA replication and causing cancer cell death [266]. Ecteinascidin 743 (trabectedin; Yondelis) (Fig. **15**), a DNA minor-groove alkylator, is used in the treatment of soft tissue sarcomas. It binds and alkylates DNA at the N2 position of guanine in the DNA minor-groove and bends the DNA toward the major-groove, thereby interfering directly with activated transcription, poisoning the transcription-coupled nucleotide excision repair complex, promoting degradation of RNA polymerase II, and generating DNA double-strand breaks [267].

It was obtained in low abundance from the sea squirt *Ecteinascidia turbinate* [268]. However, the current supply is based on a semi-synthetic procedure starting from safracin B, an antibiotic obtained by fermentation of the bacterium *Pseudomonas fluorescens* [42].

## INTRODUCTION OF NATURAL ANTI-CANCER COMPOUNDS IN CLINICAL TRIALS (DRUG DEVELOPMENT)

Phytochemicals-based clinical trials against cancer are still in their early stages, though several promising anti-neoplastic agents are under development at present. A clinical trial using phytochemicals mainly focuses on three main characteristics of cancer therapeutics:

1. looking for undesirable drug interactions with current conventional therapy,
2. with conventional cancer treatment, and
3. increasing the response of cancer cells to conventional chemotherapy and radiotherapy.

A brief description will be given of a number of phytochemicals (Table **1**) that are currently under clinical trials against different cancers.

Table 1. Anti-cancer natural compounds in clinical trials.

| Phytochemical | Chemical Structure | Type of Cancer | Assessment | ClinicalTrials.gov Identifiers |
|---|---|---|---|---|
| Curcumin (polyphenol) | | Metastatic and advanced breast cancer | Safety in combination, progression-free survival time, time to treatment failure, and quality of life | NCT03072992 |

*(Table 1) cont.....*

| Phytochemical | Chemical Structure | Type of Cancer | Assessment | ClinicalTrials.gov Identifiers |
|---|---|---|---|---|
| Berberine (alkaloid) | | Colon and rectal cancer | Prevention of recurrence | NCT03281096 |
| Sulforaphane (isothiocyanate) | | Known smokers with a high chance of developing lung cancer | Cell proliferation markers ki-67, bronchial dysplasia index, apoptosis markers including TUNEL and caspase-3 | NCT03232138 |
| Epigallocatechin (flavonoid) | | Colon and rectal cancer | Methylation pattern change in comparison to baseline | NCT02891538 |
| Lycopene (carotenoid) | | Metastatic cancer in colon and, rectum | Efficiency in decreasing the toxicity in skin alone or in combination with panitumumab | NCT03167268 |
| Resveratrol (stilbenoid) | | Low-grade GI neuroendocrine tumours | Notch-1 activation, toxicity | NCT01476592 |

Curcumin, a polyphenolic pigment, is a functional component of a familiar and widely used Indian spice called turmeric (*Curcuma longa*; Zingiberaceae) and has attracted much attention recently as a promising chemopreventive agent. A number of studies have found it to be chemotherapeutic and chemopreventive in various cancer cells, including prostate [269], ovary [270], and skin cancers [271], blood [272], breast [273], head and neck [274], and liver [275]. As an anti-cancer agent in combination with standard therapy or alone, curcumin has shown efficacy against breast [276], prostate [277], pancreatic [278, 279], colorectal [280 - 282], and haematological malignancies [283]. A recent study showed that curcumin in combination with gemcitabine in patients with locally advanced or metastatic pancreatic carcinoma improves the potency of gemcitabine without any treatment-associated toxicity [284]. A double-blind, randomized, placebo-controlled phase 2/3 trial is continuing to determine its effectiveness in combination with Paclitaxel administered once a week for 12 weeks against adva-nced or metastatic breast carcinoma (https://clinicaltrials.gov/show/NCT03072-992).

Berberine (Fig. **16**), a benzyl-tetra isoquinoline alkaloid in *Berberis* sp. (Berberidaceae), is widely known as an Ayurvedic and traditional Chinese medicine. Preclinical anti-cancer efficiency of berberine has been reported in several neoplasias of the pancreas [285], prostate [286], ovarian [287], cervical [288], colon [289], breast [290], gastrointestinal [291], oral [292], and so on. A placebo-controlled, double-blind, randomized, phase 2/3 clinical trial is underway to ascertain the effectiveness of berberine hydrochloride against the incidence of new colorectal adenomas among 1000 patients with a previous link to colorectal cancer (https://clinicaltrials.gov/show/NCT03281096).

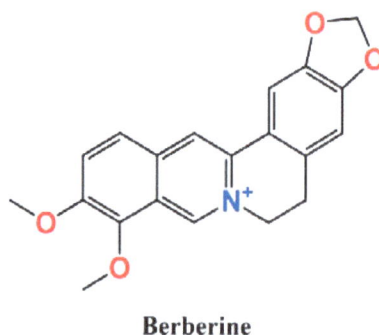

**Berberine**

**Fig. (16).** Structure of berberine.

Sulforaphane (SFN) is a nutritional isothiocyanate mainly present in cruciferous plants such as broccoli (*Brassica oleracea*, Brassicaceae). Currently, a double-blind, placebo-controlled, phase 2 clinical trial is being conducted to evaluate the chemopreventive effect of SFN tablets in former smokers with a high chance of initiation of lung cancer (https://clinicaltrials.gov/show/NCT03232138). Cipolla and colleagues conducted a double-blind, randomized, placebo-controlled clinical trial in 78 patients with augmented prostate-specific antigen (PSA) levels following radical prostatectomy. They found that oral intake of SFN for six months expressively increased the PSA doubling time (PSADT) and did not report any adverse effects compared to the placebo group [293]. Another group conducted a single-arm trial with SFN-rich broccoli sprout extracts and administered it to 20 patients for 20 weeks with prostate cancer. Despite achieving the primary endpoint, there was a noteworthy increase in the on-treatment PSADT when compared with the pre-treatment PSADT [294].

Green tea (*Camellia sinensis*; Theaceae) contains epigallocatechin (EGCG), a well-known catechin found in green tea. In a pre-surgical, placebo-controlled, randomised phase 2 pilot investigation of polyphenon E (a green tea formulation primarily containing ECGC) in bladder cancer patients, EGCG was found to be gathered in tumour tissue and decreased cell proliferation and increased apoptosis [295]. Better treatment outcomes have been reported from a combination therapy using EGCG and indole-3-carbinol in patients with advanced ovarian cancer. At present, the evaluation of chemopreventive effects is being done in an early-phase clinical trial in patients with colorectal cancer (CRC) (https://clinicaltrials.gov/show/NCT03072992).

Lycopene is a chemical compound that gives the red colour of fruits and vegetables. It is plentifully present in red tomatoes (*Solanum lycopersicum*; Solanaceae). Chen *et al.* have revealed that intake of a higher dose of lycopene had no minor effect in reducing the chance of prostate carcinoma in men [296]. A double-blinded, randomized, controlled trial in patients with HGPIN (multifocal high grade prostatic intraepithelial neoplasia) and/or atypical small acinar proliferation (ASAP), application of high dose lycopene in combination with selenium and green tea catechins (GTCs) increases the expression of prostate cancer progression associated microRNAs and the incidence of prostate cancer re-biopsy, which is indicative of avoiding the high dose of lycopene in prostate cancer patients [297]. A phase 2 clinical trial is currently underway to determine the efficacy of lycopene in reducing Panitumumab-associated skin toxicity in patients with colorectal cancer metastasis (https://clinicaltrials.gov/show/NCT-03167268).

Resveratrol (3,5,4′-trihydroxy-trans-stilbene) is a stilbenoid compound. Paller *et al.* reported that in a phase 1 trial on men, administering pulverized muscadine grape skin extract (MPX), which is rich in resveratrol, delayed the recurrence of prostate cancer by increasing the PSADT by 5.3 months [298]. In a pilot study comprising 39 women at high risk of breast tumours, trans-resveratrol decreases cancer-promoting prostaglandin E2 (PGE2) in the breast and decreases the methylation of a breast cancer-associated gene called Ras-association domain family 1 isoform A (RASSF)-1a [299]. In another pilot study in colorectal cancer patients with hepatic metastasis, resveratrol was found in the malignant hepatic tissue where the apoptosis marker caspase-3 was significantly increased [300]. A clinical trial on the efficacy of resveratrol on Notch-1 signalling in low-grade gastrointestinal neuroendocrine carcinoma has been completed, but the results have not yet been published (https://clinicaltrials.gov/show/NCT01476592).

## CONCLUSION

Many biological sources have been tested for anti-cancer activity, and a few bioactive constituents have been isolated from the advancement of modern technologies [301]. Bioassay-guided isolation is a significant way of finding new anti-cancer compounds, but it is also a long-term process. Developments in molecular biology and newly designed techniques have expanded the level of analysis for bioactivities. Natural compounds isolated so far can be accumulated in databases and assessed for anti-cancer activity. In-depth mechanistic studies of bioactive components as hits can also be evaluated. As a result, bioactive molecules can be outlined in a brief duration, and more time can be spent on further research into the modes of action. Studies show natural compounds dominate a vast majority of the chemical domain rather than synthetic substances. Identifying a variety of anti-cancer compounds from natural sources could be beneficial for drug discovery and development [302, 303].

The use of bioinformatics strategies to screen large databases of natural products could undoubtedly save time and money and aid in the detection of novel natural-based anti-cancer drug candidates. Humans have been using natural compounds derived from animals, plants, and microbes since prehistory. The treatment of cancer, in particular, has been deeply affected. Indeed, a vast number of therapeutics of natural origin have been applied to treat cancer. Hence, the list of natural products with cancer therapeutics is impressive and includes vinca alkaloids, anthracycline anti-cancer antibiotics, camptothecins, epipodophy llotoxins, rapalogs, and taxanes, to name a few. Without a doubt, entire drug families of anti-cancer agents have their roots in the secondary metabolites produced by microbes, plants, as well as marine organisms. It is now evident that the fields of cancer drug discovery and natural products are undergoing substantial change.

# CONSENT FOR PUBLICATION

Not applicable.

# CONFLICT OF INTEREST

The authors declare no conflict of interest, financial or otherwise.

# ACKNOWLEDGEMENTS

Declared none.

# REFERENCES

[1]     Fridlender, M.; Kapulnik, Y.; Koltai, H. Plant derived substances with anti-cancer activity: from folklore to practice. *Front. Plant Sci.,* **2015**, *6,* 799.
        [http://dx.doi.org/10.3389/fpls.2015.00799] [PMID: 26483815]

[2]     Kumar, A. Vincristine and vinblastine: a review. *Int. J. Med. Pharm. Sci.,* **2016**, *6*(1), 23-30.

[3]     Aslam, J.; Mujib, A.; Nasim, S.A.; Sharma, M.P. Screening of Vincristine Yield in *Ex Vitro* and *in Vitro* Somatic Embryos Derived Plantlets of Catharanthus Roseus L. (G) Don. *Sci. Hortic. (Amsterdam),* **2009**, *119*(3), 325-329.
        [http://dx.doi.org/10.1016/j.scienta.2008.08.018]

[4]     Denis, J.N.; Greene, A.E.; Guenard, D.; Gueritte-Voegelein, F.; Mangatal, L.; Potier, P. Highly Efficient, Practical Approach to Natural Taxol. *J. Am. Chem. Soc.,* **1988**, *110*(17), 5917-5919.
        [http://dx.doi.org/10.1021/ja00225a063]

[5]     Bocca, C. Taxol, a Short History of a Promising Anticancer Drug. *Minerva Biotecnol.,* **1998**, *10,* 81-83.

[6]     Holton, R.A.; Somoza, C.; Kim, H.B.; Liang, F.; Biediger, R.J.; Boatman, P.D.; Shindo, M.; Smith, C.C.; Kim, S. First Total Synthesis of Taxol. 1. Functionalization of the B Ring. *J. Am. Chem. Soc.,* **1994**, *116*(4), 1597-1598.
        [http://dx.doi.org/10.1021/ja00083a066]

[7]     Nicolaou, K.C.; Yang, Z.; Liu, J.J.; Ueno, H.; Nantermet, P.G.; Guy, R.K.; Claiborne, C.F.; Renaud, J.; Couladouros, E.A.; Paulvannan, K.; Sorensen, E.J. Total synthesis of taxol. *Nature,* **1994**, *367*(6464), 630-634.
        [http://dx.doi.org/10.1038/367630a0] [PMID: 7906395]

[8]     Holton, R.A.; Kim, H.B.; Somoza, C.; Liang, F.; Biediger, R.J.; Boatman, P.D.; Shindo, M.; Smith, C.C.; Kim, S. First Total Synthesis of Taxol. 2. Completion of the C and D Rings. *J. Am. Chem. Soc.,* **1994**, *116*(4), 1599-1600.
        [http://dx.doi.org/10.1021/ja00083a067]

[9]     Danishefsky, S.J.; Masters, J.J.; Young, W.B.; Link, J.T.; Snyder, L.B.; Magee, T.V.; Jung, D.K.; Isaacs, R.C.A.; Bornmann, W.G.; Alaimo, C.A.; Coburn, C.A.; Di Grandi, M.J. Total Synthesis of Baccatin III and Taxol. *J. Am. Chem. Soc.,* **1996**, *118*(12), 2843-2859.
        [http://dx.doi.org/10.1021/ja952692a]

[10]    Katsumata, N. Docetaxel: an alternative taxane in ovarian cancer. *Br. J. Cancer,* **2003**, *89*(S3) Suppl. 3, S9-S15.
        [http://dx.doi.org/10.1038/sj.bjc.6601495] [PMID: 14661041]

[11]    Crown, J.; O'Leary, M.; Ooi, W.S. Docetaxel and paclitaxel in the treatment of breast cancer: a review of clinical experience. *Oncologist,* **2004**, *9*(S2) Suppl. 2, 24-32.
        [http://dx.doi.org/10.1634/theoncologist.9-suppl_2-24] [PMID: 15161988]

[12]   Tiainen, L.; Tanner, M.; Lahdenperä, O.; Vihinen, P.; Jukkola, A.; Karihtala, P.; Paunu, N.; Huttunen, T.; Kellokumpu-Lehtinen, P.L. Bevacizumab Combined with Docetaxel or Paclitaxel as First-line Treatment of HER2-negative Metastatic Breast Cancer. *Anticancer Res.,* **2016**, *36*(12), 6431-6438.
[http://dx.doi.org/10.21873/anticanres.11241] [PMID: 27919965]

[13]   Khazir, J.; Mir, B.A.; Pilcher, L.; Riley, D.L. Role of Plants in Anticancer Drug Discovery. *Phytochem. Lett.,* **2014**, *7*, 173-181.
[http://dx.doi.org/10.1016/j.phytol.2013.11.010]

[14]   Stork, G.; Schultz, A.G. The total synthesis of dl-camptothecin. *J. Am. Chem. Soc.,* **1971**, *93*(16), 4074-4075.
[http://dx.doi.org/10.1021/ja00745a056] [PMID: 5138309]

[15]   Volkmann, R.; Danishefsky, S.; Eggler, J.; Solomon, D.M. Total Synthesis of (+-)-Camptothecine. *J. Am. Chem. Soc.,* **1971**, *93*(21), 5576-5577.
[http://dx.doi.org/10.1021/ja00750a045]

[16]   Ejima, A.; Terasawa, H.; Sugimori, M.; Tagawa, H. Asymmetric Synthesis of (S)-Camptothecin. *Tetrahedron Lett.,* **1989**, *30*(20), 2639-2640.
[http://dx.doi.org/10.1016/S0040-4039(00)99086-5]

[17]   Bennasar, M-L.; Juan, C.; Bosch, J. A Short Synthesis of Camptothecin *via* a 2-Fluoro-1-4-Dihydropyridine. *Chem. Commun. (Camb.),* **2000**, (24), 2459-2460.
[http://dx.doi.org/10.1039/b007814j]

[18]   Bennasar, M-L.; Zulaica, E.; Juan, C.; Alonso, Y.; Bosch, J. Addition of ester enolates to N-alkyl-2-fluoropyridinium salts: total synthesis of (+/-)-20-deoxycamptothecin and (+)-camptothecin. *J. Org. Chem.,* **2002**, *67*(21), 7465-7474.
[http://dx.doi.org/10.1021/jo026173j] [PMID: 12375981]

[19]   Zunino, F.; Dallavalleb, S.; Laccabuea, D.; Berettaa, G.; Merlinib, L.; Pratesi, G. Current status and perspectives in the development of camptothecins. *Curr. Pharm. Des.,* **2002**, *8*(27), 2505-2520.
[http://dx.doi.org/10.2174/1381612023392801] [PMID: 12369944]

[20]   Canel, C.; Moraes, R.M.; Dayan, F.E.; Ferreira, D. Podophyllotoxin. *Phytochemistry,* **2000**, *54*(2), 115-120.
[http://dx.doi.org/10.1016/S0031-9422(00)00094-7] [PMID: 10872202]

[21]   Lichota, A.; Gwozdzinski, K. Anticancer Activity of Natural Compounds from Plant and Marine Environment. *Int. J. Mol. Sci.,* **2018**, *19*(11), 3533.
[http://dx.doi.org/10.3390/ijms19113533] [PMID: 30423952]

[22]   Zhang, A.; Chang, D.; Zhang, Z.; Li, F.; Li, W.; Wang, X.; Li, Y.; Hua, Q. *In Vitro* Selection of DNA Aptamers that Binds Geniposide. *Molecules,* **2017**, *22*(3), 383.
[http://dx.doi.org/10.3390/molecules22030383] [PMID: 28264528]

[23]   Habtemariam, S.; Lentini, G. Plant-Derived Anticancer Agents: Lessons from the Pharmacology of Geniposide and Its Aglycone, Genipin. *Biomedicines,* **2018**, *6*(2), 39.
[http://dx.doi.org/10.3390/biomedicines6020039] [PMID: 29587429]

[24]   Hiranuma, S.; Hudlicky, T. Synthesis of Homoharringtonine and Its Derivative. *Tetrahedron Lett.,* **1982**, *23*(34), 3431-3434.
[http://dx.doi.org/10.1016/S0040-4039(00)87634-0]

[25]   Hansz, J. Contemporary Therapy of Chronic Myeloid Leukemia. *Postepy Nauk Med.,* **2000**, 33-29.

[26]   Woodward, R.B.; Iacobucci, G.A.; Hochstein, I.A. THE SYNTHESIS OF ELLIPTICINE. *J. Am. Chem. Soc.,* **1959**, *81*(16), 4434-4435.
[http://dx.doi.org/10.1021/ja01525a085]

[27]   Meijer, L.; Borgne, A.; Mulner, O.; Chong, J.P.J.; Blow, J.J.; Inagaki, N.; Inagaki, M.; Delcros, J-G.; Moulinoux, J-P. Biochemical and cellular effects of roscovitine, a potent and selective inhibitor of the

cyclin-dependent kinases cdc2, cdk2 and cdk5. *Eur. J. Biochem.,* **1997**, *243*(1-2), 527-536.
[http://dx.doi.org/10.1111/j.1432-1033.1997.t01-2-00527.x] [PMID: 9030781]

[28]    Corey, E.J.; Weigel, L.O.; Chamberlin, A.R.; Cho, H.; Hua, D.H. Total Synthesis of Maytansine. *J. Am. Chem. Soc.,* **1980**, *102*(21), 6613-6615.
[http://dx.doi.org/10.1021/ja00541a064]

[29]    Bhattacharyya, B.; Wolff, J. Maytansine binding to the vinblastine sites of tubulin. *FEBS Lett.,* **1977**, *75*(1), 159-162.
[http://dx.doi.org/10.1016/0014-5793(77)80075-6] [PMID: 852577]

[30]    Rogers, T.B.; Inesi, G.; Wade, R.; Lederer, W.J. Use of thapsigargin to study $Ca^{2+}$ homeostasis in cardiac cells. *Biosci. Rep.,* **1995**, *15*(5), 341-349.
[http://dx.doi.org/10.1007/BF01788366] [PMID: 8825036]

[31]    Goodyear, S.; Sharma, M.C. Roscovitine regulates invasive breast cancer cell (MDA-MB231) proliferation and survival through cell cycle regulatory protein cdk5. *Exp. Mol. Pathol.,* **2007**, *82*(1), 25-32.
[http://dx.doi.org/10.1016/j.yexmp.2006.09.002] [PMID: 17081516]

[32]    Sasaki, M.; Murae, T. A Formal Synthesis of Bruceantin. *Tetrahedron Lett.,* **1989**, *30*(3), 355-356.
[http://dx.doi.org/10.1016/S0040-4039(00)95200-6]

[33]    Cuendet, M.; Pezzuto, J.M. Antitumor activity of bruceantin: an old drug with new promise. *J. Nat. Prod.,* **2004**, *67*(2), 269-272.
[http://dx.doi.org/10.1021/np030304+] [PMID: 14987068]

[34]    Darkin-Rattray, S.J.; Gurnett, A.M.; Myers, R.W.; Dulski, P.M.; Crumley, T.M.; Allocco, J.J.; Cannova, C.; Meinke, P.T.; Colletti, S.L.; Bednarek, M.A.; Singh, S.B.; Goetz, M.A.; Dombrowski, A.W.; Polishook, J.D.; Schmatz, D.M. Apicidin: a novel antiprotozoal agent that inhibits parasite histone deacetylase. *Proc. Natl. Acad. Sci. USA,* **1996**, *93*(23), 13143-13147.
[http://dx.doi.org/10.1073/pnas.93.23.13143] [PMID: 8917558]

[35]    Hoshino, O.; Murakata, M.; Yamada, K. A Convenient Synthesis of a Bromotyrosine Derived Metabolite, Psammaplin A, from Psammaplysilla Sp. *Bioorg. Med. Chem. Lett.,* **1992**, *2*(12), 1561-1562.
[http://dx.doi.org/10.1016/S0960-894X(00)80429-1]

[36]    Simmons, T.L.; Andrianasolo, E.; McPhail, K.; Flatt, P.; Gerwick, W.H. Marine natural products as anticancer drugs. *Mol. Cancer Ther.,* **2005**, *4*(2), 333-342.
[PMID: 15713904]

[37]    Kumari, A.; Singh, R.K. Medicinal chemistry of indole derivatives: Current to future therapeutic prospectives. *Bioorg. Chem.,* **2019**, *89*, 103021.
[http://dx.doi.org/10.1016/j.bioorg.2019.103021] [PMID: 31176854]

[38]    Ramanjulu, J.M.; Ding, X.; Joullié, M.M.; Li, W-R. Synthesis of a Reduced Ring Analog of Didemnin B. *J. Org. Chem.,* **1997**, *62*(15), 4961-4969.
[http://dx.doi.org/10.1021/jo9623696]

[39]    Tomioka, K.; Kanai, M.; Koga, K. An Expeditious Synthesis of Dolastatin 10. *Tetrahedron Lett.,* **1991**, *32*(21), 2395-2398.
[http://dx.doi.org/10.1016/S0040-4039(00)79932-1]

[40]    Mita, A.C.; Hammond, L.A.; Bonate, P.L.; Weiss, G.; McCreery, H.; Syed, S.; Garrison, M.; Chu, Q.S.C.; DeBono, J.S.; Jones, C.B.; Weitman, S.; Rowinsky, E.K. Phase I and pharmacokinetic study of tasidotin hydrochloride (ILX651), a third-generation dolastatin-15 analogue, administered weekly for 3 weeks every 28 days in patients with advanced solid tumors. *Clin. Cancer Res.,* **2006**, *12*(17), 5207-5215.
[http://dx.doi.org/10.1158/1078-0432.CCR-06-0179] [PMID: 16951240]

[41]    Watanabe, J.; Minami, M.; Kobayashi, M. Antitumor activity of TZT-1027 (Soblidotin). *Anticancer*

*Res.,* **2006**, *26*(3A), 1973-1981.
[PMID: 16827132]

[42]   Cuevas, C.; Pérez, M.; Martín, M.J.; Chicharro, J.L.; Fernández-Rivas, C.; Flores, M.; Francesch, A.; Gallego, P.; Zarzuelo, M.; de La Calle, F.; García, J.; Polanco, C.; Rodríguez, I.; Manzanares, I. Synthesis of ecteinascidin ET-743 and phthalascidin Pt-650 from cyanosafracin B. *Org. Lett.,* **2000**, *2*(16), 2545-2548.
[http://dx.doi.org/10.1021/ol0062502] [PMID: 10956543]

[43]   D'Incalci, M.; Galmarini, C.M. A review of trabectedin (ET-743): a unique mechanism of action. *Mol. Cancer Ther.,* **2010**, *9*(8), 2157-2163.
[http://dx.doi.org/10.1158/1535-7163.MCT-10-0263] [PMID: 20647340]

[44]   Uemura, D.; Takahashi, K.; Yamamoto, T.; Katayama, C.; Tanaka, J.; Okumura, Y.; Hirata, Y.; Norhalichondrin, A. An Antitumor Polyether Macrolide from a Marine Sponge. *J. Am. Chem. Soc.,* **1985**, *107*(16), 4796-4798.
[http://dx.doi.org/10.1021/ja00302a042]

[45]   Bai, R.L.L.; Paull, K.D.D.; Herald, C.L.L.; Malspeis, L.; Pettit, G.R.R.; Hamel, E.; Halichondrin, B.; Homohalichondrin, B. Halichondrin B and homohalichondrin B, marine natural products binding in the vinca domain of tubulin. Discovery of tubulin-based mechanism of action by analysis of differential cytotoxicity data. *J. Biol. Chem.,* **1991**, *266*(24), 15882-15889.
[http://dx.doi.org/10.1016/S0021-9258(18)98491-7] [PMID: 1874739]

[46]   Mazumder, A.; Cerella, C.; Diederich, M. Natural scaffolds in anticancer therapy and precision medicine. *Biotechnol. Adv.,* **2018**, *36*(6), 1563-1585.
[http://dx.doi.org/10.1016/j.biotechadv.2018.04.009] [PMID: 29729870]

[47]   Sethi, N.S.; Prasad, D.N.; Singh, R.K. An Insight into the Synthesis and SAR of 2,4-Thiazolidinediones (2,4-TZD) as Multifunctional Scaffold: A Review. *Mini Rev. Med. Chem.,* **2020**, *20*(4), 308-330.
[http://dx.doi.org/10.2174/1389557519666191029102838] [PMID: 31660809]

[48]   Kumari, A.; Singh, R.K. Morpholine as ubiquitous pharmacophore in medicinal chemistry: Deep insight into the structure-activity relationship (SAR). *Bioorg. Chem.,* **2020**, *96*, 103578.
[http://dx.doi.org/10.1016/j.bioorg.2020.103578] [PMID: 31978684]

[49]   The Global Challenge of Cancer. The global challenge of cancer. *Nat. Can.,* **2020**, *1*(1), 1-2.
[http://dx.doi.org/10.1038/s43018-019-0023-9]

[50]   International Agency for Research on Cancer (IARC). **2020**.https://www.iarc.fr/news-events/lates--global-cancer-data-cancer-burden-rises-to-19-3-million-new-cases-and-10-0-million-cancer-deaths-in-2020/

[51]   Ferlay, J; Soerjomataram, I; Ervik, M; Dikshit, R; Eser, S; Mathers, C; Rebelo, M; Parkin, DM; Forman, D GLOBOCAN 2012: Estimated Cancer Incidence, Mortality and Prevalence Worldwide. **2012**.

[52]   Bray, F.; Ferlay, J.; Soerjomataram, I.; Siegel, R.L.; Torre, L.A.; Jemal, A. Global cancer statistics 2018: GLOBOCAN estimates of incidence and mortality worldwide for 36 cancers in 185 countries. *CA Cancer J. Clin.,* **2018**, *68*(6), 394-424.
[http://dx.doi.org/10.3322/caac.21492] [PMID: 30207593]

[53]   Roser, M.; Ritchie, H. *Cancer*; Our World Data, **2015**.

[54]   Wild, C.; Weiderpass, E. World Cancer Report: Cancer Research for Cancer Prevention. **2021**.

[55]   Newman, D.J.; Cragg, G.M. Natural products as sources of new drugs over the last 25 years. *J. Nat. Prod.,* **2007**, *70*(3), 461-477.
[http://dx.doi.org/10.1021/np068054v] [PMID: 17309302]

[56]   Cragg, G.M.; Grothaus, P.G.; Newman, D.J. Impact of natural products on developing new anti-cancer agents. *Chem. Rev.,* **2009**, *109*(7), 3012-3043.

[http://dx.doi.org/10.1021/cr900019j] [PMID: 19422222]

[57]   Gordaliza, M. Natural products as leads to anticancer drugs. *Clin. Transl. Oncol.,* **2007**, *9*(12), 767-776.
[http://dx.doi.org/10.1007/s12094-007-0138-9] [PMID: 18158980]

[58]   Samuelsson, G.; Bohlin, L. *Drugs of Natural Origin: A Treatise of Pharmacognosy*; 6., rev. e.; Apotekarsocieteten: Stockholm, 2009

[59]   Potente, M.; Gerhardt, H.; Carmeliet, P. Basic and therapeutic aspects of angiogenesis. *Cell,* **2011**, *146*(6), 873-887.
[http://dx.doi.org/10.1016/j.cell.2011.08.039] [PMID: 21925313]

[60]   Karamysheva, A.F. Mechanisms of angiogenesis. *Biochemistry (Mosc.),* **2008**, *73*(7), 751-762.
[http://dx.doi.org/10.1134/S0006297908070031] [PMID: 18707583]

[61]   Mercan, T.; Yamasan, B.E.; Erkan, O.; Özdemir, S. Thymoquinone Alters Ionic Currents and Decreases β Adrenergic Response in Rat Ventricle Myocytes. *J. Mol. Cell. Cardiol.,* **2018**, *120*, 22.
[http://dx.doi.org/10.1016/j.yjmcc.2018.05.074]

[62]   Peng, L.; Liu, A.; Shen, Y.; Xu, H-Z.; Yang, S.Z.; Ying, X.Z.; Liao, W.; Liu, H.X.; Lin, Z.Q.; Chen, Q.Y.; Cheng, S.W.; Shen, W.D. Antitumor and anti-angiogenesis effects of thymoquinone on osteosarcoma through the NF-κB pathway. *Oncol. Rep.,* **2013**, *29*(2), 571-578.
[http://dx.doi.org/10.3892/or.2012.2165] [PMID: 23232982]

[63]   Alobaedi, O.H.; Talib, W.H.; Basheti, I.A. Antitumor effect of thymoquinone combined with resveratrol on mice transplanted with breast cancer. *Asian Pac. J. Trop. Med.,* **2017**, *10*(4), 400-408.
[http://dx.doi.org/10.1016/j.apjtm.2017.03.026] [PMID: 28552110]

[64]   Auyeung, K.K-W.; Law, P.C.; Ko, J.K. Novel anti-angiogenic effects of formononetin in human colon cancer cells and tumor xenograft. *Oncol. Rep.,* **2012**, *28*(6), 2188-2194.
[http://dx.doi.org/10.3892/or.2012.2056] [PMID: 23023137]

[65]   Wu, Y.; Zhang, X.; Li, Z.; Yan, H.; Qin, J.; Li, T. Formononetin inhibits human bladder cancer cell proliferation and invasiveness *via* regulation of miR-21 and PTEN. *Food Funct.,* **2017**, *8*(3), 1061-1066.
[http://dx.doi.org/10.1039/C6FO01535B] [PMID: 28139790]

[66]   Elmore, S. Apoptosis: a review of programmed cell death. *Toxicol. Pathol.,* **2007**, *35*(4), 495-516.
[http://dx.doi.org/10.1080/01926230701320337] [PMID: 17562483]

[67]   Saelens, X.; Festjens, N.; Vande Walle, L.; van Gurp, M.; van Loo, G.; Vandenabeele, P. Toxic proteins released from mitochondria in cell death. *Oncogene,* **2004**, *23*(16), 2861-2874.
[http://dx.doi.org/10.1038/sj.onc.1207523] [PMID: 15077149]

[68]   Zhang, J.; Liu, L.; Wang, J.; Ren, B.; Zhang, L.; Li, W. Formononetin, an isoflavone from Astragalus membranaceus inhibits proliferation and metastasis of ovarian cancer cells. *J. Ethnopharmacol.,* **2018**, *221*, 91-99.
[http://dx.doi.org/10.1016/j.jep.2018.04.014] [PMID: 29660466]

[69]   Qi, C.; Xie, M.; Liang, J.; Li, H.; Li, Z.; Shi, S.; Yang, X.; Wang, Z.; Tang, J.; Tang, A. Formononetin Targets the MAPK and PI3K/Akt Pathways to Induce Apoptosis in Human Nasopharyngeal Carcinoma Cells *in Vitro* and *in Vivo*. *Int. J. Clin. Exp. Med.,* **2016**, *9*(2), 1180-1189.

[70]   Kim, C.; Lee, S-G.; Yang, W.M.; Arfuso, F.; Um, J-Y.; Kumar, A.P.; Bian, J.; Sethi, G.; Ahn, K.S. Formononetin-induced oxidative stress abrogates the activation of STAT3/5 signaling axis and suppresses the tumor growth in multiple myeloma preclinical model. *Cancer Lett.,* **2018**, *431*, 123-141.
[http://dx.doi.org/10.1016/j.canlet.2018.05.038] [PMID: 29857127]

[71]   Liu, Y.; He, J.; Chen, X.; Li, J.; Shen, M.; Yu, W.; Yang, Y.; Xiao, Z. The proapoptotic effect of formononetin in human osteosarcoma cells: involvement of inactivation of ERK and Akt pathways. *Cell. Physiol. Biochem.,* **2014**, *34*(3), 637-645.

[http://dx.doi.org/10.1159/000363029] [PMID: 25170541]

[72]  Yang, Y.; Zhao, Y.; Ai, X.; Cheng, B.; Lu, S. Formononetin suppresses the proliferation of human non-small cell lung cancer through induction of cell cycle arrest and apoptosis. *Int. J. Clin. Exp. Pathol.,* **2014**, *7*(12), 8453-8461.
[PMID: 25674209]

[73]  Liu, X-J.; Li, Y-Q.; Chen, Q-Y.; Xiao, S-J.; Zeng, S-E. Up-regulating of RASD1 and apoptosis of DU-145 human prostate cancer cells induced by formononetin *in vitro. Asian Pac. J. Cancer Prev.,* **2014**, *15*(6), 2835-2839.
[http://dx.doi.org/10.7314/APJCP.2014.15.6.2835] [PMID: 24761910]

[74]  Ye, Y.; Hou, R.; Chen, J.; Mo, L.; Zhang, J.; Huang, Y.; Mo, Z. Formononetin-induced apoptosis of human prostate cancer cells through ERK1/2 mitogen-activated protein kinase inactivation. *Horm. Metab. Res.,* **2012**, *44*(4), 263-267.
[http://dx.doi.org/10.1055/s-0032-1301922] [PMID: 22328166]

[75]  Huang, J.; Xie, M.; Gao, P.; Ye, Y.; Liu, Y.; Zhao, Y.; Luo, W.; Ling, Z.; Cao, Y.; Zhang, S.; Gao, F.; Tang, W. Antiproliferative Effects of Formononetin on Human Colorectal Cancer *via* Suppressing Cell Growth *in Vitro* and *in Vivo. Process Biochem.,* **2015**, *50*(6), 912-917.
[http://dx.doi.org/10.1016/j.procbio.2015.03.001]

[76]  Chen, J.; Sun, L. Formononetin-induced apoptosis by activation of Ras/p38 mitogen-activated protein kinase in estrogen receptor-positive human breast cancer cells. *Horm. Metab. Res.,* **2012**, *44*(13), 943-948.
[http://dx.doi.org/10.1055/s-0032-1321818] [PMID: 22828872]

[77]  Heiskanen, K.M.; Bhat, M.B.; Wang, H-W.; Ma, J.; Nieminen, A-L. Mitochondrial depolarization accompanies cytochrome c release during apoptosis in PC6 cells. *J. Biol. Chem.,* **1999**, *274*(9), 5654-5658.
[http://dx.doi.org/10.1074/jbc.274.9.5654] [PMID: 10026183]

[78]  Hahm, E-R.; Arlotti, J.A.; Marynowski, S.W.; Singh, S.V. Honokiol, a constituent of oriental medicinal herb magnolia officinalis, inhibits growth of PC-3 xenografts in vivo in association with apoptosis induction. *Clin. Cancer Res.,* **2008**, *14*(4), 1248-1257.
[http://dx.doi.org/10.1158/1078-0432.CCR-07-1926] [PMID: 18281560]

[79]  He, Z.; Subramaniam, D.; Ramalingam, S.; Dhar, A.; Postier, R.G.; Umar, S.; Zhang, Y.; Anant, S. Honokiol radiosensitizes colorectal cancer cells: enhanced activity in cells with mismatch repair defects. *Am. J. Physiol. Gastrointest. Liver Physiol.,* **2011**, *301*(5), G929-G937.
[http://dx.doi.org/10.1152/ajpgi.00159.2011] [PMID: 21836060]

[80]  Fan, Y.; Xue, W.; Schachner, M.; Zhao, W. Honokiol Eliminates Glioma/Glioblastoma Stem Cell-Like Cells *via* JAK-STAT3 Signaling and Inhibits Tumor Progression by Targeting Epidermal Growth Factor Receptor. *Cancers (Basel),* **2018**, *11*(1), 22.
[http://dx.doi.org/10.3390/cancers11010022] [PMID: 30587839]

[81]  Yang, S-E.; Hsieh, M-T.; Tsai, T-H.; Hsu, S-L. Down-modulation of Bcl-XL, release of cytochrome c and sequential activation of caspases during honokiol-induced apoptosis in human squamous lung cancer CH27 cells. *Biochem. Pharmacol.,* **2002**, *63*(9), 1641-1651.
[http://dx.doi.org/10.1016/S0006-2952(02)00894-8] [PMID: 12007567]

[82]  Wolf, I.; O'Kelly, J.; Wakimoto, N.; Nguyen, A.; Amblard, F.; Karlan, B.Y.; Arbiser, J.L.; Koeffler, H.P. Honokiol, a natural biphenyl, inhibits *in vitro* and *in vivo* growth of breast cancer through induction of apoptosis and cell cycle arrest. *Int. J. Oncol.,* **2007**, *30*(6), 1529-1537.
[http://dx.doi.org/10.3892/ijo.30.6.1529] [PMID: 17487375]

[83]  Garcia, A.; Zheng, Y.; Zhao, C.; Toschi, A.; Fan, J.; Shraibman, N.; Brown, H.A.; Bar-Sagi, D.; Foster, D.A.; Arbiser, J.L. Honokiol suppresses survival signals mediated by Ras-dependent phospholipase D activity in human cancer cells. *Clin. Cancer Res.,* **2008**, *14*(13), 4267-4274.
[http://dx.doi.org/10.1158/1078-0432.CCR-08-0102] [PMID: 18594009]

[84]　Fried, L.E.; Arbiser, J.L. Honokiol, a multifunctional antiangiogenic and antitumor agent. *Antioxid. Redox Signal.,* **2009,** *11*(5), 1139-1148.
[http://dx.doi.org/10.1089/ars.2009.2440] [PMID: 19203212]

[85]　Li, H-Y.; Ye, H-G.; Chen, C-Q.; Yin, L-H.; Wu, J-B.; He, L-C.; Gao, S-M. Honokiol induces cell cycle arrest and apoptosis *via* inhibiting class I histone deacetylases in acute myeloid leukemia. *J. Cell. Biochem.,* **2015,** *116*(2), 287-298.
[http://dx.doi.org/10.1002/jcb.24967] [PMID: 25187418]

[86]　Huang, K-J.; Kuo, C-H.; Chen, S-H.; Lin, C-Y.; Lee, Y-R. Honokiol inhibits *in vitro* and *in vivo* growth of oral squamous cell carcinoma through induction of apoptosis, cell cycle arrest and autophagy. *J. Cell. Mol. Med.,* **2018,** *22*(3), 1894-1908.
[http://dx.doi.org/10.1111/jcmm.13474] [PMID: 29363886]

[87]　Lv, X.; Liu, F.; Shang, Y.; Chen, S-Z. Honokiol exhibits enhanced antitumor effects with chloroquine by inducing cell death and inhibiting autophagy in human non-small cell lung cancer cells. *Oncol. Rep.,* **2015,** *34*(3), 1289-1300.
[http://dx.doi.org/10.3892/or.2015.4091] [PMID: 26136140]

[88]　Chilampalli, C.; Guillermo, R.; Kaushik, R.S.; Young, A.; Chandrasekher, G.; Fahmy, H.; Dwivedi, C. Honokiol, a chemopreventive agent against skin cancer, induces cell cycle arrest and apoptosis in human epidermoid A431 cells. *Exp. Biol. Med. (Maywood),* **2011,** *236*(11), 1351-1359.
[http://dx.doi.org/10.1258/ebm.2011.011030] [PMID: 21908486]

[89]　Deng, J.; Qian, Y.; Geng, L.; Chen, J.; Wang, X.; Xie, H.; Yan, S.; Jiang, G.; Zhou, L.; Zheng, S. Involvement of p38 mitogen-activated protein kinase pathway in honokiol-induced apoptosis in a human hepatoma cell line (hepG2). *Liver Int.,* **2008,** *28*(10), 1458-1464.
[http://dx.doi.org/10.1111/j.1478-3231.2008.01767.x] [PMID: 18507762]

[90]　Hasegawa, S.; Yonezawa, T.; Ahn, J-Y.; Cha, B-Y.; Teruya, T.; Takami, M.; Yagasaki, K.; Nagai, K.; Woo, J-T. Honokiol inhibits osteoclast differentiation and function *in vitro*. *Biol. Pharm. Bull.,* **2010,** *33*(3), 487-492.
[http://dx.doi.org/10.1248/bpb.33.487] [PMID: 20190414]

[91]　Tse, A.K-W.; Wan, C-K.; Shen, X-L.; Yang, M.; Fong, W-F. Honokiol inhibits TNF-α-stimulated NF-kappaB activation and NF-kappaB-regulated gene expression through suppression of IKK activation. *Biochem. Pharmacol.,* **2005,** *70*(10), 1443-1457.
[http://dx.doi.org/10.1016/j.bcp.2005.08.011] [PMID: 16181613]

[92]　Xu, H.L.; Tang, W.; Du, G.H.; Kokudo, N. Targeting apoptosis pathways in cancer with magnolol and honokiol, bioactive constituents of the bark of Magnolia officinalis. *Drug Discov. Ther.,* **2011,** *5*(5), 202-210.
[http://dx.doi.org/10.5582/ddt.2011.v5.5.202] [PMID: 22466367]

[93]　Zhang, R.; Humphreys, I.; Sahu, R.P.; Shi, Y.; Srivastava, S.K. *In vitro* and *in vivo* induction of apoptosis by capsaicin in pancreatic cancer cells is mediated through ROS generation and mitochondrial death pathway. *Apoptosis,* **2008,** *13*(12), 1465-1478.
[http://dx.doi.org/10.1007/s10495-008-0278-6] [PMID: 19002586]

[94]　Jung, M-Y.; Kang, H-J.; Moon, A. Capsaicin-induced apoptosis in SK-Hep-1 hepatocarcinoma cells involves Bcl-2 downregulation and caspase-3 activation. *Cancer Lett.,* **2001,** *165*(2), 139-145.
[http://dx.doi.org/10.1016/S0304-3835(01)00426-8] [PMID: 11275362]

[95]　Bozok Cetintas, V.; Tezcanli Kaymaz, B.; Aktug, H.; Oltulu, F.; Taskiran, D. Capsaicin induced apoptosis and gene expression dysregulation of human acute lymphoblastic leukemia CCRF-CEM cells. *J. BUON,* **2014,** *19*(1), 183-190.
[PMID: 24659662]

[96]　Wu, C-C.; Lin, J-P.; Yang, J-S.; Chou, S-T.; Chen, S-C.; Lin, Y-T.; Lin, H-L.; Chung, J-G. Capsaicin induced cell cycle arrest and apoptosis in human esophagus epidermoid carcinoma CE 81T/VGH cells through the elevation of intracellular reactive oxygen species and $Ca^{2+}$ productions and caspase-3

activation. *Mutat. Res.,* **2006**, *601*(1-2), 71-82.
[http://dx.doi.org/10.1016/j.mrfmmm.2006.06.015] [PMID: 16942782]

[97] Mori, A.; Lehmann, S.; O'Kelly, J.; Kumagai, T.; Desmond, J.C.; Pervan, M.; McBride, W.H.; Kizaki, M.; Koeffler, H.P. Capsaicin, a component of red peppers, inhibits the growth of androgen-independent, p53 mutant prostate cancer cells. *Cancer Res.,* **2006**, *66*(6), 3222-3229.
[http://dx.doi.org/10.1158/0008-5472.CAN-05-0087] [PMID: 16540674]

[98] Kim, J-D.; Kim, J-M.; Pyo, J-O.; Kim, S-Y.; Kim, B-S.; Yu, R.; Han, I-S. Capsaicin can alter the expression of tumor forming-related genes which might be followed by induction of apoptosis of a Korean stomach cancer cell line, SNU-1. *Cancer Lett.,* **1997**, *120*(2), 235-241.
[http://dx.doi.org/10.1016/S0304-3835(97)00321-2] [PMID: 9461043]

[99] Grimmel, M.; Backhaus, C.; Proikas-Cezanne, T. WIPI-Mediated Autophagy and Longevity. *Cells,* **2015**, *4*(2), 202-217.
[http://dx.doi.org/10.3390/cells4020202] [PMID: 26010754]

[100] Yun, C.W.; Lee, S.H. The Roles of Autophagy in Cancer. *Int. J. Mol. Sci.,* **2018**, *19*(11), 3466.
[http://dx.doi.org/10.3390/ijms19113466] [PMID: 30400561]

[101] Bao, L.; Jaramillo, M.C.; Zhang, Z.; Zheng, Y.; Yao, M.; Zhang, D.D.; Yi, X. Induction of autophagy contributes to cisplatin resistance in human ovarian cancer cells. *Mol. Med. Rep.,* **2015**, *11*(1), 91-98.
[http://dx.doi.org/10.3892/mmr.2014.2671] [PMID: 25322694]

[102] Lin, L.; Baehrecke, E.H. Autophagy, cell death, and cancer. *Mol. Cell. Oncol.,* **2015**, *2*(3), e985913.
[http://dx.doi.org/10.4161/23723556.2014.985913] [PMID: 27308466]

[103] Lu, C-H.; Chen, S-H.; Chang, Y-S.; Liu, Y-W.; Wu, J-Y.; Lim, Y-P.; Yu, H-I.; Lee, Y-R. Honokiol, a potential therapeutic agent, induces cell cycle arrest and program cell death *in vitro* and *in vivo* in human thyroid cancer cells. *Pharmacol. Res.,* **2017**, *115*, 288-298.
[http://dx.doi.org/10.1016/j.phrs.2016.11.038] [PMID: 27940017]

[104] Chio, C-C.; Chen, K-Y.; Chang, C-K.; Chuang, J-Y.; Liu, C-C.; Liu, S-H.; Chen, R-M. Improved effects of honokiol on temozolomide-induced autophagy and apoptosis of drug-sensitive and -tolerant glioma cells. *BMC Cancer,* **2018**, *18*(1), 379.
[http://dx.doi.org/10.1186/s12885-018-4267-z] [PMID: 29614990]

[105] Hahm, E-R.; Sakao, K.; Singh, S.V. Honokiol activates reactive oxygen species-mediated cytoprotective autophagy in human prostate cancer cells. *Prostate,* **2014**, *74*(12), 1209-1221.
[http://dx.doi.org/10.1002/pros.22837] [PMID: 25043291]

[106] Chang, K-H.; Yan, M-D.; Yao, C-J.; Lin, P-C.; Lai, G-M. Honokiol-induced apoptosis and autophagy in glioblastoma multiforme cells. *Oncol. Lett.,* **2013**, *6*(5), 1435-1438.
[http://dx.doi.org/10.3892/ol.2013.1548] [PMID: 24179537]

[107] Huang, K.; Chen, Y.; Zhang, R.; Wu, Y.; Ma, Y.; Fang, X.; Shen, S. Honokiol induces apoptosis and autophagy *via* the ROS/ERK1/2 signaling pathway in human osteosarcoma cells *in vitro* and *in vivo*. *Cell Death Dis.,* **2018**, *9*(2), 157.
[http://dx.doi.org/10.1038/s41419-017-0166-5] [PMID: 29410403]

[108] Kang, R.; Zhang, Q.; Zeh, H.J., III; Lotze, M.T.; Tang, D. HMGB1 in cancer: good, bad, or both? *Clin. Cancer Res.,* **2013**, *19*(15), 4046-4057.
[http://dx.doi.org/10.1158/1078-0432.CCR-13-0495] [PMID: 23723299]

[109] Tang, D.; Kang, R.; Cheh, C-W.; Livesey, K.M.; Liang, X.; Schapiro, N.E.; Benschop, R.; Sparvero, L.J.; Amoscato, A.A.; Tracey, K.J.; Zeh, H.J.; Lotze, M.T. HMGB1 release and redox regulates autophagy and apoptosis in cancer cells. *Oncogene,* **2010**, *29*(38), 5299-5310.
[http://dx.doi.org/10.1038/onc.2010.261] [PMID: 20622903]

[110] Dong, X.E.; Ito, N.; Lotze, M.T.; Demarco, R.A.; Popovic, P.; Shand, S.H.; Watkins, S.; Winikoff, S.; Brown, C.K.; Bartlett, D.L.; Zeh, H.J., III High mobility group box I (HMGB1) release from tumor cells after treatment: implications for development of targeted chemoimmunotherapy. *J. Immunother.,*

**2007**, *30*(6), 596-606.
[http://dx.doi.org/10.1097/CJI.0b013e31804efc76] [PMID: 17667523]

[111] Tang, D.; Kang, R.; Livesey, K.M.; Kroemer, G.; Billiar, T.R.; Van Houten, B.; Zeh, H.J., III; Lotze, M.T. High-mobility group box 1 is essential for mitochondrial quality control. *Cell Metab.,* **2011**, *13*(6), 701-711.
[http://dx.doi.org/10.1016/j.cmet.2011.04.008] [PMID: 21641551]

[112] Roy, M.; Liang, L.; Xiao, X.; Peng, Y.; Luo, Y.; Zhou, W.; Zhang, J.; Qiu, L.; Zhang, S.; Liu, F.; Ye, M.; Zhou, W.; Liu, J. Lycorine Downregulates HMGB1 to Inhibit Autophagy and Enhances Bortezomib Activity in Multiple Myeloma. *Theranostics,* **2016**, *6*(12), 2209-2224.
[http://dx.doi.org/10.7150/thno.15584] [PMID: 27924158]

[113] Samudio, I.; Kurinna, S.; Ruvolo, P.; Korchin, B.; Kantarjian, H.; Beran, M.; Dunner, K., Jr; Kondo, S.; Andreeff, M.; Konopleva, M. Inhibition of mitochondrial metabolism by methyl-2-cyano-3-12-dioxooleana-1,9-diene-28-oate induces apoptotic or autophagic cell death in chronic myeloid leukemia cells. *Mol. Cancer Ther.,* **2008**, *7*(5), 1130-1139.
[http://dx.doi.org/10.1158/1535-7163.MCT-07-0553] [PMID: 18483301]

[114] Wang, X-Y.; Zhang, X-H.; Peng, L.; Liu, Z.; Yang, Y-X.; He, Z-X.; Dang, H-W.; Zhou, S-F. Bardoxolone methyl (CDDO-Me or RTA402) induces cell cycle arrest, apoptosis and autophagy *via* PI3K/Akt/mTOR and p38 MAPK/Erk1/2 signaling pathways in K562 cells. *Am. J. Transl. Res.,* **2017**, *9*(10), 4652-4672.
[PMID: 29118925]

[115] Wang, Y-Y.; Yang, Y-X.; Zhao, R.; Pan, S-T.; Zhe, H.; He, Z-X.; Duan, W.; Zhang, X.; Yang, T.; Qiu, J-X.; Zhou, S.F. Bardoxolone methyl induces apoptosis and autophagy and inhibits epithelial-t--mesenchymal transition and stemness in esophageal squamous cancer cells. *Drug Des. Devel. Ther.,* **2015**, *9*, 993-1026.
[http://dx.doi.org/10.2147/DDDT.S73493] [PMID: 25733817]

[116] Duronio, R.J.; Xiong, Y. Signaling pathways that control cell proliferation. *Cold Spring Harb. Perspect. Biol.,* **2013**, *5*(3), a008904-a008904.
[http://dx.doi.org/10.1101/cshperspect.a008904] [PMID: 23457258]

[117] Park, S.; Bazer, F.W.; Lim, W.; Song, G. The O-methylated isoflavone, formononetin, inhibits human ovarian cancer cell proliferation by sub G0/G1 cell phase arrest through PI3K/AKT and ERK1/2 inactivation. *J. Cell. Biochem.,* **2018**, *119*(9), 7377-7387.
[http://dx.doi.org/10.1002/jcb.27041] [PMID: 29761845]

[118] Li, T.; Zhao, X.; Mo, Z.; Huang, W.; Yan, H.; Ling, Z.; Ye, Y. Formononetin promotes cell cycle arrest *via* downregulation of Akt/Cyclin D1/CDK4 in human prostate cancer cells. *Cell. Physiol. Biochem.,* **2014**, *34*(4), 1351-1358.
[http://dx.doi.org/10.1159/000366342] [PMID: 25301361]

[119] Chen, J.; Zeng, J.; Xin, M.; Huang, W.; Chen, X. Formononetin induces cell cycle arrest of human breast cancer cells *via* IGF1/PI3K/Akt pathways *in vitro* and *in vivo. Horm. Metab. Res.,* **2011**, *43*(10), 681-686.
[http://dx.doi.org/10.1055/s-0031-1286306] [PMID: 21932171]

[120] Kim, D-W.; Ko, S.M.; Jeon, Y-J.; Noh, Y.W.; Choi, N.J.; Cho, S.D.; Moon, H.S.; Cho, Y.S.; Shin, J.C.; Park, S.M.; Seo, K.S.; Choi, J.Y.; Chae, J.I.; Shim, J.H. Anti-proliferative effect of honokiol in oral squamous cancer through the regulation of specificity protein 1. *Int. J. Oncol.,* **2013**, *43*(4), 1103-1110.
[http://dx.doi.org/10.3892/ijo.2013.2028] [PMID: 23877711]

[121] Hahm, E-R.; Singh, K.B.; Singh, S.V. c-Myc is a novel target of cell cycle arrest by honokiol in prostate cancer cells. *Cell Cycle,* **2016**, *15*(17), 2309-2320.
[http://dx.doi.org/10.1080/15384101.2016.1201253] [PMID: 27341160]

[122] Hahm, E-R.; Singh, S.V. Honokiol causes G0-G1 phase cell cycle arrest in human prostate cancer cells

in association with suppression of retinoblastoma protein level/phosphorylation and inhibition of E2F1 transcriptional activity. *Mol. Cancer Ther.,* **2007**, *6*(10), 2686-2695.
[http://dx.doi.org/10.1158/1535-7163.MCT-07-0217] [PMID: 17938262]

[123]   Cen, M.; Yao, Y.; Cui, L.; Yang, G.; Lu, G.; Fang, L.; Bao, Z.; Zhou, J. Honokiol induces apoptosis of lung squamous cell carcinoma by targeting FGF2-FGFR1 autocrine loop. *Cancer Med.,* **2018**, *7*(12), 6205-6218.
[http://dx.doi.org/10.1002/cam4.1846] [PMID: 30515999]

[124]   Banik, K.; Ranaware, A.M.; Deshpande, V.; Nalawade, S.P.; Padmavathi, G.; Bordoloi, D.; Sailo, B.L.; Shanmugam, M.K.; Fan, L.; Arfuso, F.; Sethi, G.; Kunnumakkara, A.B. Honokiol for cancer therapeutics: A traditional medicine that can modulate multiple oncogenic targets. *Pharmacol. Res.,* **2019**, *144*, 192-209.
[http://dx.doi.org/10.1016/j.phrs.2019.04.004] [PMID: 31002949]

[125]   Guo, C.; Ma, L.; Zhao, Y.; Peng, A.; Cheng, B.; Zhou, Q.; Zheng, L.; Huang, K. Inhibitory effects of magnolol and honokiol on human calcitonin aggregation. *Sci. Rep.,* **2015**, *5*(1), 13556.
[http://dx.doi.org/10.1038/srep13556] [PMID: 26324190]

[126]   Yan, B.; Peng, Z-Y. Honokiol induces cell cycle arrest and apoptosis in human gastric carcinoma MGC-803 cell line. *Int. J. Clin. Exp. Med.,* **2015**, *8*(4), 5454-5461.
[PMID: 26131123]

[127]   Carlos-Reyes, Á.; López-González, J.S.; Meneses-Flores, M.; Gallardo-Rincón, D.; Ruíz-García, E.; Marchat, L.A.; Astudillo-de la Vega, H.; Hernández de la Cruz, O.N.; López-Camarillo, C. Dietary Compounds as Epigenetic Modulating Agents in Cancer. *Front. Genet.,* **2019**, *10*, 79.
[http://dx.doi.org/10.3389/fgene.2019.00079] [PMID: 30881375]

[128]   Perri, F.; Longo, F.; Giuliano, M.; Sabbatino, F.; Favia, G.; Ionna, F.; Addeo, R.; Della Vittoria Scarpati, G.; Di Lorenzo, G.; Pisconti, S. Epigenetic control of gene expression: Potential implications for cancer treatment. *Crit. Rev. Oncol. Hematol.,* **2017**, *111*, 166-172.
[http://dx.doi.org/10.1016/j.critrevonc.2017.01.020] [PMID: 28259291]

[129]   Uramova, S.; Kubatka, P.; Dankova, Z.; Kapinova, A.; Zolakova, B.; Samec, M.; Zubor, P.; Zulli, A.; Valentova, V.; Kwon, T.K.; Solar, P.; Kello, M.; Kajo, K.; Busselberg, D.; Pec, M.; Danko, J. Plant natural modulators in breast cancer prevention: status quo and future perspectives reinforced by predictive, preventive, and personalized medical approach. *EPMA J.,* **2018**, *9*(4), 403-419.
[http://dx.doi.org/10.1007/s13167-018-0154-6] [PMID: 30538792]

[130]   Zeng, Y.; Chen, T. DNA Methylation Reprogramming during Mammalian Development. *Genes (Basel),* **2019**, *10*(4), 257.
[http://dx.doi.org/10.3390/genes10040257] [PMID: 30934924]

[131]   Gujar, H.; Weisenberger, D.J.; Liang, G. The Roles of Human DNA Methyltransferases and Their Isoforms in Shaping the Epigenome. *Genes (Basel),* **2019**, *10*(2), 172.
[http://dx.doi.org/10.3390/genes10020172] [PMID: 30813436]

[132]   Liu, P.; Shen, J.K.; Xu, J.; Trahan, C.A.; Hornicek, F.J.; Duan, Z. Aberrant DNA methylations in chondrosarcoma. *Epigenomics,* **2016**, *8*(11), 1519-1525.
[http://dx.doi.org/10.2217/epi-2016-0071] [PMID: 27686001]

[133]   Gao, Y.; Tollefsbol, T.O. Combinational Proanthocyanidins and Resveratrol Synergistically Inhibit Human Breast Cancer Cells and Impact Epigenetic Mediating Machinery. *Int. J. Mol. Sci.,* **2018**, *19*(8), 2204.
[http://dx.doi.org/10.3390/ijms19082204] [PMID: 30060527]

[134]   Naselli, F.; Belshaw, N.J.; Gentile, C.; Tutone, M.; Tesoriere, L.; Livrea, M.A.; Caradonna, F. Phytochemical Indicaxanthin Inhibits Colon Cancer Cell Growth and Affects the DNA Methylation Status by Influencing Epigenetically Modifying Enzyme Expression and Activity. *J. Nutrigenet. Nutrigenomics,* **2015**, *8*(3), 114-127.
[http://dx.doi.org/10.1159/000439382] [PMID: 26439130]

[135]　Szarc Vel Szic, K.; Declerck, K.; Crans, R.A.J.; Diddens, J.; Scherf, D.B.; Gerhäuser, C.; Vanden Berghe, W. Epigenetic silencing of triple negative breast cancer hallmarks by Withaferin A. *Oncotarget,* **2017**, *8*(25), 40434-40453.
[http://dx.doi.org/10.18632/oncotarget.17107] [PMID: 28467815]

[136]　Moiseeva, E.P.; Almeida, G.M.; Jones, G.D.D.; Manson, M.M. Extended treatment with physiologic concentrations of dietary phytochemicals results in altered gene expression, reduced growth, and apoptosis of cancer cells. *Mol. Cancer Ther.,* **2007**, *6*(11), 3071-3079.
[http://dx.doi.org/10.1158/1535-7163.MCT-07-0117] [PMID: 18025290]

[137]　Du, L.; Xie, Z.; Wu, L.C.; Chiu, M.; Lin, J.; Chan, K.K.; Liu, S.; Liu, Z. Reactivation of RASSF1A in breast cancer cells by curcumin. *Nutr. Cancer,* **2012**, *64*(8), 1228-1235.
[http://dx.doi.org/10.1080/01635581.2012.717682] [PMID: 23145775]

[138]　Jiang, A.; Wang, X.; Shan, X.; Li, Y.; Wang, P.; Jiang, P.; Feng, Q. Curcumin Reactivates Silenced Tumor Suppressor Gene RARβ by Reducing DNA Methylation. *Phytother. Res.,* **2015**, *29*(8), 1237-1245.
[http://dx.doi.org/10.1002/ptr.5373] [PMID: 25981383]

[139]　Yu, J.; Peng, Y.; Wu, L-C.; Xie, Z.; Deng, Y.; Hughes, T.; He, S.; Mo, X.; Chiu, M.; Wang, Q-E.; He, X.; Liu, S.; Grever, M.R.; Chan, K.K.; Liu, Z. Curcumin down-regulates DNA methyltransferase 1 and plays an anti-leukemic role in acute myeloid leukemia. *PLoS One,* **2013**, *8*(2), e55934.
[http://dx.doi.org/10.1371/journal.pone.0055934] [PMID: 23457487]

[140]　Qin, W.; Zhang, K.; Clarke, K.; Weiland, T.; Sauter, E.R. Methylation and miRNA effects of resveratrol on mammary tumors *vs.* normal tissue. *Nutr. Cancer,* **2014**, *66*(2), 270-277.
[http://dx.doi.org/10.1080/01635581.2014.868910] [PMID: 24447120]

[141]　Li, H.; Xu, W.; Huang, Y.; Huang, X.; Xu, L.; Lv, Z. Genistein demethylates the promoter of CHD5 and inhibits neuroblastoma growth in vivo. *Int. J. Mol. Med.,* **2012**, *30*(5), 1081-1086.
[http://dx.doi.org/10.3892/ijmm.2012.1118] [PMID: 22960751]

[142]　Hu, P.; Ma, L.; Wang, Y.G.; Ye, F.; Wang, C.; Zhou, W-H.; Zhao, X. Genistein, a dietary soy isoflavone, exerts antidepressant-like effects in mice: Involvement of serotonergic system. *Neurochem. Int.,* **2017**, *108*, 426-435.
[http://dx.doi.org/10.1016/j.neuint.2017.06.002] [PMID: 28606822]

[143]　Porter, K.R.; Claude, A.; Fullam, E.F. A STUDY OF TISSUE CULTURE CELLS BY ELECTRON MICROSCOPY : METHODS AND PRELIMINARY OBSERVATIONS. *J. Exp. Med.,* **1945**, *81*(3), 233-246.
[http://dx.doi.org/10.1084/jem.81.3.233] [PMID: 19871454]

[144]　Oakes, S.A.; Papa, F.R. The role of endoplasmic reticulum stress in human pathology. *Annu. Rev. Pathol.,* **2015**, *10*(1), 173-194.
[http://dx.doi.org/10.1146/annurev-pathol-012513-104649] [PMID: 25387057]

[145]　Almanza, A.; Carlesso, A.; Chintha, C.; Creedican, S.; Doultsinos, D.; Leuzzi, B.; Luís, A.; McCarthy, N.; Montibeller, L.; More, S.; Papaioannou, A.; Püschel, F.; Sassano, M.L.; Skoko, J.; Agostinis, P.; de Belleroche, J.; Eriksson, L.A.; Fulda, S.; Gorman, A.M.; Healy, S.; Kozlov, A.; Muñoz-Pinedo, C.; Rehm, M.; Chevet, E.; Samali, A. Endoplasmic reticulum stress signalling - from basic mechanisms to clinical applications. *FEBS J.,* **2019**, *286*(2), 241-278.
[http://dx.doi.org/10.1111/febs.14608] [PMID: 30027602]

[146]　Kim, I.; Xu, W.; Reed, J.C. Cell death and endoplasmic reticulum stress: disease relevance and therapeutic opportunities. *Nat. Rev. Drug Discov.,* **2008**, *7*(12), 1013-1030.
[http://dx.doi.org/10.1038/nrd2755] [PMID: 19043451]

[147]　Maurel, M.; McGrath, E.P.; Mnich, K.; Healy, S.; Chevet, E.; Samali, A. Controlling the unfolded protein response-mediated life and death decisions in cancer. *Semin. Cancer Biol.,* **2015**, *33*, 57-66.
[http://dx.doi.org/10.1016/j.semcancer.2015.03.003] [PMID: 25814342]

[148]   Mori, K. The unfolded protein response: the dawn of a new field. *Proc. Jpn. Acad., Ser. B, Phys. Biol. Sci.,* **2015**, *91*(9), 469-480.
[http://dx.doi.org/10.2183/pjab.91.469] [PMID: 26560836]

[149]   Wang, M.; Law, M.E.; Castellano, R.K.; Law, B.K. The unfolded protein response as a target for anticancer therapeutics. *Crit. Rev. Oncol. Hematol.,* **2018**, *127*, 66-79.
[http://dx.doi.org/10.1016/j.critrevonc.2018.05.003] [PMID: 29891114]

[150]   Mao, X-Y.; Jin, M-Z.; Chen, J-F.; Zhou, H-H.; Jin, W-L. Live or let die: Neuroprotective and anti-cancer effects of nutraceutical antioxidants. *Pharmacol. Ther.,* **2018**, *183*, 137-151.
[http://dx.doi.org/10.1016/j.pharmthera.2017.10.012] [PMID: 29055715]

[151]   Kim, C.; Kim, B. Anti-Cancer Natural Products and Their Bioactive Compounds Inducing ER Stress-Mediated Apoptosis: A Review. *Nutrients,* **2018**, *10*(8), 1021.
[http://dx.doi.org/10.3390/nu10081021] [PMID: 30081573]

[152]   Cha, J.A.; Song, H-S.; Kang, B.; Park, M.N.; Park, K.S.; Kim, S-H.; Shim, B-S.; Kim, B. miR-211 Plays a Critical Role in Cnidium officinale Makino Extract-Induced, ROS/ER Stress-Mediated Apoptosis in U937 and U266 Cells. *Int. J. Mol. Sci.,* **2018**, *19*(3), 865.
[http://dx.doi.org/10.3390/ijms19030865] [PMID: 29543750]

[153]   Shehzad, A.; Wahid, F.; Lee, Y.S. Curcumin in cancer chemoprevention: molecular targets, pharmacokinetics, bioavailability, and clinical trials. *Arch. Pharm. (Weinheim),* **2010**, *343*(9), 489-499.
[http://dx.doi.org/10.1002/ardp.200900319] [PMID: 20726007]

[154]   Garrido-Armas, M.; Corona, J.C.; Escobar, M.L.; Torres, L.; Ordóñez-Romero, F.; Hernández-Hernández, A.; Arenas-Huertero, F. Paraptosis in human glioblastoma cell line induced by curcumin. *Toxicol. Vitr.,* **2018**, *51*, 63-73.
[http://dx.doi.org/10.1016/j.tiv.2018.04.014] [PMID: 29723631]

[155]   Huang, Y-F.; Zhu, D-J.; Chen, X-W.; Chen, Q-K.; Luo, Z-T.; Liu, C-C.; Wang, G-X.; Zhang, W-J.; Liao, N-Z. Curcumin enhances the effects of irinotecan on colorectal cancer cells through the generation of reactive oxygen species and activation of the endoplasmic reticulum stress pathway. *Oncotarget,* **2017**, *8*(25), 40264-40275.
[http://dx.doi.org/10.18632/oncotarget.16828] [PMID: 28402965]

[156]   Zheng, A.; Li, H.; Wang, X.; Feng, Z.; Xu, J.; Cao, K.; Zhou, B.; Wu, J.; Liu, J. Anticancer effect of a curcumin derivative B63: ROS production and mitochondrial dysfunction. *Curr. Cancer Drug Targets,* **2014**, *14*(2), 156-166.
[http://dx.doi.org/10.2174/1568009613666131126115444] [PMID: 24274397]

[157]   Zhang, X.; Zhang, H-Q.; Zhu, G-H.; Wang, Y-H.; Yu, X-C.; Zhu, X-B.; Liang, G.; Xiao, J.; Li, X-K. A novel mono-carbonyl analogue of curcumin induces apoptosis in ovarian carcinoma cells *via* endoplasmic reticulum stress and reactive oxygen species production. *Mol. Med. Rep.,* **2012**, *5*(3), 739-744.
[http://dx.doi.org/10.3892/mmr.2011.700] [PMID: 22159410]

[158]   Elshaer, M.; Chen, Y.; Wang, X.J.; Tang, X. Resveratrol: An overview of its anti-cancer mechanisms. *Life Sci.,* **2018**, *207*, 340-349.
[http://dx.doi.org/10.1016/j.lfs.2018.06.028] [PMID: 29959028]

[159]   Wang, F-M.; Galson, D.L.; Roodman, G.D.; Ouyang, H. Resveratrol triggers the pro-apoptotic endoplasmic reticulum stress response and represses pro-survival XBP1 signaling in human multiple myeloma cells. *Exp. Hematol.,* **2011**, *39*(10), 999-1006.
[http://dx.doi.org/10.1016/j.exphem.2011.06.007] [PMID: 21723843]

[160]   Heo, J-R.; Kim, S-M.; Hwang, K-A.; Kang, J-H.; Choi, K-C. Resveratrol induced reactive oxygen species and endoplasmic reticulum stress-mediated apoptosis, and cell cycle arrest in the A375SM malignant melanoma cell line. *Int. J. Mol. Med.,* **2018**, *42*(3), 1427-1435.
[http://dx.doi.org/10.3892/ijmm.2018.3732] [PMID: 29916532]

[161]  Révész, K.; Tütto, A.; Szelényi, P.; Konta, L. Tea flavan-3-ols as modulating factors in endoplasmic reticulum function. *Nutr. Res.,* **2011**, *31*(10), 731-740.
[http://dx.doi.org/10.1016/j.nutres.2011.09.008] [PMID: 22074797]

[162]  Rizzi, F.; Naponelli, V.; Silva, A.; Modernelli, A.; Ramazzina, I.; Bonacini, M.; Tardito, S.; Gatti, R.; Uggeri, J.; Bettuzzi, S.; Polyphenon, E. Polyphenon E(R), a standardized green tea extract, induces endoplasmic reticulum stress, leading to death of immortalized PNT1a cells by anoikis and tumorigenic PC3 by necroptosis. *Carcinogenesis,* **2014**, *35*(4), 828-839.
[http://dx.doi.org/10.1093/carcin/bgt481] [PMID: 24343359]

[163]  Modernelli, A.; Naponelli, V.; Giovanna Troglio, M.; Bonacini, M.; Ramazzina, I.; Bettuzzi, S.; Rizzi, F. EGCG antagonizes Bortezomib cytotoxicity in prostate cancer cells by an autophagic mechanism. *Sci. Rep.,* **2015**, *5*(1), 15270.
[http://dx.doi.org/10.1038/srep15270] [PMID: 26471237]

[164]  Costa, J.F.O.; Barbosa-Filho, J.M.; Maia, G.L. de A.; Guimarães, E.T.; Meira, C.S.; Ribeiro-do--Santos, R.; de Carvalho, L.C.P.; Soares, M.B.P. Potent anti-inflammatory activity of betulinic acid treatment in a model of lethal endotoxemia. *Int. Immunopharmacol.,* **2014**, *23*(2), 469-474.
[http://dx.doi.org/10.1016/j.intimp.2014.09.021] [PMID: 25281393]

[165]  Kashyap, D.; Tuli, H.S.; Sharma, A.K. Ursolic acid (UA): A metabolite with promising therapeutic potential. *Life Sci.,* **2016**, *146*, 201-213.
[http://dx.doi.org/10.1016/j.lfs.2016.01.017] [PMID: 26775565]

[166]  Jesus, J.A.; Lago, J.H.G.; Laurenti, M.D.; Yamamoto, E.S.; Passero, L.F.D. Antimicrobial activity of oleanolic and ursolic acids: an update. *Evid. Based Complement. Alternat. Med.,* **2015**, *2015*, 620472.
[http://dx.doi.org/10.1155/2015/620472] [PMID: 25793002]

[167]  Jäger, S.; Trojan, H.; Kopp, T.; Laszczyk, M.N.; Scheffler, A. Pentacyclic triterpene distribution in various plants - rich sources for a new group of multi-potent plant extracts. *Molecules,* **2009**, *14*(6), 2016-2031.
[http://dx.doi.org/10.3390/molecules14062016] [PMID: 19513002]

[168]  Xia, L.; Tan, S.; Zhou, Y.; Lin, J.; Wang, H.; Oyang, L.; Tian, Y.; Liu, L.; Su, M.; Wang, H.; Cao, D.; Liao, Q. Role of the NFκB-signaling pathway in cancer. *OncoTargets Ther.,* **2018**, *11*, 2063-2073.
[http://dx.doi.org/10.2147/OTT.S161109] [PMID: 29695914]

[169]  Xia, Y.; Shen, S.; Verma, I.M.N.F-K.B. NF-κB, an active player in human cancers. *Cancer Immunol. Res.,* **2014**, *2*(9), 823-830.
[http://dx.doi.org/10.1158/2326-6066.CIR-14-0112] [PMID: 25187272]

[170]  Averett, C.; Bhardwaj, A.; Arora, S.; Srivastava, S.K.; Khan, M.A.; Ahmad, A.; Singh, S.; Carter, J.E.; Khushman, M.; Singh, A.P. Honokiol suppresses pancreatic tumor growth, metastasis and desmoplasia by interfering with tumor-stromal cross-talk. *Carcinogenesis,* **2016**, *37*(11), 1052-1061.
[http://dx.doi.org/10.1093/carcin/bgw096] [PMID: 27609457]

[171]  Arora, S.; Singh, S.; Piazza, G.A.; Contreras, C.M.; Panyam, J.; Singh, A.P. Honokiol: a novel natural agent for cancer prevention and therapy. *Curr. Mol. Med.,* **2012**, *12*(10), 1244-1252.
[http://dx.doi.org/10.2174/156652412803833508] [PMID: 22834827]

[172]  Liu, H.; Zang, C.; Emde, A.; Planas-Silva, M.D.; Rosche, M.; Kühnl, A.; Schulz, C-O.; Elstner, E.; Possinger, K.; Eucker, J. Anti-tumor effect of honokiol alone and in combination with other anti-cancer agents in breast cancer. *Eur. J. Pharmacol.,* **2008**, *591*(1-3), 43-51.
[http://dx.doi.org/10.1016/j.ejphar.2008.06.026] [PMID: 18588872]

[173]  Wang, Z.; Zhang, X. Chemopreventive Activity of Honokiol against 7, 12 - Dimethylbenz[a]anthracene-Induced Mammary Cancer in Female Sprague Dawley Rats. *Front. Pharmacol.,* **2017**, *8*, 320.
[http://dx.doi.org/10.3389/fphar.2017.00320] [PMID: 28620301]

[174]  Hua, H.; Chen, W.; Shen, L.; Sheng, Q.; Teng, L. Honokiol augments the anti-cancer effects of

oxaliplatin in colon cancer cells. *Acta Biochim. Biophys. Sin. (Shanghai),* **2013**, *45*(9), 773-779.
[http://dx.doi.org/10.1093/abbs/gmt071] [PMID: 23786838]

[175] Tse, A.K-W.; Wan, C-K.; Shen, X-L.; Yang, M.; Fong, W-F. Honokiol inhibits TNF-alpha-stimulated NF-kappaB activation and NF-kappaB-regulated gene expression through suppression of IKK activation. *Biochem. Pharmacol.,* **2005**, *70*(10), 1443-1457.
[http://dx.doi.org/10.1016/j.bcp.2005.08.011] [PMID: 16181613]

[176] Shehzad, A.; Lee, J.; Lee, Y.S. Curcumin in various cancers. *Biofactors,* **2013**, *39*(1), 56-68.
[http://dx.doi.org/10.1002/biof.1068] [PMID: 23303705]

[177] Bemis, D.L.; Katz, A.E.; Buttyan, R. Clinical trials of natural products as chemopreventive agents for prostate cancer. *Expert Opin. Investig. Drugs,* **2006**, *15*(10), 1191-1200.
[http://dx.doi.org/10.1517/13543784.15.10.1191] [PMID: 16989596]

[178] Hatcher, H.; Planalp, R.; Cho, J.; Torti, F.M.; Torti, S.V. Curcumin: from ancient medicine to current clinical trials. *Cell. Mol. Life Sci.,* **2008**, *65*(11), 1631-1652.
[http://dx.doi.org/10.1007/s00018-008-7452-4] [PMID: 18324353]

[179] Sung, B.; Prasad, S.; Yadav, V.R.; Aggarwal, B.B. Cancer cell signaling pathways targeted by spice-derived nutraceuticals. *Nutr. Cancer,* **2012**, *64*(2), 173-197.
[http://dx.doi.org/10.1080/01635581.2012.630551] [PMID: 22149093]

[180] Aggarwal, B.B.; Vijayalekshmi, R.V.; Sung, B. Targeting inflammatory pathways for prevention and therapy of cancer: short-term friend, long-term foe. *Clin. Cancer Res.,* **2009**, *15*(2), 425-430.
[http://dx.doi.org/10.1158/1078-0432.CCR-08-0149] [PMID: 19147746]

[181] Wang, A-L.; Li, Y.; Zhao, Q.; Fan, L-Q. Formononetin inhibits colon carcinoma cell growth and invasion by microRNA□149□mediated EphB3 downregulation and inhibition of PI3K/AKT and STAT3 signaling pathways. *Mol. Med. Rep.,* **2018**, *17*(6), 7721-7729.
[http://dx.doi.org/10.3892/mmr.2018.8857] [PMID: 29620230]

[182] Zhou, R.; Xu, L.; Ye, M.; Liao, M.; Du, H.; Chen, H. Formononetin inhibits migration and invasion of MDA-MB-231 and 4T1 breast cancer cells by suppressing MMP-2 and MMP-9 through PI3K/AKT signaling pathways. *Horm. Metab. Res.,* **2014**, *46*(11), 753-760.
[http://dx.doi.org/10.1055/s-0034-1376977] [PMID: 24977660]

[183] Ly, J.D.; Grubb, D.R.; Lawen, A. The mitochondrial membrane potential (deltapsi(m)) in apoptosis; an update. *Apoptosis,* **2003**, *8*(2), 115-128.
[http://dx.doi.org/10.1023/A:1022945107762] [PMID: 12766472]

[184] Bhutani, M.; Pathak, A.K.; Nair, A.S.; Kunnumakkara, A.B.; Guha, S.; Sethi, G.; Aggarwal, B.B. Capsaicin is a novel blocker of constitutive and interleukin-6-inducible STAT3 activation. *Clin. Cancer Res.,* **2007**, *13*(10), 3024-3032.
[http://dx.doi.org/10.1158/1078-0432.CCR-06-2575] [PMID: 17505005]

[185] Wu, Y.; Starzinski-Powitz, A.; Guo, S-W. Capsaicin inhibits proliferation of endometriotic cells *in vitro. Gynecol. Obstet. Invest.,* **2008**, *66*(1), 59-62.
[http://dx.doi.org/10.1159/000124275] [PMID: 18391504]

[186] Zou, Y.; Qin, X.; Xiong, H.; Zhu, F.; Chen, T.; Wu, H. Apoptosis of human non-small-cell lung cancer A549 cells triggered by evodiamine through MTDH-dependent signaling pathway. *Tumour Biol.,* **2015**, *36*(7), 5187-5193.
[http://dx.doi.org/10.1007/s13277-015-3174-z] [PMID: 25652471]

[187] Lin, L.; Ren, L.; Wen, L.; Wang, Y.; Qi, J. Effect of evodiamine on the proliferation and apoptosis of A549 human lung cancer cells. *Mol. Med. Rep.,* **2016**, *14*(3), 2832-2838.
[http://dx.doi.org/10.3892/mmr.2016.5575] [PMID: 27485202]

[188] Pan, X.; Hartley, J.M.; Hartley, J.A.; White, K.N.; Wang, Z.; Bligh, S.W.A. Evodiamine, a dual catalytic inhibitor of type I and II topoisomerases, exhibits enhanced inhibition against camptothecin resistant cells. *Phytomedicine,* **2012**, *19*(7), 618-624.

[http://dx.doi.org/10.1016/j.phymed.2012.02.003] [PMID: 22402246]

[189]  Yang, P-M.; Tseng, H-H.; Peng, C-W.; Chen, W-S.; Chiu, S-J. Dietary flavonoid fisetin targets caspase-3-deficient human breast cancer MCF-7 cells by induction of caspase-7-associated apoptosis and inhibition of autophagy. *Int. J. Oncol.,* **2012**, *40*(2), 469-478.
       [http://dx.doi.org/10.3892/ijo.2011.1203] [PMID: 21922137]

[190]  Smith, M.L.; Murphy, K.; Doucette, C.D.; Greenshields, A.L.; Hoskin, D.W. The Dietary Flavonoid Fisetin Causes Cell Cycle Arrest, Caspase-Dependent Apoptosis, and Enhanced Cytotoxicity of Chemotherapeutic Drugs in Triple-Negative Breast Cancer Cells. *J. Cell. Biochem.,* **2016**, *117*(8), 1913-1925.
       [http://dx.doi.org/10.1002/jcb.25490] [PMID: 26755433]

[191]  Sun, X.; Ma, X.; Li, Q.; Yang, Y.; Xu, X.; Sun, J.; Yu, M.; Cao, K.; Yang, L.; Yang, G.; Zhang, G.; Wang, X. Anti-cancer effects of fisetin on mammary carcinoma cells *via* regulation of the PI3K/Akt/mTOR pathway: *In vitro and in vivo* studies. *Int. J. Mol. Med.,* **2018**, *42*(2), 811-820.
       [http://dx.doi.org/10.3892/ijmm.2018.3654] [PMID: 29749427]

[192]  Clarke, M.F.; Dick, J.E.; Dirks, P.B.; Eaves, C.J.; Jamieson, C.H.M.; Jones, D.L.; Visvader, J.; Weissman, I.L.; Wahl, G.M. Cancer stem cells--perspectives on current status and future directions: AACR Workshop on cancer stem cells. *Cancer Res.,* **2006**, *66*(19), 9339-9344.
       [http://dx.doi.org/10.1158/0008-5472.CAN-06-3126] [PMID: 16990346]

[193]  Fong, D.; Chan, M.M. Dietary Phytochemicals Target Cancer Stem Cells for Cancer Chemoprevention. In: *Mitochondria as Targets for Phytochemicals in Cancer Prevention and Therapy*; Springer New York: New York, NY, **2013**; pp. 85-125.
       [http://dx.doi.org/10.1007/978-1-4614-9326-6_5]

[194]  Panda, A.K.; Chakraborty, D.; Sarkar, I.; Khan, T.; Sa, G. New insights into therapeutic activity and anticancer properties of curcumin. *J. Exp. Pharmacol.,* **2017**, *9*, 31-45.
       [http://dx.doi.org/10.2147/JEP.S70568] [PMID: 28435333]

[195]  Norris, L.; Karmokar, A.; Howells, L.; Steward, W.P.; Gescher, A.; Brown, K. The role of cancer stem cells in the anti-carcinogenicity of curcumin. *Mol. Nutr. Food Res.,* **2013**, *57*(9), 1630-1637.
       [http://dx.doi.org/10.1002/mnfr.201300120] [PMID: 23900994]

[196]  Sordillo, P.P.; Helson, L. Curcumin and cancer stem cells: curcumin has asymmetrical effects on cancer and normal stem cells. *Anticancer Res.,* **2015**, *35*(2), 599-614.
       [PMID: 25667437]

[197]  Ramasamy, T.S.; Ayob, A.Z.; Myint, H.H.L.; Thiagarajah, S.; Amini, F. Targeting colorectal cancer stem cells using curcumin and curcumin analogues: insights into the mechanism of the therapeutic efficacy. *Cancer Cell Int.,* **2015**, *15*(1), 96.
       [http://dx.doi.org/10.1186/s12935-015-0241-x] [PMID: 26457069]

[198]  Tsai, C-F.; Hsieh, T-H.; Lee, J-N.; Hsu, C-Y.; Wang, Y-C.; Kuo, K-K.; Wu, H-L.; Chiu, C-C.; Tsai, E-M.; Kuo, P-L. Curcumin Suppresses Phthalate-Induced Metastasis and the Proportion of Cancer Stem Cell (CSC)-like Cells *via* the Inhibition of AhR/ERK/SK1 Signaling in Hepatocellular Carcinoma. *J. Agric. Food Chem.,* **2015**, *63*(48), 10388-10398.
       [http://dx.doi.org/10.1021/acs.jafc.5b04415] [PMID: 26585812]

[199]  Subramaniam, D.; Ponnurangam, S.; Ramamoorthy, P.; Standing, D.; Battafarano, R.J.; Anant, S.; Sharma, P. Curcumin induces cell death in esophageal cancer cells through modulating Notch signaling. *PLoS One,* **2012**, *7*(2), e30590.
       [http://dx.doi.org/10.1371/journal.pone.0030590] [PMID: 22363450]

[200]  Buhrmann, C.; Kraehe, P.; Lueders, C.; Shayan, P.; Goel, A.; Shakibaei, M. Curcumin suppresses crosstalk between colon cancer stem cells and stromal fibroblasts in the tumor microenvironment: potential role of EMT. *PLoS One,* **2014**, *9*(9), e107514.
       [http://dx.doi.org/10.1371/journal.pone.0107514] [PMID: 25238234]

[201]  Huang, W.; Wan, C.; Luo, Q.; Huang, Z.; Luo, Q. Genistein-inhibited cancer stem cell-like properties

and reduced chemoresistance of gastric cancer. *Int. J. Mol. Sci.,* **2014**, *15*(3), 3432-3443.
[http://dx.doi.org/10.3390/ijms15033432] [PMID: 24573253]

[202]   Fan, P.; Fan, S.; Wang, H.; Mao, J.; Shi, Y.; Ibrahim, M.M.; Ma, W.; Yu, X.; Hou, Z.; Wang, B.; Li, L. Genistein decreases the breast cancer stem-like cell population through Hedgehog pathway. *Stem Cell Res. Ther.,* **2013**, *4*(6), 146.
[http://dx.doi.org/10.1186/scrt357] [PMID: 24331293]

[203]   Zhang, L.; Li, L.; Jiao, M.; Wu, D.; Wu, K.; Li, X.; Zhu, G.; Yang, L.; Wang, X.; Hsieh, J-T.; He, D. Genistein inhibits the stemness properties of prostate cancer cells through targeting Hedgehog-Gli1 pathway. *Cancer Lett.,* **2012**, *323*(1), 48-57.
[http://dx.doi.org/10.1016/j.canlet.2012.03.037] [PMID: 22484470]

[204]   Montales, M.T.E.; Rahal, O.M.; Nakatani, H.; Matsuda, T.; Simmen, R.C.M. Repression of mammary adipogenesis by genistein limits mammosphere formation of human MCF-7 cells. *J. Endocrinol.,* **2013**, *218*(1), 135-149.
[http://dx.doi.org/10.1530/JOE-12-0520] [PMID: 23645249]

[205]   Fu, Y.; Chang, H.; Peng, X.; Bai, Q.; Yi, L.; Zhou, Y.; Zhu, J.; Mi, M. Resveratrol inhibits breast cancer stem-like cells and induces autophagy *via* suppressing Wnt/β-catenin signaling pathway. *PLoS One,* **2014**, *9*(7), e102535.
[http://dx.doi.org/10.1371/journal.pone.0102535] [PMID: 25068516]

[206]   Shankar, S.; Nall, D.; Tang, S-N.; Meeker, D.; Passarini, J.; Sharma, J.; Srivastava, R.K. Resveratrol inhibits pancreatic cancer stem cell characteristics in human and KrasG12D transgenic mice by inhibiting pluripotency maintaining factors and epithelial-mesenchymal transition. *PLoS One,* **2011**, *6*(1), e16530.
[http://dx.doi.org/10.1371/journal.pone.0016530] [PMID: 21304978]

[207]   Yang, Y-P.; Chang, Y-L.; Huang, P-I.; Chiou, G-Y.; Tseng, L-M.; Chiou, S-H.; Chen, M-H.; Chen, M-T.; Shih, Y-H.; Chang, C-H.; Hsu, C.C.; Ma, H.I.; Wang, C.T.; Tsai, L.L.; Yu, C.C.; Chang, C.J. Resveratrol suppresses tumorigenicity and enhances radiosensitivity in primary glioblastoma tumor initiating cells by inhibiting the STAT3 axis. *J. Cell. Physiol.,* **2012**, *227*(3), 976-993.
[http://dx.doi.org/10.1002/jcp.22806] [PMID: 21503893]

[208]   Pandey, P.R.; Okuda, H.; Watabe, M.; Pai, S.K.; Liu, W.; Kobayashi, A.; Xing, F.; Fukuda, K.; Hirota, S.; Sugai, T.; Wakabayashi, G.; Koeda, K.; Kashiwaba, M.; Suzuki, K.; Chiba, T.; Endo, M.; Fujioka, T.; Tanji, S.; Mo, Y.Y.; Cao, D.; Wilber, A.C.; Watabe, K. Resveratrol suppresses growth of cancer stem-like cells by inhibiting fatty acid synthase. *Breast Cancer Res. Treat.,* **2011**, *130*(2), 387-398.
[http://dx.doi.org/10.1007/s10549-010-1300-6] [PMID: 21188630]

[209]   Sayd, S.; Thirant, C.; El-Habr, E.A.; Lipecka, J.; Dubois, L.G.; Bogeas, A.; Tahiri-Jouti, N.; Chneiweiss, H.; Junier, M-P. Sirtuin-2 activity is required for glioma stem cell proliferation arrest but not necrosis induced by resveratrol. *Stem Cell Rev. Rep.,* **2014**, *10*(1), 103-113.
[http://dx.doi.org/10.1007/s12015-013-9465-0] [PMID: 23955573]

[210]   Nishimura, N.; Hartomo, T.B.; Pham, T.V.H.; Lee, M.J.; Yamamoto, T.; Morikawa, S.; Hasegawa, D.; Takeda, H.; Kawasaki, K.; Kosaka, Y.; Yamamoto, N.; Kubokawa, I.; Mori, T.; Yanai, T.; Hayakawa, A.; Takeshima, Y.; Iijima, K.; Matsuo, M.; Nishio, H. Epigallocatechin gallate inhibits sphere formation of neuroblastoma BE(2)-C cells. *Environ. Health Prev. Med.,* **2012**, *17*(3), 246-251.
[http://dx.doi.org/10.1007/s12199-011-0239-5] [PMID: 21909813]

[211]   Mineva, N.D.; Paulson, K.E.; Naber, S.P.; Yee, A.S.; Sonenshein, G.E. Epigallocatechin-3-gallate inhibits stem-like inflammatory breast cancer cells. *PLoS One,* **2013**, *8*(9), e73464.
[http://dx.doi.org/10.1371/journal.pone.0073464] [PMID: 24039951]

[212]   Fujiki, H.; Sueoka, E.; Watanabe, T.; Suganuma, M. Synergistic enhancement of anticancer effects on numerous human cancer cell lines treated with the combination of EGCG, other green tea catechins, and anticancer compounds. *J. Cancer Res. Clin. Oncol.,* **2015**, *141*(9), 1511-1522.
[http://dx.doi.org/10.1007/s00432-014-1899-5] [PMID: 25544670]

[213]   Tang, S-N.; Fu, J.; Nall, D.; Rodova, M.; Shankar, S.; Srivastava, R.K. Inhibition of sonic hedgehog pathway and pluripotency maintaining factors regulate human pancreatic cancer stem cell characteristics. *Int. J. Cancer,* **2012**, *131*(1), 30-40.
        [http://dx.doi.org/10.1002/ijc.26323] [PMID: 21796625]

[214]   Lin, C-H.; Chao, L-K.; Hung, P-H.; Chen, Y-J. EGCG inhibits the growth and tumorigenicity of nasopharyngeal tumor-initiating cells through attenuation of STAT3 activation. *Int. J. Clin. Exp. Pathol.,* **2014**, *7*(5), 2372-2381.
        [PMID: 24966947]

[215]   Newman, D. J.; Cragg, G. M. Natural Products as Sources of New Drugs from 1981 to 2014. *Journal of Natural Products,* American Chemical Society.. **2016**, 629-661.
        [http://dx.doi.org/10.1021/acs.jnatprod.5b01055]

[216]   Delgado, J.L.; Hsieh, C-M.; Chan, N-L.; Hiasa, H. Topoisomerases as anticancer targets. *Biochem. J.,* **2018**, *475*(2), 373-398.
        [http://dx.doi.org/10.1042/BCJ20160583] [PMID: 29363591]

[217]   Li, F.; Jiang, T.; Li, Q.; Ling, X. Camptothecin (CPT) and its derivatives are known to target topoisomerase I (Top1) as their mechanism of action: did we miss something in CPT analogue molecular targets for treating human disease such as cancer? *Am. J. Cancer Res.,* **2017**, *7*(12), 2350-2394.
        [PMID: 29312794]

[218]   Lynch, T. Topotecan today. *J. Clin. Oncol.,* **1996**, *14*(12), 3053-3055.
        [http://dx.doi.org/10.1200/JCO.1996.14.12.3053] [PMID: 8955649]

[219]   Hu, G.; Zekria, D.; Cai, X.; Ni, X. Current Status of CPT and Its Analogues in the Treatment of Malignancies. *Phytochem. Rev.,* **2015**, *14*(3), 429-441.
        [http://dx.doi.org/10.1007/s11101-015-9397-1]

[220]   DE Cesare, M. High Efficacy of Intravenous Gimatecan on Human Tumor Xenografts. *Anticancer Res.,* **2018**, *38*(10), 5783-5790.
        [http://dx.doi.org/10.21873/anticanres.12917] [PMID: 30275200]

[221]   Xu, H.; Lv, M.; Tian, X. A review on hemisynthesis, biosynthesis, biological activities, mode of action, and structure-activity relationship of podophyllotoxins: 2003-2007. *Curr. Med. Chem.,* **2009**, *16*(3), 327-349.
        [http://dx.doi.org/10.2174/092986709787002682] [PMID: 19149581]

[222]   Pommier, Y.; Leo, E.; Zhang, H.; Marchand, C. DNA topoisomerases and their poisoning by anticancer and antibacterial drugs. *Chem. Biol.,* **2010**, *17*(5), 421-433.
        [http://dx.doi.org/10.1016/j.chembiol.2010.04.012] [PMID: 20534341]

[223]   Nitiss, J.L. Targeting DNA topoisomerase II in cancer chemotherapy. *Nat. Rev. Cancer,* **2009**, *9*(5), 338-350.
        [http://dx.doi.org/10.1038/nrc2607] [PMID: 19377506]

[224]   Wu, C-C.; Li, T-K.; Farh, L.; Lin, L-Y.; Lin, T-S.; Yu, Y-J.; Yen, T-J.; Chiang, C-W.; Chan, N-L. Structural basis of type II topoisomerase inhibition by the anticancer drug etoposide. *Science,* **2011**, *333*(6041), 459-462.
        [http://dx.doi.org/10.1126/science.1204117] [PMID: 21778401]

[225]   Staker, B.L.; Feese, M.D.; Cushman, M.; Pommier, Y.; Zembower, D.; Stewart, L.; Burgin, A.B. Structures of three classes of anticancer agents bound to the human topoisomerase I-DNA covalent complex. *J. Med. Chem.,* **2005**, *48*(7), 2336-2345.
        [http://dx.doi.org/10.1021/jm049146p] [PMID: 15801827]

[226]   Staker, B.L.; Hjerrild, K.; Feese, M.D.; Behnke, C.A.; Burgin, A.B., Jr; Stewart, L. The mechanism of topoisomerase I poisoning by a camptothecin analog. *Proc. Natl. Acad. Sci. USA,* **2002**, *99*(24), 15387-15392.

[http://dx.doi.org/10.1073/pnas.242259599] [PMID: 12426403]

[227] Rowinsky, E.K. The development and clinical utility of the taxane class of antimicrotubule chemotherapy agents. *Annu. Rev. Med.,* **1997**, *48*, 353-374.
[http://dx.doi.org/10.1146/annurev.med.48.1.353] [PMID: 9046968]

[228] Tsao, C-K.; Cutting, E.; Martin, J.; Oh, W.K. The role of cabazitaxel in the treatment of metastatic castration-resistant prostate cancer. *Ther. Adv. Urol.,* **2014**, *6*(3), 97-104.
[http://dx.doi.org/10.1177/1756287214528557] [PMID: 24883107]

[229] Jordan, M.A.; Wilson, L. Microtubules as a target for anticancer drugs. *Nat. Rev. Cancer,* **2004**, *4*(4), 253-265.
[http://dx.doi.org/10.1038/nrc1317] [PMID: 15057285]

[230] Kellogg, E.H.; Hejab, N.M.A.; Howes, S.; Northcote, P.; Miller, J.H.; Díaz, J.F.; Downing, K.H.; Nogales, E. Insights into the Distinct Mechanisms of Action of Taxane and Non-Taxane Microtubule Stabilizers from Cryo-EM Structures. *J. Mol. Biol.,* **2017**, *429*(5), 633-646.
[http://dx.doi.org/10.1016/j.jmb.2017.01.001] [PMID: 28104363]

[231] Waight, A.B.; Bargsten, K.; Doronina, S.; Steinmetz, M.O.; Sussman, D.; Prota, A.E. Structural Basis of Microtubule Destabilization by Potent Auristatin Anti-Mitotics. *PLoS One,* **2016**, *11*(8), e0160890.
[http://dx.doi.org/10.1371/journal.pone.0160890] [PMID: 27518442]

[232] Ravelli, R.B.G.; Gigant, B.; Curmi, P.A.; Jourdain, I.; Lachkar, S.; Sobel, A.; Knossow, M. Insight into tubulin regulation from a complex with colchicine and a stathmin-like domain. *Nature,* **2004**, *428*(6979), 198-202.
[http://dx.doi.org/10.1038/nature02393] [PMID: 15014504]

[233] Doodhi, H.; Prota, A.E.; Rodríguez-García, R.; Xiao, H.; Custar, D.W.; Bargsten, K.; Katrukha, E.A.; Hilbert, M.; Hua, S.; Jiang, K.; Grigoriev, I.; Yang, C.H.; Cox, D.; Horwitz, S.B.; Kapitein, L.C.; Akhmanova, A.; Steinmetz, M.O. Termination of Protofilament Elongation by Eribulin Induces Lattice Defects that Promote Microtubule Catastrophes. *Curr. Biol.,* **2016**, *26*(13), 1713-1721.
[http://dx.doi.org/10.1016/j.cub.2016.04.053] [PMID: 27321995]

[234] van Der Heijden, R.; Jacobs, D.I.; Snoeijer, W.; Hallard, D.; Verpoorte, R. The Catharanthus alkaloids: pharmacognosy and biotechnology. *Curr. Med. Chem.,* **2004**, *11*(5), 607-628.
[http://dx.doi.org/10.2174/0929867043455846] [PMID: 15032608]

[235] Keglevich, P.; Hazai, L.; Kalaus, G.; Szántay, C. Modifications on the basic skeletons of vinblastine and vincristine. *Molecules,* **2012**, *17*(5), 5893-5914.
[http://dx.doi.org/10.3390/molecules17055893] [PMID: 22609781]

[236] Umezawa, H.; Maeda, K.; Takeuchi, T.; Okami, Y. New antibiotics, bleomycin A and B. *J. Antibiot. (Tokyo),* **1966**, *19*(5), 200-209.
[PMID: 5953301]

[237] Fujii, A.; Takita, T.; Shimada, N.; Umezawa, H. Biosyntheses of new bleomycins. *J. Antibiot. (Tokyo),* **1974**, *27*(1), 73-77.
[http://dx.doi.org/10.7164/antibiotics.27.73] [PMID: 4135574]

[238] Joint Formulary Committee. *(Great Britain). BNF 80: September 2020 - March 2021.; BMJ Group*; Pharmaceutical Press: London, **2020**.

[239] Petering, D.H.; Mao, Q.; Li, W.; DeRose, E.; Antholine, W.E. Metallobleomycin-DNA interactions: structures and reactions related to bleomycin-induced DNA damage. *Met. Ions Biol. Syst.,* **1996**, *33*, 619-648.
[PMID: 8742858]

[240] Stubbe, J.; Kozarich, J.W.; Wu, W.; Vanderwall, D.E. Bleomycins: A Structural Model for Specificity, Binding, and Double Strand Cleavage. *Acc. Chem. Res.,* **1996**, *29*(7), 322-330.
[http://dx.doi.org/10.1021/ar9501333]

[241] Kong, J.; Yi, L.; Xiong, Y.; Huang, Y.; Yang, D.; Yan, X.; Shen, B.; Duan, Y.; Zhu, X. The discovery

and development of microbial bleomycin analogues. *Appl. Microbiol. Biotechnol.,* **2018**, *102*(16), 6791-6798.
[http://dx.doi.org/10.1007/s00253-018-9129-8] [PMID: 29876605]

[242] Zhao, C.; Xia, C.; Mao, Q.; Försterling, H.; DeRose, E.; Antholine, W.E.; Subczynski, W.K.; Petering, D.H. Structures of HO(2)-Co(III)bleomycin A(2) bound to d(GAGCTC)(2) and d(GGAAGCTTCC)(2): structure-reactivity relationships of Co and Fe bleomycins. *J. Inorg. Biochem.,* **2002**, *91*(1), 259-268.
[http://dx.doi.org/10.1016/S0162-0134(02)00420-8] [PMID: 12121784]

[243] D'Angio, G.J.; Evans, A.; Breslow, N.; Beckwith, B.; Bishop, H.; Farewell, V.; Goodwin, W.; Leape, L.; Palmer, N.; Sinks, L.; Sutow, W.; Tefft, M.; Wolff, J. The treatment of Wilms' tumor: results of the Second National Wilms' Tumor Study. *Cancer,* **1981**, *47*(9), 2302-2311.
[http://dx.doi.org/10.1002/1097-0142(19810501)47:9<2302::AID-CNCR2820470933>3.0.CO;2-K] [PMID: 6164480]

[244] Khatua, S.; Nair, C.N.; Ghosh, K. Immune-mediated thrombocytopenia following dactinomycin therapy in a child with alveolar rhabdomyosarcoma: the unresolved issues. *J. Pediatr. Hematol. Oncol.,* **2004**, *26*(11), 777-779.
[http://dx.doi.org/10.1097/00043426-200411000-00020] [PMID: 15543019]

[245] Jaffe, N.; Paed, D.; Traggis, D.; Salian, S.; Cassady, J.R. Improved outlook for Ewing's sarcoma with combination chemotherapy (vincristine, actinomycin D and cyclophosphamide) and radiation therapy. *Cancer,* **1976**, *38*(5), 1925-1930.
[http://dx.doi.org/10.1002/1097-0142(197611)38:5<1925::AID-CNCR2820380510>3.0.CO;2-J] [PMID: 991106]

[246] Turan, T.; Karacay, O.; Tulunay, G.; Boran, N.; Koc, S.; Bozok, S.; Kose, M.F. Results with EMA/CO (etoposide, methotrexate, actinomycin D, cyclophosphamide, vincristine) chemotherapy in gestational trophoblastic neoplasia. *Int. J. Gynecol. Cancer,* **2006**, *16*(3), 1432-1438.
[http://dx.doi.org/10.1136/ijgc-00009577-200605000-00074] [PMID: 16803542]

[247] Sobell, H.M. Actinomycin and DNA transcription. *Proc. Natl. Acad. Sci. USA,* **1985**, *82*(16), 5328-5331.
[http://dx.doi.org/10.1073/pnas.82.16.5328] [PMID: 2410919]

[248] Waksman, S.A.; Woodruff, H.B. Bacteriostatic and Bactericidal Substances Produced by a Soil Actinomyces. *Exp. Biol. Med. (Maywood),* **1940**, *45*(2), 609-614.
[http://dx.doi.org/10.3181/00379727-45-11768]

[249] Satange, R.; Chuang, C-Y.; Neidle, S.; Hou, M-H. Polymorphic G:G mismatches act as hotspots for inducing right-handed Z DNA by DNA intercalation. *Nucleic Acids Res.,* **2019**, *47*(16), 8899-8912.
[http://dx.doi.org/10.1093/nar/gkz653] [PMID: 31361900]

[250] Fujiwara, A.; Hoshino, T.; Westley, J.W. Anthracycline Antibiotics. *Crit. Rev. Biotechnol.,* **1985**, *3*(2), 133-157.
[http://dx.doi.org/10.3109/07388558509150782]

[251] Minotti, G.; Menna, P.; Salvatorelli, E.; Cairo, G.; Gianni, L. Anthracyclines: molecular advances and pharmacologic developments in antitumor activity and cardiotoxicity. *Pharmacol. Rev.,* **2004**, *56*(2), 185-229.
[http://dx.doi.org/10.1124/pr.56.2.6] [PMID: 15169927]

[252] Peng, X.; Chen, B.; Lim, C.C.; Sawyer, D.B. The cardiotoxicology of anthracycline chemotherapeutics: translating molecular mechanism into preventative medicine. *Mol. Interv.,* **2005**, *5*(3), 163-171.
[http://dx.doi.org/10.1124/mi.5.3.6] [PMID: 15994456]

[253] Weiss, R.B. The anthracyclines: will we ever find a better doxorubicin? *Semin. Oncol.,* **1992**, *19*(6), 670-686.
[PMID: 1462166]

[254]  Howerton, S.B.; Nagpal, A.; Williams, L.D. Surprising roles of electrostatic interactions in DNA-ligand complexes. *Biopolymers,* **2003**, *69*(1), 87-99.
[http://dx.doi.org/10.1002/bip.10319] [PMID: 12717724]

[255]  Simůnek, T.; Stérba, M.; Popelová, O.; Adamcová, M.; Hrdina, R.; Gersl, V. Anthracycline-induced cardiotoxicity: overview of studies examining the roles of oxidative stress and free cellular iron. *Pharmacol. Rep.,* **2009**, *61*(1), 154-171.
[http://dx.doi.org/10.1016/S1734-1140(09)70018-0] [PMID: 19307704]

[256]  Shi, K.; Pan, B.; Sundaralingam, M. Structure of a B-form DNA/RNA chimera (dC)(rG)d(ATCG) complexed with daunomycin at 1.5 A resolution. *Acta Crystallogr. D Biol. Crystallogr.,* **2003**, *59*(Pt 8), 1377-1383.
[http://dx.doi.org/10.1107/S0907444903011788] [PMID: 12876339]

[257]  Langlois d'Estaintot, B.; Gallois, B.; Brown, T.; Hunter, W.N. The molecular structure of a 4'-epiadriamycin complex with d(TGATCA) at 1.7A resolution: comparison with the structure of 4'-epiadriamycin d(TGTACA) and d(CGATCG) complexes. *Nucleic Acids Res.,* **1992**, *20*(14), 3561-3566.
[http://dx.doi.org/10.1093/nar/20.14.3561] [PMID: 1641324]

[258]  Milazzo, G.; Mercatelli, D.; Di Muzio, G.; Triboli, L.; De Rosa, P.; Perini, G.; Giorgi, F.M. Histone Deacetylases (HDACs): Evolution, Specificity, Role in Transcriptional Complexes, and Pharmacological Actionability. *Genes (Basel),* **2020**, *11*(5), E556.
[http://dx.doi.org/10.3390/genes11050556] [PMID: 32429325]

[259]  Nakajima, H.; Kim, Y.B.; Terano, H.; Yoshida, M.; Horinouchi, S. FR901228, a potent antitumor antibiotic, is a novel histone deacetylase inhibitor. *Exp. Cell Res.,* **1998**, *241*(1), 126-133.
[http://dx.doi.org/10.1006/excr.1998.4027] [PMID: 9633520]

[260]  Greshock, T.J.; Johns, D.M.; Noguchi, Y.; Williams, R.M. Improved total synthesis of the potent HDAC inhibitor FK228 (FR-901228). *Org. Lett.,* **2008**, *10*(4), 613-616.
[http://dx.doi.org/10.1021/ol702957z] [PMID: 18205373]

[261]  Pópulo, H.; Lopes, J.M.; Soares, P. The mTOR signalling pathway in human cancer. *Int. J. Mol. Sci.,* **2012**, *13*(2), 1886-1918.
[http://dx.doi.org/10.3390/ijms13021886] [PMID: 22408430]

[262]  Bellmunt, J.; Szczylik, C.; Feingold, J.; Strahs, A.; Berkenblit, A. Temsirolimus safety profile and management of toxic effects in patients with advanced renal cell carcinoma and poor prognostic features. *Ann. Oncol.,* **2008**, *19*(8), 1387-1392.
[http://dx.doi.org/10.1093/annonc/mdn066] [PMID: 18385198]

[263]  Dosio, F.; Brusa, P.; Cattel, L. Immunotoxins and anticancer drug conjugate assemblies: the role of the linkage between components. *Toxins (Basel),* **2011**, *3*(7), 848-883.
[http://dx.doi.org/10.3390/toxins3070848] [PMID: 22069744]

[264]  Towle, M.J.; Salvato, K.A.; Budrow, J.; Wels, B.F.; Kuznetsov, G.; Aalfs, K.K.; Welsh, S.; Zheng, W.; Seletsky, B.M.; Palme, M.H.; Habgood, G.J.; Singer, L.A.; Dipietro, L.V.; Wang, Y.; Chen, J.J.; Quincy, D.A.; Davis, A.; Yoshimatsu, K.; Kishi, Y.; Yu, M.J.; Littlefield, B.A. *In vitro* and *in vivo* anticancer activities of synthetic macrocyclic ketone analogues of halichondrin B. *Cancer Res.,* **2001**, *61*(3), 1013-1021.
[PMID: 11221827]

[265]  Okouneva, T.; Azarenko, O.; Wilson, L.; Littlefield, B.A.; Jordan, M.A. Inhibition of centromere dynamics by eribulin (E7389) during mitotic metaphase. *Mol. Cancer Ther.,* **2008**, *7*(7), 2003-2011.
[http://dx.doi.org/10.1158/1535-7163.MCT-08-0095] [PMID: 18645010]

[266]  Singh, R.K.; Kumar, S.; Prasad, D.N.; Bhardwaj, T.R. Therapeutic journery of nitrogen mustard as alkylating anticancer agents: Historic to future perspectives. *Eur. J. Med. Chem.,* **2018**, *151*, 401-433.
[http://dx.doi.org/10.1016/j.ejmech.2018.04.001] [PMID: 29649739]

[267]   Grohar, P.J.; Griffin, L.B.; Yeung, C.; Chen, Q-R.; Pommier, Y.; Khanna, C.; Khan, J.; Helman, L.J. Ecteinascidin 743 interferes with the activity of EWS-FLI1 in Ewing sarcoma cells. *Neoplasia,* **2011**, *13*(2), 145-153.
[http://dx.doi.org/10.1593/neo.101202] [PMID: 21403840]

[268]   Rath, C.M.; Janto, B.; Earl, J.; Ahmed, A.; Hu, F.Z.; Hiller, L.; Dahlgren, M.; Kreft, R.; Yu, F.; Wolff, J.J.; Kweon, H.K.; Christiansen, M.A.; Håkansson, K.; Williams, R.M.; Ehrlich, G.D.; Sherman, D.H. Meta-omic characterization of the marine invertebrate microbial consortium that produces the chemotherapeutic natural product ET-743. *ACS Chem. Biol.,* **2011**, *6*(11), 1244-1256.
[http://dx.doi.org/10.1021/cb200244t] [PMID: 21875091]

[269]   Nakamura, K.; Yasunaga, Y.; Segawa, T.; Ko, D.; Moul, J.W.; Srivastava, S.; Rhim, J.S. Curcumin down-regulates AR gene expression and activation in prostate cancer cell lines. *Int. J. Oncol.,* **2002**, *21*(4), 825-830.
[http://dx.doi.org/10.3892/ijo.21.4.825] [PMID: 12239622]

[270]   Yallapu, M.M.; Maher, D.M.; Sundram, V.; Bell, M.C.; Jaggi, M.; Chauhan, S.C. Curcumin induces chemo/radio-sensitization in ovarian cancer cells and curcumin nanoparticles inhibit ovarian cancer cell growth. *J. Ovarian Res.,* **2010**, *3*(1), 11.
[http://dx.doi.org/10.1186/1757-2215-3-11] [PMID: 20429876]

[271]   Huang, M.T.; Newmark, H.L.; Frenkel, K. Inhibitory effects of curcumin on tumorigenesis in mice. *J. Cell. Biochem. Suppl.,* **1997**, *27*(S27), 26-34.
[http://dx.doi.org/10.1002/(SICI)1097-4644(1997)27+<26::AID-JCB7>3.0.CO;2-3] [PMID: 9591190]

[272]   Taverna, S.; Giallombardo, M.; Pucci, M.; Flugy, A.; Manno, M.; Raccosta, S.; Rolfo, C.; De Leo, G.; Alessandro, R. Curcumin inhibits *in vitro* and *in vivo* chronic myelogenous leukemia cells growth: a possible role for exosomal disposal of miR-21. *Oncotarget,* **2015**, *6*(26), 21918-21933.
[http://dx.doi.org/10.18632/oncotarget.4204] [PMID: 26116834]

[273]   Mock, C.D.; Jordan, B.C.; Selvam, C. Recent Advances of Curcumin and its Analogues in Breast Cancer Prevention and Treatment. *RSC Advances,* **2015**, *5*(92), 75575-75588.
[http://dx.doi.org/10.1039/C5RA14925H] [PMID: 27103993]

[274]   Wilken, R.; Veena, M.S.; Wang, M.B.; Srivatsan, E.S. Curcumin: A review of anti-cancer properties and therapeutic activity in head and neck squamous cell carcinoma. *Mol. Cancer,* **2011**, *10*(1), 12.
[http://dx.doi.org/10.1186/1476-4598-10-12] [PMID: 21299897]

[275]   Darvesh, A.S.; Aggarwal, B.B.; Bishayee, A. Curcumin and liver cancer: a review. *Curr. Pharm. Biotechnol.,* **2012**, *13*(1), 218-228.
[http://dx.doi.org/10.2174/138920112798868791] [PMID: 21466422]

[276]   Bayet-Robert, M.; Kwiatkowski, F.; Leheurteur, M.; Gachon, F.; Planchat, E.; Abrial, C.; Mouret-Reynier, M-A.; Durando, X.; Barthomeuf, C.; Chollet, P.; Phase, I. Phase I dose escalation trial of docetaxel plus curcumin in patients with advanced and metastatic breast cancer. *Cancer Biol. Ther.,* **2010**, *9*(1), 8-14.
[http://dx.doi.org/10.4161/cbt.9.1.10392] [PMID: 19901561]

[277]   Mahammedi, H.; Planchat, E.; Pouget, M.; Durando, X.; Curé, H.; Guy, L.; Van-Praagh, I.; Savareux, L.; Atger, M.; Bayet-Robert, M.; Gadea, E.; Abrial, C.; Thivat, E.; Chollet, P.; Eymard, J.C. The New Combination Docetaxel, Prednisone and Curcumin in Patients with Castration-Resistant Prostate Cancer: A Pilot Phase II Study. *Oncology,* **2016**, *90*(2), 69-78.
[http://dx.doi.org/10.1159/000441148] [PMID: 26771576]

[278]   Epelbaum, R.; Schaffer, M.; Vizel, B.; Badmaev, V.; Bar-Sela, G. Curcumin and gemcitabine in patients with advanced pancreatic cancer. *Nutr. Cancer,* **2010**, *62*(8), 1137-1141.
[http://dx.doi.org/10.1080/01635581.2010.513802] [PMID: 21058202]

[279]   Kanai, M.; Otsuka, Y.; Otsuka, K.; Sato, M.; Nishimura, T.; Mori, Y.; Kawaguchi, M.; Hatano, E.; Kodama, Y.; Matsumoto, S.; Murakami, Y.; Imaizumi, A.; Chiba, T.; Nishihira, J.; Shibata, H. A phase I study investigating the safety and pharmacokinetics of highly bioavailable curcumin

(Theracurmin) in cancer patients. *Cancer Chemother. Pharmacol.,* **2013**, *71*(6), 1521-1530.
[http://dx.doi.org/10.1007/s00280-013-2151-8] [PMID: 23543271]

[280] Carroll, R.E.; Benya, R.V.; Turgeon, D.K.; Vareed, S.; Neuman, M.; Rodriguez, L.; Kakarala, M.; Carpenter, P.M.; McLaren, C.; Meyskens, F.L., Jr; Brenner, D.E. Phase IIa clinical trial of curcumin for the prevention of colorectal neoplasia. *Cancer Prev. Res. (Phila.),* **2011**, *4*(3), 354-364.
[http://dx.doi.org/10.1158/1940-6207.CAPR-10-0098] [PMID: 21372035]

[281] Irving, G.R.; Iwuji, C.O.; Morgan, B.; Berry, D.P.; Steward, W.P.; Thomas, A.; Brown, K.; Howells, L.M. Combining curcumin (C3-complex, Sabinsa) with standard care FOLFOX chemotherapy in patients with inoperable colorectal cancer (CUFOX): study protocol for a randomised control trial. *Trials,* **2015**, *16*(1), 110.
[http://dx.doi.org/10.1186/s13063-015-0641-1] [PMID: 25872567]

[282] James, M.I.; Iwuji, C.; Irving, G.; Karmokar, A.; Higgins, J.A.; Griffin-Teal, N.; Thomas, A.; Greaves, P.; Cai, H.; Patel, S.R.; Morgan, B.; Dennison, A.; Metcalfe, M.; Garcea, G.; Lloyd, D.M.; Berry, D.P.; Steward, W.P.; Howells, L.M.; Brown, K. Curcumin inhibits cancer stem cell phenotypes in ex vivo models of colorectal liver metastases, and is clinically safe and tolerable in combination with FOLFOX chemotherapy. *Cancer Lett.,* **2015**, *364*(2), 135-141.
[http://dx.doi.org/10.1016/j.canlet.2015.05.005] [PMID: 25979230]

[283] Ghalaut, V.S.; Sangwan, L.; Dahiya, K.; Ghalaut, P.S.; Dhankhar, R.; Saharan, R. Effect of imatinib therapy with and without turmeric powder on nitric oxide levels in chronic myeloid leukemia. *J. Oncol. Pharm. Pract.,* **2012**, *18*(2), 186-190.
[http://dx.doi.org/10.1177/1078155211416530] [PMID: 21844132]

[284] Pastorelli, D.; Fabricio, A.S.C.; Giovanis, P.; D'Ippolito, S.; Fiduccia, P.; Soldà, C.; Buda, A.; Sperti, C.; Bardini, R.; Da Dalt, G.; Rainato, G.; Gion, M.; Ursini, F. Phytosome complex of curcumin as complementary therapy of advanced pancreatic cancer improves safety and efficacy of gemcitabine: Results of a prospective phase II trial. *Pharmacol. Res.,* **2018**, *132*, 72-79.
[http://dx.doi.org/10.1016/j.phrs.2018.03.013] [PMID: 29614381]

[285] Abrams, S.L.; Follo, M.Y.; Steelman, L.S.; Lertpiriyapong, K.; Cocco, L.; Ratti, S.; Martelli, A.M.; Candido, S.; Libra, M.; Murata, R.M.; Rosalen, P.L.; Montalto, G.; Cervello, M.; Gizak, A.; Rakus, D.; Mao, W.; Lombardi, P.; McCubrey, J.A. Abilities of berberine and chemically modified berberines to inhibit proliferation of pancreatic cancer cells. *Adv. Biol. Regul.,* **2019**, *71*, 172-182.
[http://dx.doi.org/10.1016/j.jbior.2018.10.003] [PMID: 30361003]

[286] Youn, D-H.; Park, J.; Kim, H-L.; Jung, Y.; Kang, J.; Lim, S.; Song, G.; Kwak, H.J.; Um, J-Y. Berberine Improves Benign Prostatic Hyperplasia *via* Suppression of 5 Alpha Reductase and Extracellular Signal-Regulated Kinase *in Vivo* and *in Vitro*. *Front. Pharmacol.,* **2018**, *9*, 773.
[http://dx.doi.org/10.3389/fphar.2018.00773] [PMID: 30061836]

[287] Hou, D.; Xu, G.; Zhang, C.; Li, B.; Qin, J.; Hao, X.; Liu, Q.; Zhang, X.; Liu, J.; Wei, J.; Gong, Y.; Liu, Z.; Shao, C. Berberine induces oxidative DNA damage and impairs homologous recombination repair in ovarian cancer cells to confer increased sensitivity to PARP inhibition. *Cell Death Dis.,* **2017**, *8*(10), e3070.
[http://dx.doi.org/10.1038/cddis.2017.471] [PMID: 28981112]

[288] Mahata, S.; Bharti, A.C.; Shukla, S.; Tyagi, A.; Husain, S.A.; Das, B.C. Berberine modulates AP-1 activity to suppress HPV transcription and downstream signaling to induce growth arrest and apoptosis in cervical cancer cells. *Mol. Cancer,* **2011**, *10*(1), 39.
[http://dx.doi.org/10.1186/1476-4598-10-39] [PMID: 21496227]

[289] Mao, L.; Chen, Q.; Gong, K.; Xu, X.; Xie, Y.; Zhang, W.; Cao, H.; Hu, T.; Hong, X.; Zhan, Y-Y. Berberine decelerates glucose metabolism *via* suppression of mTOR-dependent HIF-1α protein synthesis in colon cancer cells. *Oncol. Rep.,* **2018**, *39*(5), 2436-2442.
[http://dx.doi.org/10.3892/or.2018.6318] [PMID: 29565467]

[290] Zhao, Y.; Jing, Z.; Lv, J.; Zhang, Z.; Lin, J.; Cao, X.; Zhao, Z.; Liu, P.; Mao, W. Berberine activates caspase-9/cytochrome c-mediated apoptosis to suppress triple-negative breast cancer cells *in vitro* and

*in vivo*. Biomed. Pharmacother., **2017**, *95*, 18-24.
[http://dx.doi.org/10.1016/j.biopha.2017.08.045] [PMID: 28826092]

[291]  Hesari, A.; Ghasemi, F.; Cicero, A.F.G.; Mohajeri, M.; Rezaei, O.; Hayat, S.M.G.; Sahebkar, A. Berberine: A potential adjunct for the treatment of gastrointestinal cancers? *J. Cell. Biochem.*, **2018**, *119*(12), 9655-9663.
[http://dx.doi.org/10.1002/jcb.27392] [PMID: 30125974]

[292]  Lin, C-Y.; Hsieh, P-L.; Liao, Y-W.; Peng, C-Y.; Lu, M-Y.; Yang, C-H.; Yu, C-C.; Liu, C-M. Berberine-targeted miR-21 chemosensitizes oral carcinomas stem cells. *Oncotarget*, **2017**, *8*(46), 80900-80908.
[http://dx.doi.org/10.18632/oncotarget.20723] [PMID: 29113353]

[293]  Cipolla, B.G.; Mandron, E.; Lefort, J.M.; Coadou, Y.; Della Negra, E.; Corbel, L.; Le Scodan, R.; Azzouzi, A.R.; Mottet, N. Effect of Sulforaphane in Men with Biochemical Recurrence after Radical Prostatectomy. *Cancer Prev. Res. (Phila.)*, **2015**, *8*(8), 712-719.
[http://dx.doi.org/10.1158/1940-6207.CAPR-14-0459] [PMID: 25968598]

[294]  Alumkal, J.J.; Slottke, R.; Schwartzman, J.; Cherala, G.; Munar, M.; Graff, J.N.; Beer, T.M.; Ryan, C.W.; Koop, D.R.; Gibbs, A.; Gao, L.; Flamiatos, J.F.; Tucker, E.; Kleinschmidt, R.; Mori, M. A phase II study of sulforaphane-rich broccoli sprout extracts in men with recurrent prostate cancer. *Invest. New Drugs*, **2015**, *33*(2), 480-489.
[http://dx.doi.org/10.1007/s10637-014-0189-z] [PMID: 25431127]

[295]  Gee, J.R.; Saltzstein, D.R.; Kim, K.; Kolesar, J.; Huang, W.; Havighurst, T.C.; Wollmer, B.W.; Stublaski, J.; Downs, T.; Mukhtar, H.; House, M.G.; Parnes, H.L.; Bailey, H.H. A Phase II Randomized, Double-blind, Presurgical Trial of Polyphenon E in Bladder Cancer Patients to Evaluate Pharmacodynamics and Bladder Tissue Biomarkers. *Cancer Prev. Res. (Phila.)*, **2017**, *10*(5), 298-307.
[http://dx.doi.org/10.1158/1940-6207.CAPR-16-0167] [PMID: 28325826]

[296]  Chen, J.; Song, Y.; Zhang, L. Lycopene/tomato consumption and the risk of prostate cancer: a systematic review and meta-analysis of prospective studies. *J. Nutr. Sci. Vitaminol. (Tokyo)*, **2013**, *59*(3), 213-223.
[http://dx.doi.org/10.3177/jnsv.59.213] [PMID: 23883692]

[297]  Gontero, P.; Marra, G.; Soria, F.; Oderda, M.; Zitella, A.; Baratta, F.; Chiorino, G.; Gregnanin, I.; Daniele, L.; Cattel, L.; Frea, B.; Brusa, P. A randomized double-blind placebo controlled phase I-II study on clinical and molecular effects of dietary supplements in men with precancerous prostatic lesions. Chemoprevention or "chemopromotion"? *Prostate*, **2015**, *75*(11), 1177-1186.
[http://dx.doi.org/10.1002/pros.22999] [PMID: 25893930]

[298]  Paller, C.J.; Rudek, M.A.; Zhou, X.C.; Wagner, W.D.; Hudson, T.S.; Anders, N.; Hammers, H.J.; Dowling, D.; King, S.; Antonarakis, E.S.; Drake, C.G.; Eisenberger, M.A.; Denmeade, S.R.; Rosner, G.L.; Carducci, M.A. A phase I study of muscadine grape skin extract in men with biochemically recurrent prostate cancer: Safety, tolerability, and dose determination. *Prostate*, **2015**, *75*(14), 1518-1525.
[http://dx.doi.org/10.1002/pros.23024] [PMID: 26012728]

[299]  Zhu, W.; Qin, W.; Zhang, K.; Rottinghaus, G.E.; Chen, Y-C.; Kliethermes, B.; Sauter, E.R. Trans-resveratrol alters mammary promoter hypermethylation in women at increased risk for breast cancer. *Nutr. Cancer*, **2012**, *64*(3), 393-400.
[http://dx.doi.org/10.1080/01635581.2012.654926] [PMID: 22332908]

[300]  Howells, L.M.; Berry, D.P.; Elliott, P.J.; Jacobson, E.W.; Hoffmann, E.; Hegarty, B.; Brown, K.; Steward, W.P.; Gescher, A.J.; Phase, I. Phase I randomized, double-blind pilot study of micronized resveratrol (SRT501) in patients with hepatic metastases--safety, pharmacokinetics, and pharmacodynamics. *Cancer Prev. Res. (Phila.)*, **2011**, *4*(9), 1419-1425.
[http://dx.doi.org/10.1158/1940-6207.CAPR-11-0148] [PMID: 21680702]

[301]  Shoemaker, R.H. The NCI60 human tumour cell line anticancer drug screen. *Nat. Rev. Cancer*, **2006**, *6*(10), 813-823.

[http://dx.doi.org/10.1038/nrc1951] [PMID: 16990858]

[302]  Rosén, J.; Gottfries, J.; Muresan, S.; Backlund, A.; Oprea, T.I. Novel chemical space exploration *via* natural products. *J. Med. Chem.,* **2009**, *52*(7), 1953-1962.
[http://dx.doi.org/10.1021/jm801514w] [PMID: 19265440]

[303]  Harvey, A.L.; Clark, R.L.; Mackay, S.P.; Johnston, B.F. Current strategies for drug discovery through natural products. *Expert Opin. Drug Discov.,* **2010**, *5*(6), 559-568.
[http://dx.doi.org/10.1517/17460441.2010.488263] [PMID: 22823167]

# CHAPTER 2

# Role of Terpenoids as Anticancer Compounds: An Insight into Prevention and Treatment

**Bhawna Chopra**[*, 1], **Ashwani Dhingra**[1], **Kanaya Lal Dhar**[2], **Kunal Nepali**[3] and **Deo Nandan Prasad**[4]

[1] *Guru Gobind Singh College of Pharmacy, Yamuna Nagar-135001, Haryana, India*

[2] *Emeritus Scientist, Indian Institute of Integrative Medicine, CSIR, Jammu-180016, India*

[3] *Taipei Medical University, Taiwan*

[4] *Shivalik College of Pharmacy, Nangal-140124, Punjab, India*

**Abstract:** The human population is affected by the wide range of malignant cancers. Several cancer treatment options, including surgery, radiation, chemotherapy, immunotherapy, and others, are available or within our reach. However, the excessive toxic effects that assimilate the negative impact on patients and thus impede progress in cancer treatment have yet to be identified. Recent efforts in the research and development of anticancer drugs derived from natural products have led to the identification of numerous heterocyclic terpenes that inhibit cell proliferation, metastasis, apoptosis, and other mechanisms. The anticancer activity of the terpenoids is quite promising, and it could lead to more opportunities for cancer therapy. The current chapter provides an overview of recent developments in the field of heterocyclic terpenes and their analogues as anticancer compounds. As a result, this provides an overview of the progress made in developing terpenes and analogues as potential anticancer agents, including their synthetic modification, SAR, and action mechanisms. The current studies are hoped to help researchers in increasing their chances of gaining breakthrough insights in the field that can be used in cancer therapeutic practise.

**Keywords:** Biological activity, Cancer, History, Isoprene, Pathology, Terpenes.

## INTRODUCTION

In today's era, natural products are the richest source of components with enormous structural diversity, and their potential in drug discovery and development has also been explored. They were successful as outstanding leads for the production of numerous pharmaceuticals.

---
[*] **Corresponding author Bhawna Chopra and Rajesh Kumar:** Guru Gobind Singh College of Pharmacy, Yamuna Nagar-135001, Haryana, India; Tel:+919034051015; E-mails: bhawna8486@gmail.com

Several life-threatening diseases, along with drug resistance, are now affecting the world on a colossal scale. Therefore, further exploration of natural bioactive components is required. It was particularly evident in the field of cancer, where more than 50% of the approved drugs were of natural origin for the last two decades. Despite the tremendous progress made in the past decades, there is an increasing demand for access, discovery, and development of novel molecular entities or scaffolds [1]. Literature suggests that terpenoids consist of approximately 25,000 chemical structures that have found potential practical applications in the fragrance and flavour industries since ancient times. They are utilized in many pharmaceutical and chemical industries [2]. Terpenoids, or isoprenoids, are the prenyl lipid subclasses that are the oldest and most widelyspread in natural bioactive components [3 - 5]. Terpenoids can be classified based on the number of carbon atoms formed by the linear arrangement of the isoprene units [6, 7], such as with one isoprene unit-hemiterpenoids, with two isoprene units-monoterpenoids, with three units-sesquiterpenoids, four isoprene units-diterpenoids, five isoprene units-sesterterpenoids, six isoprene units-triterpenoids, and compounds exhibiting a large number of isoprene units-polyterpenoids. The classification of terpenoids with examples is shown in Fig. (**1**).

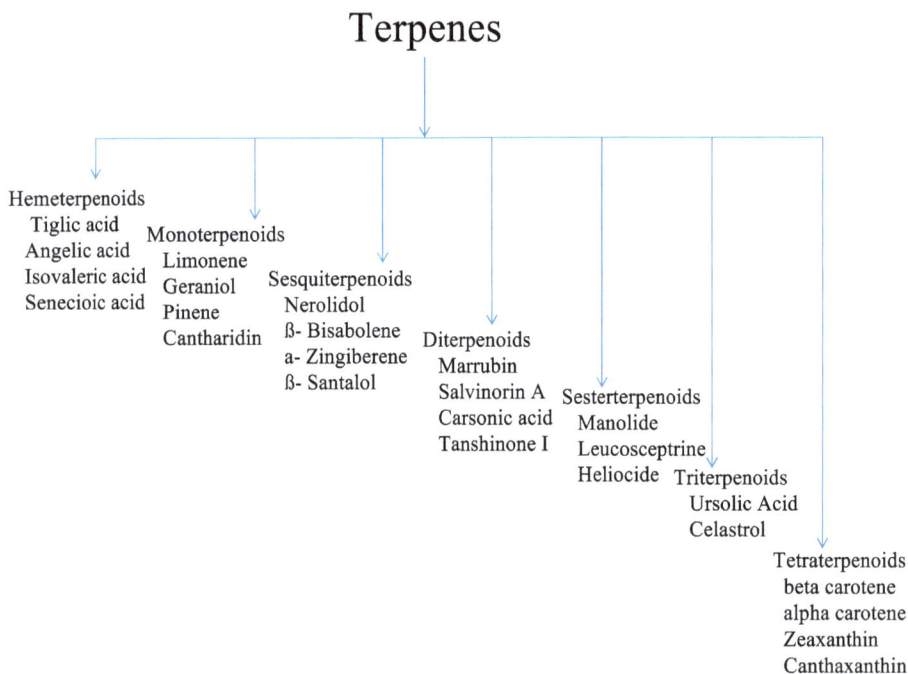

**Fig. (1).** Classification of terpenoids with examples.

Terpenoids were known to possess anti-inflammatory, antibacterial, antiviral, antimalarial, antitumour, and anti-ageing properties. They found application as an insect repellant, immunoregulator, and neuroprotective agent acting *via* a variant mechanism of action [8]. Various *in-vitro* and *in-vivo* studies report the number of pathways responsible for the anticancer activity: inhibition of cell proliferation and tumour growth, activation of apoptosis, cell cycle arrest at different phases, suppression of NF-kB and the ubiquitin-proteasome pathway, and many more. Thus, we can say that a diverse era of terpenoids acts on the variable targets, channels (TRPV1), or receptor sites against cancer [9]. However, terpenes are marketed as pharmaceuticals, such as menthol, a monoterpene used as a topical analgesic and sold as an over-the-counter (OTC) drug named Salonpas, having a varying menthol composition [10].

At present, many terpenoids are clinically explored as anticancer agents. Many new terpenoids exhibit cytotoxicity against various tumour cells [11 - 14] and are found to be cancer-preventive and possess efficacy as anticancer agents in pre-clinical animal models. It is quite hopeful that they will be able to translate their pre-clinical promise into clinical potential and be able to overcome multidrug resistance or enhance efficacy, which may also help in decreasing the level of adverse effects associated with both the drug and terpenoid molecule. Keeping this in view, the chapter focuses on the naturally occurring terpenoids and their analogues possessing anticancer activity. By modifying the parent nucleus, the chapter demonstrated the potency and efficacy of terpenoidal molecules, shedding more light on their cancer therapy potential.

## Hemiterpenoids

Hemeterpenoids are the simplest class of terpenoids. The most prominent hemiterpene was collected from the leaves of popular oaks and willows. It was also obtained from herbs, such as *Hamamelis japonica* [15]. Other plant hemeterpenoids [16] include tiglic acid, angelic acid, isovaleric acid, senecioic acid, and isoamyl alcohol, as shown in Fig. (**2**). The literature doesn't conclude with any extensive reports related to their anticancer effects.

## Monoterpenoids

Defensive resins of aromatic plants, floral scents, and essential oils constitute the majority of the monoterpenes [17, 18]. Complex monoterpenes were also obtained from the polyketide 1, 3, 6, 8,-tetrahydroxynaphthalene (THN) produced by *Streptomyces* bacteria. However, further studies are required to explore the enzymes that can be utilized as highly selective biocatalysts to overcome the limitations of chemical compounds [19]. These terpenes were non-nutritive, like essential oils of citrus fruits, cherries, mint, and herbs. Various terpene cyclasescatalyze the formation of monoterpenes. These terpenes exhibit physical and chemical properties with numerous biological potentials, such as in cancer [20 - 24]. These monoterpenes are further classified as acyclic, monocyclic, or bicyclic, depending upon their chemical nature. Some of them describing their biological potential are listed in Table **1**, and some monoterpenes with greater anticancer activity are discussed in this section.

a. ***Limonene***: It is a monocyclic monoterpene used in the industry for various cleaning products and as an additive (flavouring agent). It possesses different biological properties like antioxidant, anti-inflammatory, antinociceptive, insecticidal and many more [25]. It gains significance because it was a well-known validated chemopreventive agent against several pancreatic, stomach, colon, skin, and liver cancers [26]. Limonene and its metabolite, perillyl alcohol (POH), have been shown to have numerous biochemical benefits as a chemotherapeutic agent.It can cause apoptosis by increasing pro-apoptotic factors while decreasing anti-apoptotic factors [27, 28]. It was also involved in the inhibition of small G protein isoprenylation [29] and $Na^+ /K^+ATPase$ [30], induction of proto-oncogenes [29], disruption of various regulatory protein complexes [31], suppression of 3-hydroxy-3-methylglutanyl coenzyme reductase [32], resulting in inhibition of the protein isoprenylation. It also exerts its effects on B cell lymphoma associated X protein, cytochrome c release, cysteine-aspartic proteases (caspase)-3, 9, TGF- β and Bcl-2 [27]. Thus, limonene inhibits tumour growth, metastasis *via* anti-angiogenic, pro-apoptotic and antioxidant effects.

b. ***Perillyl alcohol:*** It occurs naturally and is known to be the major limonene metabolite, with significant antitumour activity [33]. Research proves that it can be employed in cancer prevention and treatment, thus gaining emerging interest in it due to its initial evaluation in phase I and phase II clinical trials for the treatment of breast, ovarian, and prostate cancer [34]. Due to this, various derivatives were prepared after its structure modification, like carbamates, esters, glucosides, and amino-modified POH derivatives of POH [35 - 40]. It also shows its subsequent failure in clinical effect in a phase II metastatic colon cancer trial conducted by the University of Wisconsin. Administration of 1-2g/kg of perillyl alcohol to rats reduces the incidence and multiplicity of invasive colonic adenocarcinoma and the dose of 75mg/kg thrice a week (i.p.) inhibits lung tumour formation [33]. In another study, tumour growth inhibition was reported to be 35.33% and 45.4% at a dose of 100 and 200 mg/kg/day, respectively, with no toxic effects [41]. Reports also conclude that perillyl alcohol exerts a cytotoxic effect against OVCAR-8, HCT-116, HepG2 and SF-295 cell lines [42, 43]. Perillyl alcohol can also be obtained from *Citrus sinensis, Citrus limon, Citrus aurantifolia, Citrus* *reticulate, Citrus paradise and* were known to exhibitanti-inflammatory, chemopreventive and other biological properties [44, 45].

c. ***Geraniol:*** Itis an acyclic monoterpene and can be obtained from *Cinnamomum tenuipilum, Valeriana officinalis* and has been proven to be used as antitumour, anti-inflammatory, antioxidative, antimicrobial activities, hepatoprotective, cardioprotective, neuroprotective [46 - 48]. It can also be used to treat various types of cancer, such as lung, colon, prostate, pancreatic, and liver cancer [49 - 53]. Geraniol is also known to have significant pharmacological potential, such as antioxidant, anti-inflammatory, anti-microbial, and anti-microbial properties [54]. It was proved in *in-vitro* studies that geraniol inhibits the growth of HepG2 human carcinoma cells by decreasing the HMG-CoA reductase level in mammals, thus it can be employed in liver cancer cells [55]. Studies demonstrate that it regulates a variety of signalling molecules and therefore participates in the cell cycle, cell proliferation, apoptosis, autophagy, and metabolism, which thus reveals geraniol as a multitarget drug candidate to treat cancer [56]. Studies also report that it has been used in the treatment of endometrial carcinoma and skin cancer by inhibiting the oncogenes and thus activating the tumour suppressor genes. It suppresses the Ras/Raf/ERK1/2 signalling pathway and thus induces apoptosis in DMBA/TPA-mediated skin tumourogenesis [54, 57]. It also prevents the G1 phase of MCF-7 breast cancer cell lines [58]. Kim *et al.* conclude in their study that it effectively induces apoptosis and autophagy in tumour cells, activates (AMPK) and inhibits (mTOR) the signalling pathway, and thus is found to be most effective in the treatment of prostate cancer [59].

d. ***Cantharidin:*** It is a monoterpene isolated from blister beetles that has been widely used in TCM to treat a variety of ailments and cancer (hepatoma and oesophagal carcinoma) [60]. The cantharidin's anticancer property demonstrates its spectrum against cancer cells of leukaemia, colorectal bladder, and breast [61 - 63]. It has been proven that it potentially inhibits the protein phosphatase 2A (PP2A) and heat shock transcription factor (HSF-1) [64]. Studies report that PP2A inhibition triggers cancer cell apoptosis in an IKKa/IKBa/p65 Nf-kB pathway dependent manner, leading to the subsequent activation of the TNF-alpha TRAIL R1 and TRAIL R2 extrinsic apoptotic signalling [65]. Thus, the research suggests that it can act by repressing cancerous cell growth and proliferation, inducing apoptosis in cancer cells (both extrinsic and intrinsic pathways), DNA damage and repair associated proteins, cell cycle arrest and metastasis, and by autophagy [60]. It also exerts cytotoxic effects [60]. Various clinical reports explore its potential, but still, its use is limited due to its severe side effects and extremely high toxicity level.

Thousands of new derivatives were synthesized, including norcantharidin, norcantharimide, cantharidinamides, anhydride-modified derivatives, and *N*-hydroxycantharidine [66, 67].

e. ***Camptothecin***: Camptothecin was discovered to be an amazing modified monoterpene indole alkaloid with anticancer activity in preliminary clinical trial studies [68, 69]. It is effective in both colon and gastric tumours, with the enzyme DNA topoisomerase one thought to be the primary cellular target [70]. As a result, various derivatives were developed. Topotecan, irinotecan, and belotecan were the most important, and they were approved for cancer therapy [68, 69].

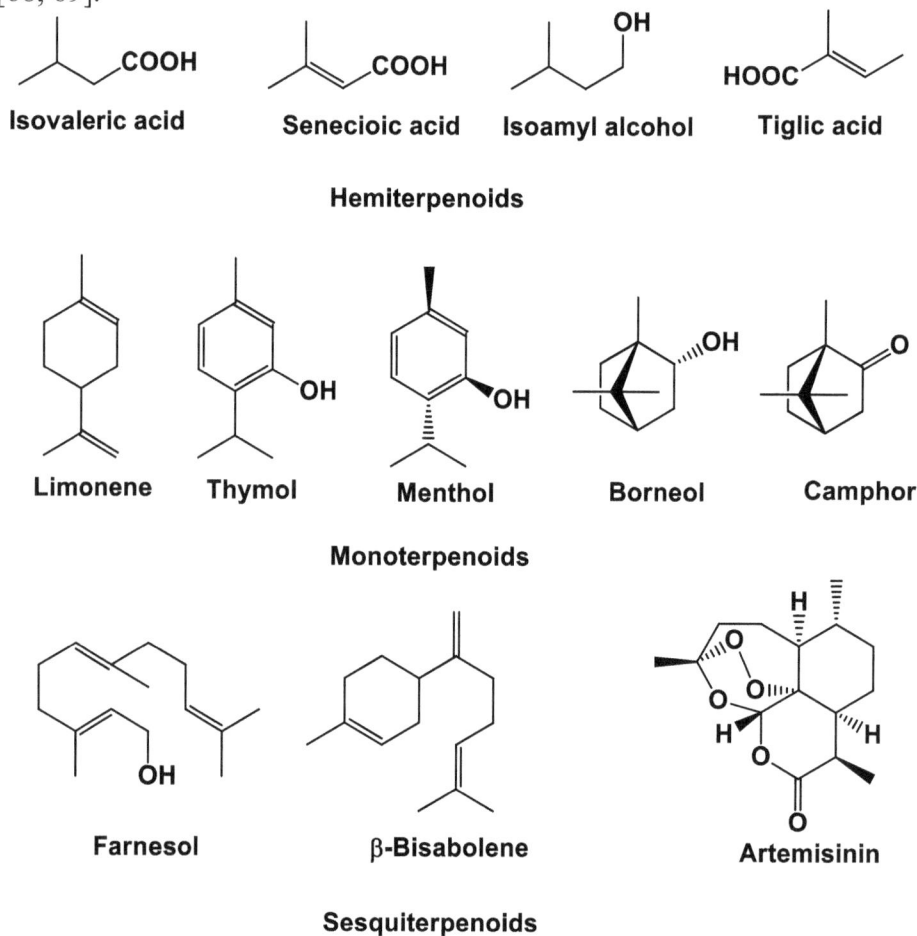

Isovaleric acid    Senecioic acid    Isoamyl alcohol    Tiglic acid

**Hemiterpenoids**

Limonene    Thymol    Menthol    Borneol    Camphor

**Monoterpenoids**

Farnesol    β-Bisabolene    Artemisinin

**Sesquiterpenoids**

**Fig. (2).** Chemical structure of Hemi, mono and sesquiterpenoids.

**Table 1. Monoterpenoids with their anticancer potential.**

| Name | Resource | Medicinal Properties | Refs. |
|---|---|---|---|
| Myrcene | *Lippiacitriodora, Laurus nobilis* | Antibacterial, cardiotonic, diuretic | [71] |
| Citral | *Cymbopogon flexuosus* | Antibacterial, antiviral, cytotoxic, anti-inflammatory | [71] |
| Linalool | *Cinnamomum camphora, Coriandrum sativum* | Antibacterial, antimycoplasmal, antiviral, anti-inflammatory, anti-edematous | [71] |
| Thymol | *Thymus vulgaris* L. | Antibacterial, anticancer | [71] |
| Carvone | *Carum carvi* L., *Mentha spicata* L. | Antibacterial, anticancer | [71] |
| Pinene | *Pinus palustris* (α-pinene), *Pinus caribaea* (β-pinene) and *P. pinaster* | Antibacterial, antiviral, antifungal, hypotensive | [71] |
| Limonene | *Citrus sinensis, Citrus limon, Citrus Aurantifolia, Citrus reticulate, Citrus paradise* | Antimicrobial, antioxidant, antinociceptive, insecticidal | [26, 72] |
| Menthol | *Mentha piperita* L. | Antibacterial, antispasmodic, antiseptic, antiulcer activity | [73, 74] |
| Eucalyptol | *Eucalyptus globulus, Rosmarinus officinalis* | Expectorant against bronchial catarrh (asthma), antiulcer activity | [73, 75] |
| Cantharidin | *Mylabrisphalerata* or *Mylabriscichorii, Cantharis vesicatoris* | Antiparasitic, anticancer | [47, 48, 76, 77] |
| Camphor | *Cinnamomum camphora* | Insecticidal, analgesic, antiviral, antimicrobial, anticoccidial, antinociceptive, anticancer, antitussive | [78] |

## Sesquiterpenoids

Sesquiterpenes are a type of terpene that is less volatile than monoterpenes and consists of three isoprene units with the molecular formula $C_{15}H_{24}$ (shown in Fig. (**2**)). They may be acyclic, monocyclic, bicyclic, or tricyclic or contain rings having unique combinations of sesquiterpene lactones. Among these, lactones are widely distributed in marine and terrestrial organisms, showing biological potential. Biological modification such as oxidation or rearrangement generates related sesquiterpenoids that serve as defensive agents or pheromones [79]. In the current era, there is an increasing demand for sesquiterpene lactones due to their high therapeutic potential as cytotoxic and anticancer agents [80]. Several sesquiterpenoids exist in nature, farnesol, β-nerolidol, β-bisabolene, α-zingiberene, α-humulene, β-santalol, β-caryophyllene, δ-cadinene, alantolactone, chamazulene, nootkatone, khushimol, thujopsene, patchoulol, zerumbone and vernodalinol. They exhibit antibacterial, antimicrobial, antiviral, antiprotozoal, cytotoxic activity and many more [80]. Some examples with anticancer potential were described in this section.

a. ***Artemisinin:*** It is a trioxane sesquiterpene lactone obtained from *Artemisia annua*. It is an important antimalarial drug with no significant side effects [81] or clinical resistance, although some tolerance has been reported [82]. This compound contains an endoperoxide ring nucleus, which was essential for the antimalarial activity. Artemisinin and its derivatives have also been used in immunosuppression, schistosomiasis, and cancer therapy [83 - 87]. Its derivatives like dihydroartemisinin and artesunate can be utilized in the treatment of cancer and are thus reported to inhibit various types of cancer [88 - 91]. Dihydroartemisinin, a metabolite of artemisinin derivatives and artesunate, a semisynthetic derivative, explores anticancer potential [92]. Artemisinin and its derivatives inhibit angiogenesis, metastasis, and invasion by regulating the levels of urokinase plasminogen activator, matrix metalloproteinase, avb3 integrins, and vascular endothelial growth factor [93 - 96]. Thus, it can be concluded that artemisinin presents a useful pharmacophore in the discovery of novel drugs against cancer. Various studies also demonstrate that artemisinin and its monomer analogues possess low toxicity and a short half-life, thus not being effective against cancer [97]. Comparative analyses were performed between monomeric compounds and artemisinin-derived dimmers and concluded that the dimeric form was more active than the corresponding monomers in both *in-vivo* and *in-vitro* studies, revealing their highest potential as anticancer drugs [98 - 100]. SAR studies demonstrate that the linkers (alkyl, aromatic ring, carbonate, carbamide, ester, and ether linkers) between the two artemisinin moieties have a significant influence on the anticancer activity. Research studies also made evident that the anticancer activities of artemisinin derivatives are likely to be mediated by multiple cellular events like cyclin D, cyclin E, CDK 2, CDK 4, p21, p27, and NF-KB [89, 90, 101 - 103], which induce apoptosis *via* activating p38 MAPK and caspases [89, 101, 104 - 109].

b. ***Dehydrocostuslactone (DHE):***It also belongs to the sesquiterpene lactone family and possesses antitumour activity. It acts against the human hepatoma cell lines, namely HepG2 and PLC/PRF/5, involving the apoptotic death of cancer cells in the liver through the mitochondrial pathway due to increased levels of different proteins like pro-apoptotic proteins, caspase-3, 4, apoptosis-inducing factor and endonuclease G, and decreased levels of anti-apoptotic proteins. It also causes an alteration in protein kinases and affects the regulation of CHOP/GADD153, splicing of X-box transcription factor-1 mRNA and the process of caspase-4 activation [110]. Thus, it concludes that it can act by several mechanisms: inhibiting proliferation, metastasis, invasion, telomerase, inducing cell apoptosis and angiogenesis, modulating ROS generation, f transporters, FPTase, and eIF4E [111].

c. *α-Bisabolbol:* It is a naturally occurring sesquiterpene alcohol isolated in 1951 by Isaac and collaborators from the blossoms of chamomile, *Matricaria chamomilla*. It exists in four possible stereoisomers and has been widely used as an ingredient in dermatological and cosmetic formulations. It has analgesic, anticancer, anti-inflammatory, anti-irritant, antibacterial, and other pharmacological properties [112]. It induces apoptosis through the intrinsic and extrinsic pathways by acting on or increasing the level of associated proteins with a concomitant decrease in the level of Bcl-2 [113]. It decreases the cell proliferation and *via*bility in pancreatic cancer cell lines [114] and induces cytotoxicity in HepG2 cells [113].

d. *Furanodiene*: Furanodiene, a sesquiterpene isolated from the Chinese medicinal plant, *Curcuma wenyujin*. It inhibits the proliferation and increases the LDH release in cell lines in a dose-dependent manner and causes cell arrest at the $G_0/G_1$ phase and suppresses the cancer cell growth in the breast [115]. It exhibits the antiproliferative effects by causing inhibition of HepG2 cells, inducing apoptosis which results in depolarization of mitochondrial transmembrane, p38 and caspase-3 activation, the release of cystic, activation of caspase-3, cleavage of PARP and inactivation of ERK1/2 MAPK signalling cascades [116]. Another study carried out by Maio and its coworkers in 2008 concludes that a plant, *Cremanthodium discoideum* contains two highly oxygenated bisabolane type sesquiterpenes named HOBS 1 and HOBS 2, which shows antiproliferative effects along with redifferentiation process in SMMC-7721 human hepatoma cells. These sesquiterpenes arrest the cell growth in the $G_1$ phase and increase the activity of tyrosine-α-ketoglutarate and GFsimultaneously decreases the level of α-fetoprotein (AFP) and γ-glutamyl transferase [117].

e. *Costunolide:* Costunolide, a sesquiterpene lactone, was obtained as an important active constituent from the plant *Aucklandialappa*. According to the literature, it can be used to treat bladder [118], ovarian [119], leukemia [120], and prostate cancer [121, 122] by inhibiting cancer cell proliferation and angiogenesis, inducing apoptosis and differentiation of cancer cells, and inhibiting metastasis and invasion of cancer cells.

f. *Others:* Many other examples like Zerumbone and vernodalinol were known to possess anticancer potential. Zerumbone possesses antiproliferative potential due to apoptosis, increased Bax level and decreased level of Bcl-2 [123], whereas Vernodalinol shows anticancer as well as a cytotoxic effect due to DNA inhibition [124].

## Diterpenoids

Among other terpene classes, diterpenes are in the spotlight due to their excellent biological properties, such as their ability to act against inflammation, microbes, cancer, and many other disorders. It belongs to the C20 class of terpenoids, having $C_{20}H_{32}$ and commonly exists in a polyoxygenated form with keto and hydroxyl groups, esterified by small-sized aliphatic or aromatic acids. The bioactive diterpenes such as grayanotoxin, forskolin, eleganolone, marrubenol, 4-deoxyandrographolide, crotogoudin, crotobarin, sideritol, (-)-atiserene, (-)isoatiserene, eriocatisin A, Kaurane and pimarane-type diterpenes, and ent-Atisane natural diterpenoid [125 - 127] have anticancer and other pharmacological properties. Some examples are listed in Tables **2** and **3** with their anticancer mechanisms, and their chemical structures are shown in Fig. (**3**).

**Table 2. Anticancer mechanism of diterpenes.**

| Diterpene and its Derivatives | Biological Source | Cell Lines | Action and Strength | Refs. |
|---|---|---|---|---|
| Alcyonolide | *Cespitularia species.* | HCT 116 cells | IC50 bet 5.85 - 91.4 µM | [128] |
| Neocaesalpin AA, AB, AC, AD, AE, 12α-methoxyl, 5α,14βdihydroxy-1α,6α,7βtriacetoxycass-13(15)-en-16,12-olide Neocaesalpin AA, AB, AC, AD, AE, 12α-methoxyl,5α, | *Caesalpinia minax* | Hela, HCT-8, HepG-2, MCF-7, A549 cell lines | Moderate activity having IC50 values from 18.4-83.9 µM | [129] |
| Eryngiolide A | *Pleurotuseryngii* | HeLa, HepG2 | Moderate activity with IC50 values 20.6 and 28.6 µM | [130] |
| Cavernenes A-D, KalihinenesEand F | *Acanthella cavernosa* | HCT116,A549,QGY-7701, HeLa, MDA-MB-231 | IC50 of 6–18 µM | [131] |
| Neocaesalpin MR | *Caesalpinia minax* | HeLa, HCT-8 | Mild (IC50: 36.8 and 45.2 µg/mL respectively) | [132] |
| Tomocinon, Tomocinol A and B | *Caesalpinia sappan* | PANC-1 | IC50 values between 34.7 and 42.4 µM | [133] |
| Pachydictyols B and C | *Dictyotadichotoma* | Human tumour cell lines | Weak action having mean IC of >30.0 µM | [134] |
| VitextrifolinsA-G | *Vitex trifolia* | A549, HCT116, HL-60, ZR-75-30 | IC50 > 5 µg/mL | [135] |
| Leptoclalin A | *Sinularialeptoclados* | K-562, T-47 D | Weak (IC50:12.8 and 15.4 µg/mL respectively) | [136] |
| Podoimbricatin A and B | *Podocarpus imbricatus* | A549, NCI-H292 | IC50 range- 9.5 - 47.8 µM | [137] |
| Sarcophytolol and sarcophytolide B and C | *Sarcophyton glaucum* | HepG2, MCF-7, PC-3 | IC50 range - 9.3 - 25 µM | [138] |
| Aphanamixins A–F | *Aphanamixispolystachya* | HepG2, AGS, MCF-7 and A-549 cancer cell lines | Weak, IC50 > 10 µM | [139] |
| Trichodelphinines A–E | *Delphinium trichophorum* | A549 cancer cells | IC50 values ranged from 12.03 to 52.79 µM | [140] |

(Table 2) cont.....

| Diterpene and its Derivatives | Biological Source | Cell Lines | Action and Strength | Refs. |
|---|---|---|---|---|
| Henrin A | *Pteris henryi* | KB, HCT116, MCF-7, A549 | Cytotoxicity, >20 μg/mL | [141] |
| Tomocins A–H | *Vietnamese Caesalpinia* | PANC-1 | PC50 between 51 and 75 μM | [142] |
| Oridonin | *Rabdosiarubescens* | HEp-2 cells, OCM-1, UM2B, BxPC-3 | apoptosis (5–20 μM conc.), Fas and Bcl-2 mediated apoptosis, Caspase-mediated apoptosis | [143-145] |
| Gramaderins A-D | *Grangeamaderapatana* | FMLP/CB-induced human neutrophils | ROS generation and elastase release inhibition, C50 range- 4.70 and >10 μM | [146] |
| Tripchlorolide | *Tripterygium wilfordii* | A549 cells | Autophagy | [147] |
| Eriocalyxin B | *Isodoneriocalyx* | PANC-1, SW1990, CAPAN-1& 2 | Apoptosis and cell cycle arrest | [148] |
| Tanshinone IIA | *Salvia miltiorrhiza* | CaSki, SiHa, HeLa, C33a | Cell cycle arrest, apoptosis | [149] |
| Triptolide | *Tripterygium wilfordii* | Colon cancer cell lines HCT116 and HT29 | Cell cycle arrest at G1 phase | [150] |
| Sclareol | *Salvia sclarea* | MG63 | Apoptosis, cell cycle arrest, loss of ΛΨm | [151] |
| Ponicidin | *Isodonadenolomus* | HT29 colorectal cancer cell line | Cell cycle arrest, upregulation of caspase 3 and Bax | [152] |
| Carnosic acid | *Rosemarinus officinalis* | HepG2 cells | Autophagic cell death through inhibition of the Akt/mTOR pathway | [153] |
| Jaridonin | *Isodonrubescens* | MGC- 803 | Upregulation of ATM, Chk1, Chk2, phosphorylated Cdc2 and CDK2, Cell cycle arrest | [154] |

a. ***Tanshinone IIA***: It demonstrates its anticancer properties in *in vitro* and *in vivo* studies in significant human carcinoma cell lines of breast and colon cancer [155 - 158]. It also acts as a DNA minor grove binder and thus causes inhibition of binding of RNAPII to DNA. It also helps in the initiation process of RNAPII phosphorylation, down-regulates the various transcription factors and up-regulates the many other processes contributing to the anticancer mechanism [157, 158]. Tanshinone IIA inhibits multiple types of cancer cells [159 - 161] and thus effects the invasion and metastasis of cancer, reducing the levels of several proteins and increasing the levels of MMP 1 and 2 [162, 163]. Other related tanshinones are tanshinone I, cryptotanshinon and dihydrotanshinone, all found to be anticancer [164 - 166].

b. ***Triptolide:*** Triptolide was known to be a promising gene transcriptioninhibitor [167].The $Ca^{++}$ channel polycystin-2 [167], an unknown 90-kDa nucleoprotein [168], and a subunit of the transcription factor TFIIH-XPB [169] were among the molecular targets of triptolide. It binds to XPB *via* covalent bonds, inhibiting XPB ATPase activity and proving to be the primary molecular target of triptolide. It also causes DNA damage by inducing nucleotide excision repair as a result of XPB inhibition. Triptolide inhibits transcriptional activity and helps in the mediation of its role in cancer treatment [170]. Assuming that proteins do, to some extent, mediate anticancer effects, further research was required.

c. ***Pseudolaric Acid B***: It has antifungal and anti-angiogenic properties. It was obtained from *Pseudolarix kaempferi*. It was intensively evaluated as an anticancer and was known to have broad-spectrum cytotoxicity against cancer cell lines with an $IC_{50}$ of 1 μM [171]. Research revealed that the cytotoxicity is due to the destabilization of microtubules and is thus responsible for the microtubule blockage in tumour cytostatic and angiogenic effects [172, 173]. Pseudolaric acid B bypasses P-gp and has the potential to be used against cancer, particularly for resistant anticancer drugs [174]. It directly inhibits endothelial cell growth, induces apoptosis and autophagy, and antagonizes the VEGF-stimulated cellular events [175 - 177].

d. ***Andrographolide***: It also exhibits anticancer potential by inhibiting cancer cell growth by inducing apoptosis, thereby activating the kinase pathways like mitogen-activated protein kinase and thus exerting a cytotoxic effect [178]. It shows a pronounced therapeutic effect by blocking Nf-kB signalling due to the covalent bond formation of reduced cysteine in the oligonucleotide binding pocket of p50 [179]. It also exerts protective effects on beta cells by inhibiting NF-kB, reducing the phosphorylation of p65 and IkBa at serine units and promoting the proliferation and apoptosis of cancer cells [180]. Thus, it acts on various cyclins, cyclin-dependent kinases, metalloproteinases, growth factors, and tumour suppressor proteins, thus mediating anticancer activity *via* inhibition of cancer cell proliferation and the survival process of metastasis [181].

e. ***Oridonin***: Itis obtained from the *Rabdosiarubescens* and has been found to have therapeutic use for solid tumours. It is known to inhibit T cell leukaemia's growth, acute and chronic lymphocytic leukaemia [181], and induce apoptosis, leading to cell death [182]. It exerts cytotoxic effects *via* the generation of reactive oxygen species, affecting various apoptotic proteins and tumour suppressor genes [183]. Treatment with oridonin helps in the downregulation of PI2K/Akt signaling, thereby contributing to the induction of cancer cell apoptosis [184]. Research also concludes that autophagy enhances various pathways' signalling processes and inhibits ROS-mediated apoptosis [185]. In addition to that, oridonin induces autophagy and apoptosis in HeLa cells and was significantly reduced by *N*-acetylcysteine administration [186]. The reasons for these discrepancies are still unknown. It is possible that this was due to the geographical factors of various species' existences or possibly the heterogenicity of cancer cells.

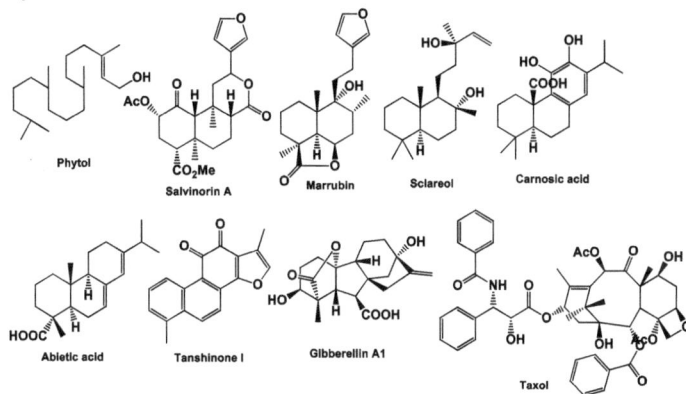

**Fig. (3).** Chemical structures of diterpenoids.

**Table 3. Resource, medicinal properties and anticancer mechanism of diterpenoids.**

| Name | Resource | Medicinal Properties | Anticancer Mechanism | Refs. |
|---|---|---|---|---|
| Phytol | Ester attachment in the chlorophyll molecule | Antimicrobial, cytotoxic, antioxidant, anti-convulsant, anxiolytic, induce apoptosis, anti-inflammatory. | - | [187] |
| Excisanin A | *Isodonmacrocalyxin D* | Anticancer | Apoptosis, inhibition of AKT signalling pathway | [188] |
| Paclitaxel | *Texusbrevifolia* | Anticancer | - | [189] |
| Triptolide | *Tripterygium wilfordii* | Anti-inflammatory, anti-immune disorders, antiproliferative, anticancer | effects the DNA binding affinity, interferes with NF-kB, p53, NF-AT, HSF-1, inhibition of RNA polymerase I and II | [168, 190 - 194] |
| α-Terpineol | *Salvia libanotica* | Antitumour, cytotoxic | suppresses NF-kB signaling. | [195, 196] |
| Gnidimacrin | *Stellerachamaejasme* | Anticancer | inhibits the growth of protein kinase C, suppression of cdc2 transcription, increases the level of cyclin dependantkinase -1 | [197, 198] |

a. ***Other diterpenoids:*** Many others, such as marrubin, salvinorin A, carsonic acid, tanshinone I, and taxol [199 - 204] have known to exibhit anticancer and other multifunctional pharmacological properties.

## Sesterterpenoids

Sesterterpenoids constitute five isoprene units to form a carbon backbone containing molecules and exist in different frameworks [205, 206]. Some examples of these were hippolode E, manolide, leucosceptrine, heliocide, nitiol, and sestertatin, possessing numerous pharmacological activities. These typical examples with their chemical structures are shown in Fig. (**4**)

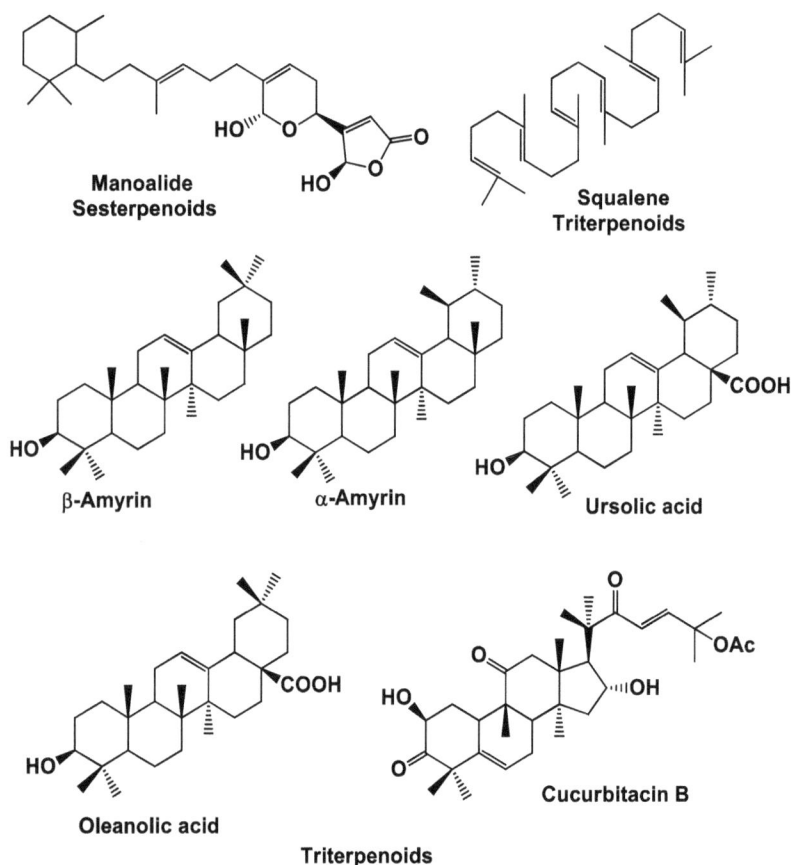

**Fig. (4).** Chemical structure of sesquiterpenoids and triterpenoids.

## Triterpenoids

These are the naturally occurring molecules of vegetable, animal, and fungal origin, comprising the carbon skeleton of six isoprene units named triterpenoids

[207, 208]. They contain a cyclopentane perhydrophenanthrene ring system, and their important representatives are squalene, dammarane, lanostane, oleane, lupine, ursane, or triterpenoid sapogenin [209]. Table **4** illustrates the types of triterpenes with their neoplastic cell line effects. Some examples of having anticancer potential were discussed in this section and are also listed in Table **5**.

**Table 4. Examples of neoplastic cell lines sensitive to cytotoxic properties of triterpenes.**

| Triterpene | Type of Neoplasm |
|---|---|
| Squalene derivatives | Leukemia, melanoma, sarcoma, lung, colon breast, ovary, prostate & kidney cancer |
| Dammarane derivatives | Lung, ovarian, colorectal, colon glioma cancer |
| Lanostane and its derivatives | Leukemia, melanoma, glioma, gastric, pancreas, colon, hepatic, lung and breast cancer |
| Oleanane and its derivatives | Thyroid, ovarian, breast, colorectal and glioma cancer |
| Lupane and its derivatives | Lung, prostate, breast, prostate, ovarian, cervical, thyroid and colon cancer |
| Ursane and its derivatives | Pancreas, prostate, cervical, hepatic, breast, colorectal, leukemia and colon adenocarcinoma |

a. ***Celastrol:*** It gains tremendous interest against variant disorders like cancer, inflammation, arthritis, asthma, Alzheimer's, and lupus [210 - 212]. It was employed as an anticancer, but its mechanism based on the molecular basis remains unclear. Variant reports conclude that it may act by causing direct inhibition of IKKA, b kinases, proteasomes, and AKT/mTOR/P70S6K signalling, inactivation of Cdc37, p23, or by activation of HSF1. It was also concluded from various studies that the anticancer effect was due to the presence of the quinone methide structure, which undergoes reaction with the thiol groups of the cysteine residues to form protein adducts [213 - 215]. Celastrol is also a proteasome inhibitor, as evidenced by *in vitro* and *in vivo* studies. It is highly susceptible to nucleophilic attack because it contains ketone carbons on the B ring of the parent molecule [215, 216].

b. ***Oleanolic acid***: It is a triterpene that possesses chemotherapeutic properties against cancer cell lines and shows concentration-dependent inhibition of intercellular adhesion molecules, thus treating liver cancer cells [217]. It is also known to be an effective antiproliferative agent because it induces apoptosis associated with alteration in protein and downregulates the level of Bcl-2 family proteins [218]. It exhibits anti-tumour, anti-hepatoma, and antiproliferative action. It was known to induce apoptosis, cell cycle arrest, up and downregulation of enzymes, decrease the level of Bcl-2 and surviving; inhibition of various signaling pathways; activation of Wnt/-catenin signalling [219] were found to be underlying molecular mechanisms of UA action [217,

218]. It also helps to protect the hepatoma cells and thus reduces the HBx-mediated autophagy through modulation of Ras homolog gene family member A [220]. Ursolic acid effects the process of glycolysis and thus helps in promoting anticancer action [221]. According to reports [222, 223], ursolic acid nanoparticles can be used as anticancer agents with improved activity and bioavailability.

c. ***Cucurbitacins:*** They were an oxygenated triterpene group found in many plants [224] and had been reported to be anti-tumour agent.Among the group, cucurbitacin B effectively acts against cancer by decreasing the viability of cell lines through apoptosis, suppressing the transcription factor signal transducer and activating transcription-3 phosphorylation with a cell-killing effect [225]. Cucurbitacin B was also notified of growth inhibitory effects by induction of cell cycle arrest at the S phase and apoptosis associated with downregulation of cyclin D1 and CDC-2 [194]. It also mediates the inhibitory action of c-Raf activation without causing possible alterations in STAT3 phosphorylation [226, 227]. Cucurbitacins significantly inhibit the proliferation of multiple tumour line cells and induce cell cycle arrest at the G and S phases and differentiation in several cell lines [228 - 230]. Cucurbitacin D and I were isolated from the *Elaeocarpus hainanensis* and evaluated as anticancer and cytotoxic activity [231, 232]. A combination of cucurbitacin D and E with X rays was found to be protective and effective in treating cancer [233]. Because of this, combination therapy is gaining much more importance and has become the focus of current research. Other molecular targets were F-actin, STAT 3, cellular dysfunction, and signal transduction [234, 235].

d. ***Ginsenosides*** suppress the growth and inhibition of various targets. Cell cycle arrest suppresses the growth of cells by cell cycle arrest [236]. Ginsenoside–Rh2 inhibits DNA synthesis by downregulating the cyclin-dependent kinase activity [237] and by apoptosis through activation of caspase-3 followed by proteolytic cleavage of PARP [238]. The case of ginsenoside Rk1 revealed that it induces apoptosis through activation of caspase 8 and 3 by decreasing the level of Fas-associated death domain expression [239]. Kim *et al.* [240] reported the growth-suppressive effect of ginsenoside Rs3 in SK-Hep-1 cells by apoptosis and cell cycle arrest in the $G_1$/S phase.

**Table 5. Resource, medicinal properties and anticancer mechanism of triterpenoids.**

| Name | Resource | Medicinal Properties | Anticancer Mechanism | Refs. |
|---|---|---|---|---|
| Squalene | *Carcharhinus amblyrhynchos Olea europaea* | Emollient, skin hydration, antioxidant, antitumour | - | [241] |

*(Table 5) cont.....*

| Name | Resource | Medicinal Properties | Anticancer Mechanism | Refs. |
|------|----------|---------------------|----------------------|-------|
| α-Amyrin | *Bursera and Protium* species, *Taraxacum officinale* | Antimicrobial, antifungal, anti-inflammatory, antiulcer | Inhibit NF-KB, IL-1 β, COX-2, CREB, ERK, PKC, p38 MAPK | [242] |
| β-Amyrin | *Nelumbo nucifera, Amphipterygiumadstringens* | | Inhibit NF-κB, IL-1β, COX-2, CREB, ERK, PKC, P38 MAPK | |
| Ursolic acid | *Ocimum sanctum, Vaccinum myrtillus L., Rosmarinus officinalis* | Antiproliferative, cytotoxic, anticancer, neuroprotective, antitumour, antihypertensive, antihyperuricemic, antihyperlipidemic, antioxidant, antibacterial, antihistaminic | Anti-mutagenic, Anti-tumour, Inhibition of cell proliferation, Displayed cytotoxicity cancer cells by ↑apoptosis, ↓Bcl-2, PARP cleavage, GR modulation. Growth inhibitory effect by decreasing $O_2$ consumption | [243] |
| Boswellic acid and its derivatives | *Boswellia serrata* | Anti-inflammatory, anticancer | Antiproliferative reduces apoptosis and leads to the activation of Caspase-3,8 and 9 | [244] |
| Lupeol | *Tamarindus indica, Allanblackiamonticola, Himatanthussucuuba* | Anti-inflammatory, anticancer, hepatoprotective, cardioprotective | Growth inhibition of SMMC7721 cells *via* activation of caspase - 3 | [245] |
| Alisol and its derivatives | *Alisma orientalis* | Antihypertensive, Antihyperlipidemic, treatment of urological disorders, anticancer | Induces the autophagy and apoptosis, cell cycle arrest | [246, 247] |
| Pachymic acid | *Poriacocos* | Anti-inflammatory, anticancer | Induces apoptosis, activation of PARP, caspase-3 and 9, DNA Topoisomerase I and II inhibition, suppresses invasion of MDA-MB-231 and MCF-7, decreases the secretion of MMP9, reduces the NF-kB activity | [248 - 251] |

| Name | Resource | Medicinal Properties | Anticancer Mechanism | Refs. |
|---|---|---|---|---|
| Acetin | *Actaea recemosa* | Anticancer | Inhibits the growth of HepG2 cells | [252] |
| Ardisiacrispin (A+B) | *Ardisia crenta* | Cytotoxic, antiproliferative | Pro-apoptotic, microtubule disruptive function | [253] |
| Astragaloside IV | *Radix astragali* | Anticancer | Growth inhibition decreases oncogene level VAV3.1 and increases the level of BIP/GRP78, HSP70, HSPAIA, and HSPA8. | [254] |
| Asiatic acid | *Centella asiatica* | Anticancer | Apoptotic increases the level of calcium | [255] |
| Betulinic acid | *Triphyophyllumpeltatum, Ancistrocladusheyneanus* | Anticancer, cytotoxic | Induces apoptosis, inhibits the phosphatidylinositol 3 kinase/AKT pathway, increases the level of Bcl-2 | [256] |
| Echinocystic acid | *Luffa cylindrical* | Antiproliferative, antimicrobial | DNA fragmentation, activation of caspase-3, 8, 9, JNK pathway and p38, truncation of Bid, reduces the level of Bcl-2 | [257] |
| Escin | *Aesculus wilsonii* | Anticancer | Disruption in G1/S phase progression | [258] |
| Ganodermic acid | *Ganoderma lucidum* | Anticancer | Blocks G1 to S phase | [259] |
| Ganoderiol F | *Ganoderiolambonense* | Antiproliferative | Inhibition of DNA synthesis, cell cycle arrest | [260] |
| 24- Hydroxyursolic acid | *The derivative of ursolic acid* | Anticancer | Inhibit cell proliferation, Induce cellular apoptosis by activation of PARP, caspase-3, and phosphorylation of p53 at Ser15. Activate AMPK, inhibition of COX-2 induces DNA fragmentation in cancer cells | [261] |

*(Table 5) cont.....*

| Name | Resource | Medicinal Properties | Anticancer Mechanism | Refs. |
|---|---|---|---|---|
| Corosolic acid | *Lagerstroemia speciosa* | antidiabetic, anti-inflammatory, antiproliferative, protein kinase C inhibitor | Suppress cell proliferation, ↓NF-κB, ↓proteasomal activity | [262, 263] |
| Oleanolic acid | *Olea europaea, Calendula officinalis* | Anticancer, antitumour, antidiabetic, antimicrobial, hepatoprotective, antioxidant, antihypertensive, anti-inflammatory, antiparasitic | Cytotoxicity, inhibit angiogenesis | [264] |
| Pomolic acid | *Paulownia tomentosa* | Antimalarial, anticancer, hypertensive | Cytotoxicity, Inhibit DNA polymerase β, Activate AMPK | [265, 266] |
| Pristimerin | *Celastrushypoleucus* | Antifungal, Anticytomegalovirus, anticancer | Induce cell apoptosis, inhibit cell viability, angiogenesisand tumour cell proliferation, induce caspase-dependent apoptosis, inhibit NF-kB, proteasome activity | [265, 267, 268] |
| Taraxerol | *Clitoreaternatea, Mangifera indica* | Anti-Alzheimer's, Anti-Parkinsonism, antimicrobial, anticancer, antiallergic, anti-inflammatory, antidiabetic | Inhibitory action on cancer cell | [269] |
| Gypenosides | *Gynostemnapentaphyllum* | Cytotoxic | Alteration in apoptosis mediated proteins | [270] |
| IH-901 | Metabolite of *Ginseng* | Cytotoxic, Antiproliferative, apoptotic | Induces apoptosis, leads to the activation of caspase -9 and 3, release of cyt. C | [271, 272] |
| Kalopanaxsaponins A and I | *Nigella glanulifera* | Cytotoxic | - | [273] |

(Table 5) cont.....

| Name | Resource | Medicinal Properties | Anticancer Mechanism | Refs. |
|---|---|---|---|---|
| Lucidenic acid A, B, C and N | *Ganoderma lucidum* | Antiproliferative, antivasive | Inhibition of matrix metalloproteinase-9, and kinases, suppression of NF-kB- DNA binding activities | [274, 275] |
| 25-methoxyhispidol A | *Poncirustrifolata* | Antiproliferative | Apoptosis, cell cycle arrest at G phase, downregulation and upregulation of different proteins | [276] |
| Waltonitone | *Gentian waltonii* | Anticancer | Apoptosis, upregulation of mRNA expressions of caspases, protease factor and other proteins | [277] |
| Triterpenoid saponins | *Androsace umbellate* | Antitumour, cytotoxic | - | [278] |
| Betulinic acid | *Betula pubescens* | Anticancer, anti-HIV, antimalarial, antibacterial, anthelmintic, anti-inflammatory | Apoptosis inducer, Cytotoxic, ↑Apoptosis, Caspase activation, Inhibit cell proliferation through ↓Bcl-2, ↓cyclin D1, ↑Bax | [279, 280] |
| Cucurbitacin B | Various species from Cucurbitaceae family | Anti-inflammatory, antioxidant, antiviral, antipyretic, analgesic and antimalarial, anticancer | - | [281] |
| Asiatic acid | *Centella asiatica* | Anti-inflammatory and wound healing, anticancer, antioxidant, hepatoprotective, antidiabetic, anti-hepatitis C virus | Apoptosis inducer *via* caspase-3 activation and ROS, Growth inhibition by ↑apoptosis, increases Bax, p38 & ERK ½ | [282] |

*(Table 5) cont.....*

| Name | Resource | Medicinal Properties | Anticancer Mechanism | Refs. |
|---|---|---|---|---|
| Betulin | *Betula* Species | Anticancer, antiviral, antibacterial | Apoptosis, anti-angiogenic, Antioxidant, cell differentiation enhancer. Inhibit ROS generation, Fas upregulation, caspase-8- dependent BID activation with successive inhibition of the mitochondrial pathway | [282] |
| Friedelin | *Cassia tora* | Anti-inflammatory, antiviral, antibacterial, suppression of tumour promotion activities | Suppress cell proliferation and topoisomerase | [282] |
| Glycyrrhetinic acid | *Glycyrrhiza glabra* | Anti-inflammatory, antitumour, antiulcer, anticancer, antibacterial, antiviral, antileishmanial | Induce apoptosis, the release of cytochrome, caspase-8 activation, Bcl-2, Bcl-xL(anti-apoptotic) downregulation | [282] |
| Lantadene A and B | *Lantana camara* | Anti-inflammatory, antitumour, antiulcer, anticancer, antimicrobial, antiviral, Anti TB | Induces apoptosis by activating the caspase-3, regulates Bcl-2, Bax expression, downregulation of AP-1 and NF-κB (p65) | [282] |
| Maslinic acid | *Crataegus oxyacantha* | Anti-colonic cancer, anti-diabetogenic, antioxidant, antiviral, and anti-inflammation, inhibits TNF signalling | Reduces cell proliferation, induce apoptosis, increased release of cytochrome c | [282] |
| Sitosterol | *Urtica dioica, Nigella sativa* | Anti-inflammatory, chemopreventive, hypocholesterolemic, angiogenic, anthelmintic, antimutagenic, immunomodulator, anticancer, neuroprotective, antidiabetic, antioxidant | Angiogenesis and metastasis inhibition decreases the level of $Bcl_2$, AKT, Increase Caspase-3, MAPK family | [283] |

*(Table 5) cont.....*

| Name | Resource | Medicinal Properties | Anticancer Mechanism | Refs. |
|------|----------|----------------------|----------------------|-------|
| Stigmasterol | *Physostigmavenenosum, Brassica napus* L. | Anti-osteoarthritic, antitumour, cytotoxic, anti-hypercholesterolemic, antioxidant, antimutagenic, anti-inflammatory | Angiogenesis and metastasis inhibition decrease the level of Bcl$_2$, AKT, Increase Caspase-3, MAPK family | [284] |

## Tetraterpenoids

Tetraterpenoids are one of the significant classes of terpenoids which includes mainly carotenoids. Carotenoids are natural fat-soluble pigments that provide colouration to the plant and animal species [285]. Lycopene contains eight isoprene units joined head to tail to give a conjugated system responsible for producing colour. This conjugated system provides a chromophoric character to the molecule. Nowadays, these carotenoids find their utilization in reducing cancer risk and are thus employed as dietary intake. Pre-clinical studies reveal the utilization of carotenoids (β-carotene, α-carotene, zeaxanthin and canthaxanthin) as anticarcinogenic [286]. Some carotenoids are discussed further below, and the chemical structures of tetraterpenoids are depicted in Fig. (**5**).

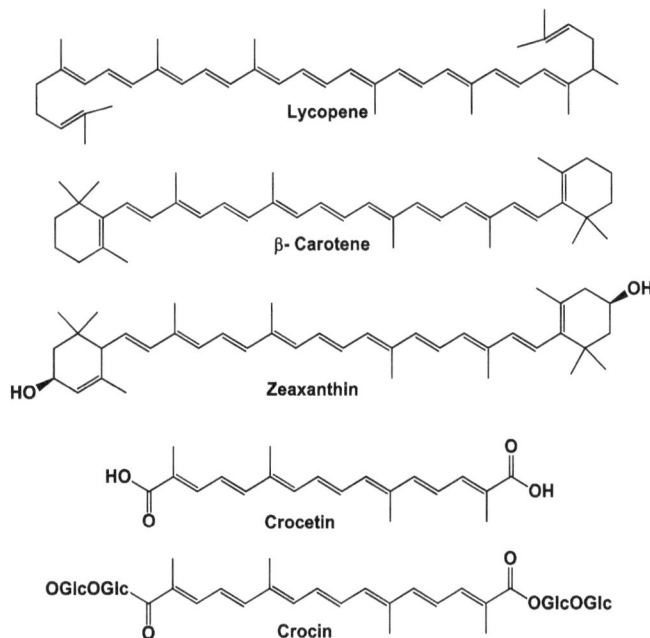

**Fig. (5).** Chemical structure of tetraterpenoids.

a. ***Fucoxanthin:*** Chemically, it is an oxygenated carotenoid present in *Laminaria japonica, Undaria pinnatifida and Hijikia fusiformis*. It is used to treat cancer by inhibiting the growth of cancer cells like HepG2 by causing cell arrest at the G phase. It also decreases the levels of cyclin proteins D1, D3 and cdk4. It also shows the antiproliferative effect [287, 288].

b. ***Lycopene:***It is an open-chain linear hydrocarbon containing conjugated and non-conjugated double bonds intheir chemical structure [289]. It inhibits the Hep3B cells by arresting the cell cycle and damaging DNA. It effectively shows its antimigration and antivasive properties against highly invasive Sk Hep-1 cells [290]. It mediates their cation *via* NF-kB inhibition, leading to a decreased level of MMP-9 [291]. It is also used in combination or with soy isoflavones to lower serum PSA levels in men with prostate cancer [289]. It attributes the anti-angiogenic effect by attenuating the MMP-2 and uPA activity [292 - 294]. Proteomic analysis revealed that lycopene modulates the expression of a broad range of proteins [295]. This approach may represent a powerful strategy to gain mechanistic insights into the mode of action of lycopene.

c. ***β-carotene***: It plays an intensive role in treating cancer by decreasing the proliferation and differentiation of cells with increased albumin expression, haptoglobin and fibrinogen [296]. It also induces apoptosis and necrosis to produce genotoxic and cytotoxic effects in HepG2 cells. It also upregulates the peroxime proliferator-activated receptor gamma by inducing apoptosis and can be employed in treating breast cancer [297]. Despite the several reports, studies are still required to explore the potential of β-carotene and develop the method to select the carotenoid to modulate drug resistance [298].

d. ***Others:*** Other carotenoids like lutein, antheraxanthin, violaxanthin, fucoxanthin and canthaxanthin were also used to produce moderate effects on tumour cells. It was believed that carotenoids enhance chemotherapy's effectiveness by competing with anticancer drugs [299]. It was well investigated that the combination of carotenoids with different cytotoxic agents synergistically enhances the cytotoxicity in Caco-2 cells [300].

## ANALOGS OF TERPENOIDS

The IIIM research group synthesized a terpenoidal-based vasicine analogue, according to the literature. The prepared lactams exhibit antitussive potential vis-a-vis the parent monoterpenoids. The other synthetic analogue of vasicine, 7, 8, 9, 10-tetrahydroazepino[2,1-b]quinazolon-12(6*H*)-one found to be 6-10 folds more potent. The objective was to synthesize a novel analogue of vasicine by replacing ring C of C-1 with the lactam prepared by nitrogen insertion in the structure of menthol to design a molecule with better antitussive activity than the previously synthesized analogue while preserving bronchodilatory potential. The study proves that newer analogues can be prepared with better pharmacological potential by structure modification [301].

## STRUCTURE MODIFICATION IN TERPENOIDS

**Marrubin**: Literature reports that the lactone ring's opening by refluxing with potassium hydroxide yields an active marrubiinic acid (70%). It was found to be 11 times more active than the other standard drugs. Further, modifying this molecule gives another component named marrubenol. Marrubernol was obtained after the reduction of marrubiinic acid with reducing agents and was, therefore, screened as a vasorelaxant. Blocking the free acidic groups in marrubinic acid, on the other hand, reduced its biological activities [302].

**Tanshinone I**: Modification in the ring B of the parent nucleus generates the active analogues as lactam derivatives with improved anticancer effects and good bioavailability [303].

**Andrographolide:** Chemoselective functionalization at C14 hydroxy of the parent molecule has been evaluated as cytotoxic against leukaemia cell lines. Studies prove that the α-alkylidene-γ-butyrolactone moiety of andrographolide plays a vital role in the molecule's biological potential [304].

**Betulinic acid:** Hydrogenation of the parent molecule yields dihydrobetulinic acid, and its amide derivatives are more potent anti-HIV agents. When coupled with amino acids at the C-28 carboxylic acid portion, it produces conjugates with a cytotoxicity profile. Following esterification, methyl ester derivative components were obtained with comparable cytotoxicity results. Some are less cytotoxic than others (methyl ester derivatives of phenylalanine, leucine, glutamic acid, and valine analogues), while others are more cytotoxic (methyl ester derivatives of glycine, methionine, tryptophan, and alanine analogues) [305].

**Artemisinin:** Dimerization of two-parent molecules by the linker (alkyl, aromatic ring, carbonate, carbamide, ester, and ether linkers) results in active analogues as anticancer. The introduction of the hydroxyl group onto the linker results in a loss of activity. The action is reduced when the aromatic ring on the linker is replaced rather than the alkyl moiety, but it is enhanced when the alkyl group is extended.In addition to this, bis-substituted dimers were more potent than monosubstituted dimers [306].

## CONCLUSION

Terpenes are natural compounds that constitute the largest class of natural bioactive components and nowadays are proven to have a rich reservoir of compounds that might help drug discovery and the development of newer drug entities to cure deadly diseases. The chapter aims to explore the anticancer terpenoidal components that may promise and will potentially open new opportunities for cancer therapy. However, current research studies are somehow restricted to descriptive findings and lack mechanistic insight and SAR studies. There is a requirement for more efforts to identify the new targets, which may increase the chances of gaining breakthrough insights into cancer. It is still required to understand the gene functions that could be the novel components of new pathways to overcome life-threatening diseases, which may give more contemporary insights for many pharmaceutical industries. Terpenoids, thus prove to be an important help drug entity for the pharmaceutical and biotechnological industries. It may also help in the development of products that regulate the immune system of the tumour microenvironment, proving to be a novel cancer treatment in the future.

## CONSENT FOR PUBLICATION

Not applicable.

## CONFLICT OF INTEREST

The authors declare no conflict of interest, financial or otherwise.

## ACKNOWLEDGEMENT

The authors extend their heartful thanks to Principal, Guru Gobind Singh College of Pharmacy, Yamuna Nagar, for valuable suggestions and moral support.

## REFERENCES

[1]    Newman, D.J.; Cragg, G.M.; Snader, K.M. Natural products as sources of new drugs over the period 1981-2002. *J. Nat. Prod.,* **2003**, *66*(7), 1022-1037.
[http://dx.doi.org/10.1021/np030096l] [PMID: 12880330]

[2]    Gershenzon, J.; Dudareva, N. The function of terpene natural products in the natural world. *Nat. Chem. Biol.,* **2007**, *3*(7), 408-414.
[http://dx.doi.org/10.1038/nchembio.2007.5] [PMID: 17576428]

[3]    Sacchettini, J.C.; Poulter, C.D. Creating isoprenoid diversity. *Science,* **1997**, *277*(5333), 1788-1789.
[http://dx.doi.org/10.1126/science.277.5333.1788] [PMID: 9324768]

[4]    Peñuelas, J.; Munné-Bosch, S. Isoprenoids: an evolutionary pool for photoprotection. *Trends Plant Sci.,* **2005**, *10*(4), 166-169.
[http://dx.doi.org/10.1016/j.tplants.2005.02.005] [PMID: 15817417]

[5]    Withers, S.T.; Keasling, J.D. Biosynthesis and engineering of isoprenoid small molecules. *Appl. Microbiol. Biotechnol.,* **2007**, *73*(5), 980-990.
[http://dx.doi.org/10.1007/s00253-006-0593-1] [PMID: 17115212]

[6]    Eschenmoser, A.; Ruzicka, L.; Jeger, O. A stereochemical interpretation of the biogenetic isoprene rule of the triterpenes. *Helv. Chem. Ada,* **1955**, *38*, 1890-1904.

[http://dx.doi.org/10.1002/hlca.19550380728]

[7]     Ruzicka, L. Perspektiven der biogenese und der chemie der terpene. *Pure Appl. Chem.,* **1963**, *6*, 493-523.
[http://dx.doi.org/10.1351/pac196306040493]

[8]     Yang, W.; Chen, X.; Li, Y. Advances in Pharmacological Activities of Terpenoids. *Nat. Prod. Commun.,* **2020**, *15*(3), 1-13.
[http://dx.doi.org/10.1177/1934578X20903555]

[9]     Bujak, J.K.; Kosmala, D.; Szopa, I.M.; Majchrzak, K.; Bednarczyk, P. Inflammation, cancer and immunity-implication of TRPV1 channel. *Front. Oncol.,* **2019**, *9*, 1087.
[http://dx.doi.org/10.3389/fonc.2019.01087] [PMID: 31681615]

[10]    Feucht, C.L.; Patel, D.R. Analgesics and anti-inflammatory medications in sports: use and abuse. *Pediatr. Clin. North Am.,* **2010**, *57*(3), 751-774.
[http://dx.doi.org/10.1016/j.pcl.2010.02.004] [PMID: 20538155]

[11]    Prakash, V. Terpenoids as Cytotoxic Compounds: A Perspective. *Phcog. Rev,* **2018**, *12*, 166-176.
[http://dx.doi.org/10.4103/phrev.phrev_3_18]

[12]    Shin, S.A.; Moon, S.Y.; Kim, W.Y.; Paek, S.M.; Park, H.H.; Lee, C.S. Structure-Based Classification and Anti-Cancer Effects of Plant Metabolites. *Int. J. Mol. Sci.,* **2018**, *19*(9), 2651.
[http://dx.doi.org/10.3390/ijms19092651] [PMID: 30200668]

[13]    Chopra, B.; Dhingra, A.K.; Dhar, K.L.; Nepali, K. Emerging role of terpenoids for the treatment of cancer: A review. *Mini Rev. Med. Chem.,* **2021**, *21*(16), 2300-2336.
[http://dx.doi.org/10.2174/1389557521666210112143024] [PMID: 33438537]

[14]    Ansari, I.A.; Akhtar, M.S. Current Insights on the Role of Terpenoids as Anticancer Agents: A Perspective on Cancer Prevention and Treatment.*Natural Bio-active Compounds*; Swamy, M.; Akhtar, M., Eds.; Springer: Singapore, **2019**.
[http://dx.doi.org/10.1007/978-981-13-7205-6_3]

[15]    Croteau, R.; Johnsos, M.A. Biosynthesis of terpenoid wood extractives.*Biosynthesis and biodegradation of wood components*; Higuchi, T., Ed.; Academic Press: Orlando, FL, **1985**, pp. 379-439.
[http://dx.doi.org/10.1016/B978-0-12-347880-1.50019-2]

[16]    Brielmann, H.L.; Setzer, W.N.; Kaufmann, P.B. Phytochemicals: The chemical components of plants.*Natural Products from Plants,* 2nd ed; Cseke, L.J., Ed.; CRC Press: Boca Raton, FL, **2006**, pp. 1-50.

[17]    Loza-Tavera, H. Monoterpenes in essential oils. Biosynthesis and properties. *Adv. Exp. Med. Biol.,* **1999**, *464*, 49-62.
[http://dx.doi.org/10.1007/978-1-4615-4729-7_5] [PMID: 10335385]

[18]    Little, D.B.; Croteau, R. Biochemistry of essential oil plants: a thirty year overview. IN: Teranishi R, Wick EL, Hornstein I, Ed.; Flavor Chemistry: Thirty years of progress: Kulwer Academic Plenum. Flavor Chemistry: Thirty years of progress. Kulwer Academic Plenum, **1999**.

[19]    Murray, L.A.M.; McKinnie, S.M.K.; Moore, B.S.; George, J.H. Meroterpenoid natural products from Streptomyces bacteria - the evolution of chemoenzymatic syntheses. *Nat. Prod. Rep.,* **2020**, *37*(10), 1334-1366.
[http://dx.doi.org/10.1039/D0NP00018C] [PMID: 32602506]

[20]    Ninemets, U.; Hauff, K.; Bertin, N. Monoterpene emissions in relation to foliar photosynthetic and structural variables in Mediterranean evergreen *Quercus* species. *New Phytol.,* **2002**, *153*(2), 243-256.
[http://dx.doi.org/10.1046/j.0028-646X.2001.00323.x]

[21]    Sharkey, T.D.; Yeh, S. Isoprene emission from plants. *Annu. Rev. Plant Physiol. Plant Mol. Biol.,* **2001**, *52*, 407-436.
[http://dx.doi.org/10.1146/annurev.arplant.52.1.407] [PMID: 11337404]

[22]  Davis, E.M.; Croteau, R. Cyclization enzymes in the biosynthesis of monoterpenes, sesquiterpenes and diterpenes. *Biosynth. Arom. Polyket. Isopre. Alkal.,* **2000**, *20*, 53-95.
[http://dx.doi.org/10.1007/3-540-48146-X_2]

[23]  Crowell, P.L. Prevention and therapy of cancer by dietary monoterpenes. *J. Nutr.,* **1999**, *129*(3), 775S-778S.
[http://dx.doi.org/10.1093/jn/129.3.775S] [PMID: 10082788]

[24]  Wagner, K.H.; Elmadfa, I. Biological relevance of terpenoids. Overview focusing on mono-, di- and tetraterpenes. *Ann. Nutr. Metab.,* **2003**, *47*(3-4), 95-106.
[http://dx.doi.org/10.1159/000070030] [PMID: 12743459]

[25]  Erasto, P.; Alvaro, M.V. Limonene - A Review: Biosynthetic, Ecological and Pharmacological Relevance. *Nat. Prod. Commun.,* **2008**, *3*(7), 1193-1202.
[http://dx.doi.org/10.1177/1934578X0800300728]

[26]  Sun, J. D-Limonene: safety and clinical applications. *Altern. Med. Rev.,* **2007**, *12*(3), 259-264.
[PMID: 18072821]

[27]  Jia, S.S.; Xi, G.P.; Zhang, M.; Chen, Y.B.; Lei, B.; Dong, X.S.; Yang, Y.M. Induction of apoptosis by D-limonene is mediated by inactivation of Akt in LS174T human colon cancer cells. *Oncol. Rep.,* **2013**, *29*(1), 349-354.
[http://dx.doi.org/10.3892/or.2012.2093] [PMID: 23117412]

[28]  Ariazi, E.A.; Satomi, Y.; Ellis, M.J.; Haag, J.D.; Shi, W.; Sattler, C.A.; Gould, M.N. Activation of the transforming growth factor beta signaling pathway and induction of cytostasis and apoptosis in mammary carcinomas treated with the anticancer agent perillyl alcohol. *Cancer Res.,* **1999**, *59*(8), 1917-1928.
[PMID: 10213501]

[29]  Satomi, Y.; Miyamoto, S.; Gould, M.N. Induction of AP-1 activity by perillyl alcohol in breast cancer cells. *Carcinogenesis,* **1999**, *20*(10), 1957-1961.
[http://dx.doi.org/10.1093/carcin/20.10.1957] [PMID: 10506111]

[30]  Garcia, D.G.; Amorim, L.M.; de Castro Faria, M.V.; Freire, A.S.; Santelli, R.E.; Da Fonseca, C.O.; Quirico-Santos, T.; Burth, P. The anticancer drug perillyl alcohol is a Na/K-ATPase inhibitor. *Mol. Cell. Biochem.,* **2010**, *345*(1-2), 29-34.
[http://dx.doi.org/10.1007/s11010-010-0556-9] [PMID: 20689980]

[31]  Sundin, T.; Peffley, D.M.; Hentosh, P. Disruption of an hTERT-mTOR-RAPTOR protein complex by a phytochemical perillyl alcohol and rapamycin. *Mol. Cell. Biochem.,* **2013**, *375*(1-2), 97-104.
[http://dx.doi.org/10.1007/s11010-012-1532-3] [PMID: 23283642]

[32]  Kawata, S.; Nagase, T.; Yamasaki, E.; Ishiguro, H.; Matsuzawa, Y. Modulation of the mevalonate pathway and cell growth by pravastatin and d-limonene in a human hepatoma cell line (Hep G2). *Br. J. Cancer,* **1994**, *69*(6), 1015-1020.
[http://dx.doi.org/10.1038/bjc.1994.199] [PMID: 8198962]

[33]  Chen, T.C.; Fonseca, C.O.D.; Schönthal, A.H. Preclinical development and clinical use of perillyl alcohol for chemoprevention and cancer therapy. *Am. J. Cancer Res.,* **2015**, *5*(5), 1580-1593.
[PMID: 26175929]

[34]  Mukhtar, Y.M.; Adu-Frimpong, M.; Xu, X.; Yu, J. Biochemical significance of limonene and its metabolites: future prospects for designing and developing highly potent anticancer drugs. *Biosci. Rep.,* **2018**, *38*(6), BSR20181253.
[http://dx.doi.org/10.1042/BSR20181253] [PMID: 30287506]

[35]  Chen, T.; Levin, D.; Pupalli, S. Pharmaceutical compositions comprising POH derivatives. *US Patents 580372,* **2012**.

[36]  Eummer, J.T.; Gibbs, B.S.; Zahn, T.J.; Sebolt-Leopold, J.S.; Gibbs, R.A. Novel limonene phosphonate and farnesyl diphosphate analogues: design, synthesis, and evaluation as potential protein-farnesyl

transferase inhibitors. *Bioorg. Med. Chem.,* **1999**, *7*(2), 241-250.
[http://dx.doi.org/10.1016/S0968-0896(98)00202-8] [PMID: 10218815]

[37] Das, B.C.; Mahalingam, S.M.; Panda, L.; Wang, B.; Campbell, P.; Evans, T. Design and synthesis of potential new apoptosis agents: hybrid compounds containing perillyl alcohol and new constrained retinoids. *Tetrahedron Lett.,* **2010**, *51*(11), 1462-1466.
[http://dx.doi.org/10.1016/j.tetlet.2010.01.003] [PMID: 20379349]

[38] Xanthakis, E.; Magkouta, S.; Loutrari, H. Enzymatic synthesis of perillyl alcohol derivatives and investigation of their antiproliferative activity. *Biocatal. Biotransform.,* **2009**, *27*, 170-178.
[http://dx.doi.org/10.1080/10242420902811089]

[39] Nandurkar, N.S.; Zhang, J.; Ye, Q.; Ponomareva, L.V.; She, Q.B.; Thorson, J.S. The identification of perillyl alcohol glycosides with improved antiproliferative activity. *J. Med. Chem.,* **2014**, *57*(17), 7478-7484.
[http://dx.doi.org/10.1021/jm500870u] [PMID: 25121720]

[40] Hui, Z.; Zhang, M.; Cong, L.; Xia, M.; Dong, J. Synthesis and antiproliferative effects of amino-modified perillyl alcohol derivatives. *Molecules,* **2014**, *19*(5), 6671-6682.
[http://dx.doi.org/10.3390/molecules19056671] [PMID: 24858099]

[41] Andrade, L.N.; Amaral, R.G.; Dória, G.A.; Fonseca, C.S.; da Silva, T.K.; Albuquerque Júnior, R.L.; Thomazzi, S.M.; do Nascimento, L.G.; Carvalho, A.A.; de Sousa, D.P. *In vivo* anti-tumour activity and toxicological evaluations of perillaldehyde 8,9-epoxide, a derivative of perillyl alcohol. *Int. J. Mol. Sci.,* **2016**, *17*(1), 32-11.
[http://dx.doi.org/10.3390/ijms17010032] [PMID: 26742032]

[42] Andrade, L.N.; Lima, T.C.; Amaral, R.G.; Pessoa, Cdo.Ó.; Filho, M.O.; Soares, B.M.; Nascimento, L.G.; Carvalho, A.A.; de Sousa, D.P. Evaluation of the cytotoxicity of structurally correlated p-menthane derivatives. *Molecules,* **2015**, *20*(7), 13264-13280.
[http://dx.doi.org/10.3390/molecules200713264] [PMID: 26197313]

[43] Oturanel, C.E.; Kıran, İ.; Özşen, Ö.; Çiftçi, G.A.; Atlı, Ö. Cytotoxic AO. Cytotoxic, antiproliferative and apoptotic effects of perillyl alcohol and its biotransformation metabolite on A549 and HepG2 cancer cell lines. *Anticancer. Agents Med. Chem.,* **2017**, *17*(9), 1243-1250.
[http://dx.doi.org/10.2174/1871520617666170103093923] [PMID: 28044940]

[44] Simonsen, J.L.; Owen, L.N.; Barton, D.H.R. *The Terpenes*; University Press: Cambridge, **1947**.

[45] Kelloff, G.J.; Boone, C.W.; Crowell, J.A.; Steele, V.E.; Lubet, R.A.; Doody, L.A.; Malone, W.F.; Hawk, E.T.; Sigman, C.C. New agents for cancer chemoprevention. *J. Cell. Biochem. Suppl.,* **1996**, *26*, 1-28.
[http://dx.doi.org/10.1002/(SICI)1097-4644(1996)25+<1::AID-JCB1>3.0.CO;2-4] [PMID: 9154166]

[46] Chen, W.; Viljoen, A.M. Geraniol — A review of a commercially important fragrance material. *S. Afr. J. Bot.,* **2010**, *76*, 643-651.
[http://dx.doi.org/10.1016/j.sajb.2010.05.008]

[47] Maria, H. P. de L. Antimicrobial activity of geraniol: an integrative review. *J. Essent. Oil Res.,* **2020**, *2020*
[http://dx.doi.org/10.1080/10412905.2020.1745697]

[48] Pavan, B.; Dalpiaz, A.; Marani, L.; Beggiato, S.; Ferraro, L.; Canistro, D.; Paolini, M.; Vivarelli, F.; Valerii, M.C.; Comparone, A.; De Fazio, L.; Spisni, E. Geraniol Pharmacokinetics, Bioavailability and Its Multiple Effects on the Liver Antioxidant and Xenobiotic-Metabolizing Enzymes. *Front. Pharmacol.,* **2018**, *9*, 18.
[http://dx.doi.org/10.3389/fphar.2018.00018] [PMID: 29422862]

[49] Galle, M.; Crespo, R.; Kladniew, B.R.; Villegas, S.M.; Polo, M.; de Bravo, M.G. Suppression by geraniol of the growth of A549 human lung adenocarcinoma cells and inhibition of the mevalonate pathway in culture and *in vivo*: potential use in cancer chemotherapy. *Nutr. Cancer,* **2014**, *66*(5), 888-895.

[http://dx.doi.org/10.1080/01635581.2014.916320] [PMID: 24875281]

[50]   Carnesecchi, S.; Schneider, Y.; Ceraline, J.; Duranton, B.; Gosse, F.; Seiler, N.; Raul, F. Geraniol, a component of plant essential oils, inhibits growth and polyamine biosynthesis in human colon cancer cells. *J. Pharmacol. Exp. Ther.,* **2001**, *298*(1), 197-200.
[PMID: 11408542]

[51]   Kim, S.H.; Bae, H.C.; Park, E.J.; Lee, C.R.; Kim, B.J.; Lee, S.; Park, H.H.; Kim, S.J.; So, I.; Kim, T.W.; Jeon, J.H. Geraniol inhibits prostate cancer growth by targeting cell cycle and apoptosis pathways. *Biochem. Biophys. Res. Commun.,* **2011**, *407*(1), 129-134.
[http://dx.doi.org/10.1016/j.bbrc.2011.02.124] [PMID: 21371438]

[52]   Burke, Y.D.; Stark, M.J.; Roach, S.L.; Sen, S.E.; Crowell, P.L. Inhibition of pancreatic cancer growth by the dietary isoprenoids farnesol and geraniol. *Lipids,* **1997**, *32*(2), 151-156.
[http://dx.doi.org/10.1007/s11745-997-0019-y] [PMID: 9075204]

[53]   Ong, T.P.; Heidor, R.; de Conti, A.; Dagli, M.L.; Moreno, F.S. Farnesol and geraniol chemopreventive activities during the initial phases of hepatocarcinogenesis involve similar actions on cell proliferation and DNA damage, but distinct actions on apoptosis, plasma cholesterol and HMGCoA reductase. *Carcinogenesis,* **2006**, *27*(6), 1194-1203.
[http://dx.doi.org/10.1093/carcin/bgi291] [PMID: 16332721]

[54]   Lei, Y.; Fu, P.; Jun, X.; Cheng, P. Pharmacological Properties of Geraniol - A Review. *Planta Med.,* **2019**, *85*(1), 48-55.
[http://dx.doi.org/10.1055/a-0750-6907] [PMID: 30308694]

[55]   Polo, M.P.; de Bravo, M.G. Effect of geraniol on fatty-acid and mevalonate metabolism in the human hepatoma cell line Hep G2. *Biochem. Cell Biol.,* **2006**, *84*(1), 102-111.
[http://dx.doi.org/10.1139/o05-160] [PMID: 16462894]

[56]   Mączka, W.; Wińska, K.; Grabarczyk, M. One Hundred Faces of Geraniol. *Molecules,* **2020**, *25*(14), 3303.
[http://dx.doi.org/10.3390/molecules25143303] [PMID: 32708169]

[57]   Chaudhary, S.C.; Siddiqui, M.S.; Athar, M.; Alam, M.S. Geraniol inhibits murine skin tumorigenesis by modulating COX-2 expression, Ras-ERK1/2 signaling pathway and apoptosis. *J. Appl. Toxicol.,* **2013**, *33*(8), 828-837.
[http://dx.doi.org/10.1002/jat.2739] [PMID: 22760862]

[58]   Cho, M.; So, I.; Chun, J.N.; Jeon, J.H. The antitumor effects of geraniol: Modulation of cancer hallmark pathways (Review). *Int. J. Oncol.,* **2016**, *48*(5), 1772-1782. [review].
[http://dx.doi.org/10.3892/ijo.2016.3427] [PMID: 26983575]

[59]   Kim, S.H.; Park, E.J.; Lee, C.R.; Chun, J.N.; Cho, N.H.; Kim, I.G.; Lee, S.; Kim, T.W.; Park, H.H.; So, I.; Jeon, J.H. Geraniol induces cooperative interaction of apoptosis and autophagy to elicit cell death in PC-3 prostate cancer cells. *Int. J. Oncol.,* **2012**, *40*(5), 1683-1690.
[PMID: 22200837]

[60]   Naz, F.; Wu, Y.; Zhang, N.; Yang, Z.; Yu, C. Anticancer Attributes of Cantharidin: Involved Molecular Mechanisms and Pathways. *Molecules,* **2020**, *25*(14), 3279.
[http://dx.doi.org/10.3390/molecules25143279] [PMID: 32707651]

[61]   Chen, Y.N.; Chen, J.C.; Yin, S.C.; Wang, G.S.; Tsauer, W.; Hsu, S.F.; Hsu, S.L. Effector mechanisms of norcantharidin-induced mitotic arrest and apoptosis in human hepatoma cells. *Int. J. Cancer,* **2002**, *100*(2), 158-165.
[http://dx.doi.org/10.1002/ijc.10479] [PMID: 12115564]

[62]   Huan, S.K.; Lee, H.H.; Liu, D.Z.; Wu, C.C.; Wang, C.C. Cantharidin-induced cytotoxicity and cyclooxygenase 2 expression in human bladder carcinoma cell line. *Toxicology,* **2006**, *223*(1-2), 136-143.
[http://dx.doi.org/10.1016/j.tox.2006.03.012] [PMID: 16697099]

[63]   Huh, J.E.; Kang, K.S.; Chae, C.; Kim, H.M.; Ahn, K.S.; Kim, S.H. Roles of p38 and JNK mitogen-activated protein kinase pathways during cantharidin-induced apoptosis in U937 cells. *Biochem. Pharmacol.,* **2004**, *67*(10), 1811-1818.
[http://dx.doi.org/10.1016/j.bcp.2003.12.025] [PMID: 15130758]

[64]   Honkanen, R.E. Cantharidin, another natural toxin that inhibits the activity of serine/threonine protein phosphatases types 1 and 2A. *FEBS Lett.,* **1993**, *330*(3), 283-286.
[http://dx.doi.org/10.1016/0014-5793(93)80889-3] [PMID: 8397101]

[65]   Li, W.; Chen, Z.; Zong, Y.; Gong, F.; Zhu, Y.; Zhu, Y.; Lv, J.; Zhang, J.; Xie, L.; Sun, Y.; Miao, Y.; Tao, M.; Han, X.; Xu, Z. PP2A inhibitors induce apoptosis in pancreatic cancer cell line PANC-1 through persistent phosphorylation of IKKα and sustained activation of the NF-κB pathway. *Cancer Lett.,* **2011**, *304*(2), 117-127.
[http://dx.doi.org/10.1016/j.canlet.2011.02.009] [PMID: 21376459]

[66]   Deng, L.P.; Dong, J.; Cai, H.; Wang, W. Cantharidin as an antitumor agent: a retrospective review. *Curr. Med. Chem.,* **2013**, *20*(2), 159-166.
[http://dx.doi.org/10.2174/092986713804806711] [PMID: 23210849]

[67]   Wang, G.; Dong, J.; Deng, L. Overview of Cantharidin and its Analogues. *Curr. Med. Chem.,* **2018**, *25*(17), 2034-2044.
[http://dx.doi.org/10.2174/0929867324666170414165253] [PMID: 28413963]

[68]   Li, F.; Jiang, T.; Li, Q.; Ling, X. Camptothecin (CPT) and its derivatives are known to target topoisomerase I (Top1) as their mechanism of action: did we miss something in CPT analogue molecular targets for treating human disease such as cancer? *Am. J. Cancer Res.,* **2017**, *7*(12), 2350-2394.
[PMID: 29312794]

[69]   Kacprzak, K.M. Chemistry and Biology of Camptothecin and its Derivatives.*Natural Products*; Ramawat, K.; Mérillon, J.M., Eds.; Springer: Berlin, Heidelberg, **2013**, pp. 643-682.
[http://dx.doi.org/10.1007/978-3-642-22144-6_26]

[70]   Basili, S.; Moro, S. Novel camptothecin derivatives as topoisomerase I inhibitors. *Expert Opin. Ther. Pat.,* **2009**, *19*(5), 555-574.
[http://dx.doi.org/10.1517/13543770902773437] [PMID: 19441934]

[71]   Kozioł, A.; Stryjewska, A.; Librowski, T.; Sałat, K.; Gaweł, M.; Moniczewski, A.; Lochyński, S. An overview of the pharmacological properties and potential applications of natural monoterpenes. *Mini Rev. Med. Chem.,* **2014**, *14*(14), 1156-1168.
[http://dx.doi.org/10.2174/1389557514666141127145820] [PMID: 25429661]

[72]   Erasto, P.; Viljoen, A.M. Limonene - A Review: Biosynthetic, Ecological and Pharmacological Relevance. *Nat. Prod. Commun.,* **2008**, *3*(7), 1193-1202.
[http://dx.doi.org/10.1177/1934578X0800300728]

[73]   Oliveira, Fde.A.; Andrade, L.N.; de Sousa, É.B.V.; de Sousa, D.P. Anti-ulcer activity of essential oil constituents. *Molecules,* **2014**, *19*(5), 5717-5747.
[http://dx.doi.org/10.3390/molecules19055717] [PMID: 24802985]

[74]   a) Schäfer, B. Menthol: Minze *versus* Tagasako-Prozess. *Chem. Unserer Zeit,* **2013**, *47*, 174-182.
[http://dx.doi.org/10.1002/ciuz.201300599] b) Kamatou, G.P.P.; Vermaak, I.; Viljoen, A.M.; Lawrence, B.M. Menthol: a simple monoterpene with remarkable biological properties. *Phytochemistry,* **2013**, *96*, 15-25.
[http://dx.doi.org/10.1016/j.phytochem.2013.08.005] [PMID: 24054028] c) Sachan, A.K.; Das, D.R.; Shuaib, M.D. An overview on Menthaepiperitae (peppermint oil). *Int. J. Pharm. Chem. Biol. Sci.,* **2013**, *3*, 834-838.

[75]   a) Cameron, G.C; Stuart, E Eucalyptol. *Perf. Flav.,* **2000**, *25*, 6-16.b) Worth, H.; Schacher, C.; Dethlefsen, U. Concomitant therapy with Cineole (Eucalyptole) reduces exacerbations in COPD: a placebo-controlled double-blind trial. *Respir. Res.,* **2009**, *10*, 69.

[http://dx.doi.org/10.1186/1465-9921-10-69] [PMID: 19624838]

[76]    Whitman, D.W.; Andrés, M.F.; Martínez-Díaz, R.A.; Ibáñez-Escribano, A.; Olmeda, A.S.; González-Coloma, A. Antiparasitic Properties of Cantharidin and the Blister Beetle *Berberomeloe majalis* (Coleoptera: Meloidae). *Toxins (Basel),* **2019,** *11*(4), 234.
[http://dx.doi.org/10.3390/toxins11040234] [PMID: 31013660]

[77]    Naz, F.; Wu, Y.; Zhang, N.; Yang, Z.; Yu, C. Anticancer Attributes of Cantharidin: Involved Molecular Mechanisms and Pathways. *Molecules,* **2020,** *25*(14), 3279.
[http://dx.doi.org/10.3390/molecules25143279] [PMID: 32707651]

[78]    Zielińska-Błajet, M.; Feder-Kubis, J. Monoterpenes and Their Derivatives-Recent Development in Biological and Medical Applications. *Int. J. Mol. Sci.,* **2020,** *21*(19), 707.
[http://dx.doi.org/10.3390/ijms21197078] [PMID: 32992914]

[79]    Sharma, A.; Bajpai, V.K.; Shukla, S. *Sequiterpenes and cytotoxicity. Ramawat KG, Me'rillon JM*; Products, N.; Heidelberg, S-V.B., Eds.; , **2013.**

[80]    Petrovic, S.; Maksimovic, Z.; Kundakovic, T. *Prirucnik za teorijskuiprakti cnunastavui zpredmeta Farmakognozija*; Faculty of Pharmacy, University of Belgrade, **2009.**

[81]    Gordi, T.; Lepist, E.I. Artemisinin derivatives: toxic for laboratory animals, safe for humans? *Toxicol. Lett.,* **2004,** *147*(2), 99-107.
[http://dx.doi.org/10.1016/j.toxlet.2003.12.009] [PMID: 14757313]

[82]    Dondorp, A.M.; Nosten, F.; Yi, P.; Das, D.; Phyo, A.P.; Tarning, J.; Lwin, K.M.; Ariey, F.; Hanpithakpong, W.; Lee, S.J.; Ringwald, P.; Silamut, K.; Imwong, M.; Chotivanich, K.; Lim, P.; Herdman, T.; An, S.S.; Yeung, S.; Singhasivanon, P.; Day, N.P.; Lindegardh, N.; Socheat, D.; White, N.J. Artemisinin resistance in *Plasmodium falciparum* malaria. *N. Engl. J. Med.,* **2009,** *361*(5), 455-467.
[http://dx.doi.org/10.1056/NEJMoa0808859] [PMID: 19641202]

[83]    Meshnick, S.R. Artemisinin antimalarials: mechanisms of action and resistance. *Med. Trop. (Mars.),* **1998,** *58*(3) Suppl., 13-17.
[PMID: 10212891]

[84]    Burrows, J.N.; Chibale, K.; Wells, T.N. The state of the art in anti-malarial drug discovery and development. *Curr. Top. Med. Chem.,* **2011,** *11*(10), 1226-1254.
[http://dx.doi.org/10.2174/156802611795429194] [PMID: 21401508]

[85]    Liu, R.; Dong, H.F.; Jiang, M.S. Artemisinin: the gifts from traditional Chinese medicine not only for malaria control but also for schistosomiasis control. *Parasitol. Res.,* **2012,** *110*(5), 2071-2074.
[http://dx.doi.org/10.1007/s00436-011-2707-7] [PMID: 22033738]

[86]    Kumar, S.; Singh, R.K.; Patial, B.; Goyal, S.; Bhardwaj, T.R. Recent advances in novel heterocyclic scaffolds for the treatment of drug-resistant malaria. *J. Enzyme Inhib. Med. Chem.,* **2016,** *31*(2), 173-186.
[http://dx.doi.org/10.3109/14756366.2015.1016513] [PMID: 25775094]

[87]    Firestone, G.L.; Sundar, S.N. Anticancer activities of artemisinin and its bioactive derivatives. *Expert Rev. Mol. Med.,* **2009,** *11*, e32.
[http://dx.doi.org/10.1017/S1462399409001239] [PMID: 19883518]

[88]    Jiao, Y.; Ge, C.M.; Meng, Q.H.; Cao, J.P.; Tong, J.; Fan, S.J. Dihydroartemisinin is an inhibitor of ovarian cancer cell growth. *Acta Pharmacol. Sin.,* **2007,** *28*(7), 1045-1056.
[http://dx.doi.org/10.1111/j.1745-7254.2007.00612.x] [PMID: 17588342]

[89]    Chen, H.; Sun, B.; Pan, S.; Jiang, H.; Sun, X. Dihydroartemisinin inhibits growth of pancreatic cancer cells *in vitro* and *in vivo. Anticancer Drugs,* **2009,** *20*(2), 131-140.
[http://dx.doi.org/10.1097/CAD.0b013e3283212ade] [PMID: 19209030]

[90]    Li, S.; Xue, F.; Cheng, Z.; Yang, X.; Wang, S.; Geng, F.; Pan, L. Effect of artesunate on inhibiting proliferation and inducing apoptosis of SP2/0 myeloma cells through affecting NFkappaB p65. *Int. J.*

*Hematol.,* **2009**, *90*(4), 513-521.
[http://dx.doi.org/10.1007/s12185-009-0409-z] [PMID: 19728025]

[91]   Efferth, T.; Dunstan, H.; Sauerbrey, A.; Miyachi, H.; Chitambar, C.R. The anti-malarial artesunate is also active against cancer. *Int. J. Oncol.,* **2001**, *18*(4), 767-773.
[http://dx.doi.org/10.3892/ijo.18.4.767] [PMID: 11251172]

[92]   Chaturvedi, D.; Goswami, A.; Saikia, P.P.; Barua, N.C.; Rao, P.G. Artemisinin and its derivatives: a novel class of anti-malarial and anti-cancer agents. *Chem. Soc. Rev.,* **2010**, *39*(2), 435-454.
[http://dx.doi.org/10.1039/B816679J] [PMID: 20111769]

[93]   Rasheed, S.A.; Efferth, T.; Asangani, I.A.; Allgayer, H. First evidence that the antimalarial drug artesunate inhibits invasion and *in vivo* metastasis in lung cancer by targeting essential extracellular proteases. *Int. J. Cancer,* **2010**, *127*(6), 1475-1485.
[http://dx.doi.org/10.1002/ijc.25315] [PMID: 20232396]

[94]   Hwang, Y.P.; Yun, H.J.; Kim, H.G.; Han, E.H.; Lee, G.W.; Jeong, H.G. Suppression of PMA-induced tumor cell invasion by dihydroartemisinin *via* inhibition of PKCalpha/Raf/MAPKs and NF-kappaB/AP-1-dependent mechanisms. *Biochem. Pharmacol.,* **2010**, *79*(12), 1714-1726.
[http://dx.doi.org/10.1016/j.bcp.2010.02.003] [PMID: 20152819]

[95]   Chen, H.H.; Zhou, H.J.; Wang, W.Q.; Wu, G.D. Antimalarial dihydroartemisinin also inhibits angiogenesis. *Cancer Chemother. Pharmacol.,* **2004**, *53*(5), 423-432.
[http://dx.doi.org/10.1007/s00280-003-0751-4] [PMID: 15132130]

[96]   Buommino, E.; Baroni, A.; Canozo, N.; Petrazzuolo, M.; Nicoletti, R.; Vozza, A.; Tufano, M.A. Artemisinin reduces human melanoma cell migration by down-regulating alpha V beta 3 integrin and reducing metalloproteinase 2 production. *Invest. New Drugs,* **2009**, *27*(5), 412-418.
[http://dx.doi.org/10.1007/s10637-008-9188-2] [PMID: 18956140]

[97]   Lai, H.C.; Singh, N.P.; Sasaki, T. Development of artemisinin compounds for cancer treatment. *Invest. New Drugs,* **2013**, *31*(1), 230-246.
[http://dx.doi.org/10.1007/s10637-012-9873-z] [PMID: 22935909]

[98]   Chu, X.M.; Wang, C.; Liu, W.; Liang, L.L.; Gong, K.K.; Zhao, C.Y.; Sun, K.L. Quinoline and quinolone dimers and their biological activities: An overview. *Eur. J. Med. Chem.,* **2019**, *161*, 101-117.
[http://dx.doi.org/10.1016/j.ejmech.2018.10.035] [PMID: 30343191]

[99]   Ren, Q.C.; Gao, C.; Xu, Z.; Feng, L.S.; Liu, M.L.; Wu, X.; Zhao, F. Bis-coumarin Derivatives and Their Biological Activities. *Curr. Top. Med. Chem.,* **2018**, *18*(2), 101-113.
[http://dx.doi.org/10.2174/1568026618666180221114515] [PMID: 29473509]

[100]  Fröhlich, T.; Çapcı Karagöz, A.; Reiter, C.; Tsogoeva, S.B. Artemisinin-Derived Dimers: Potent Antimalarial and Anticancer Agents. *J. Med. Chem.,* **2016**, *59*(16), 7360-7388.
[http://dx.doi.org/10.1021/acs.jmedchem.5b01380] [PMID: 27010926]

[101]  Hou, J.; Wang, D.; Zhang, R.; Wang, H. Experimental therapy of hepatoma with artemisinin and its derivatives: *in vitro* and *in vivo* activity, chemosensitization, and mechanisms of action. *Clin. Cancer Res.,* **2008**, *14*(17), 5519-5530.
[http://dx.doi.org/10.1158/1078-0432.CCR-08-0197] [PMID: 18765544]

[102]  Willoughby, J.A., Sr; Sundar, S.N.; Cheung, M.; Tin, A.S.; Modiano, J.; Firestone, G.L. Artemisinin blocks prostate cancer growth and cell cycle progression by disrupting Sp1 interactions with the cyclin-dependent kinase-4 (CDK4) promoter and inhibiting CDK4 gene expression. *J. Biol. Chem.,* **2009**, *284*(4), 2203-2213.
[http://dx.doi.org/10.1074/jbc.M804491200] [PMID: 19017637]

[103]  Chen, H.; Sun, B.; Wang, S.; Pan, S.; Gao, Y.; Bai, X.; Xue, D. Growth inhibitory effects of dihydroartemisinin on pancreatic cancer cells: involvement of cell cycle arrest and inactivation of nuclear factor-kappaB. *J. Cancer Res. Clin. Oncol.,* **2010**, *136*(6), 897-903.
[http://dx.doi.org/10.1007/s00432-009-0731-0] [PMID: 19941148]

[104]  Lu, J.J.; Meng, L.H.; Cai, Y.J.; Chen, Q.; Tong, L.J.; Lin, L.P.; Ding, J. Dihydroartemisinin induces apoptosis in HL-60 leukemia cells dependent of iron and p38 mitogen-activated protein kinase activation but independent of reactive oxygen species. *Cancer Biol. Ther.,* **2008**, *7*(7), 1017-1023.
[http://dx.doi.org/10.4161/cbt.7.7.6035] [PMID: 18414062]

[105]  Wang, S.J.; Gao, Y.; Chen, H.; Kong, R.; Jiang, H.C.; Pan, S.H.; Xue, D.B.; Bai, X.W.; Sun, B. Dihydroartemisinin inactivates NF-kappaB and potentiates the anti-tumor effect of gemcitabine on pancreatic cancer both *in vitro* and *in vivo*. *Cancer Lett.,* **2010**, *293*(1), 99-108.
[http://dx.doi.org/10.1016/j.canlet.2010.01.001] [PMID: 20137856]

[106]  Michaelis, M.; Kleinschmidt, M.C.; Barth, S.; Rothweiler, F.; Geiler, J.; Breitling, R.; Mayer, B.; Deubzer, H.; Witt, O.; Kreuter, J.; Doerr, H.W.; Cinatl, J.; Cinatl, J., Jr Anti-cancer effects of artesunate in a panel of chemoresistant neuroblastoma cell lines. *Biochem. Pharmacol.,* **2010**, *79*(2), 130-136.
[http://dx.doi.org/10.1016/j.bcp.2009.08.013] [PMID: 19698702]

[107]  Chen, T.; Li, M.; Zhang, R.; Wang, H. Dihydroartemisinin induces apoptosis and sensitizes human ovarian cancer cells to carboplatin therapy. *J. Cell. Mol. Med.,* **2009**, *13*(7), 1358-1370.
[http://dx.doi.org/10.1111/j.1582-4934.2008.00360.x] [PMID: 18466355]

[108]  Mu, D.; Zhang, W.; Chu, D.; Liu, T.; Xie, Y.; Fu, E.; Jin, F. The role of calcium, P38 MAPK in dihydroartemisinin-induced apoptosis of lung cancer PC-14 cells. *Cancer Chemother. Pharmacol.,* **2008**, *61*(4), 639-645.
[http://dx.doi.org/10.1007/s00280-007-0517-5] [PMID: 17609948]

[109]  Handrick, R.; Ontikatze, T.; Bauer, K.D.; Freier, F.; Rübel, A.; Dürig, J.; Belka, C.; Jendrossek, V. Dihydroartemisinin induces apoptosis by a Bak-dependent intrinsic pathway. *Mol. Cancer Ther.,* **2010**, *9*(9), 2497-2510.
[http://dx.doi.org/10.1158/1535-7163.MCT-10-0051] [PMID: 20663933]

[110]  Hsu, Y.L.; Wu, L.Y.; Kuo, P.L. Dehydrocostuslactone, a medicinal plant-derived sesquiterpene lactone, induces apoptosis coupled to endoplasmic reticulum stress in liver cancer cells. *J. Pharmacol. Exp. Ther.,* **2009**, *329*(2), 808-819.
[http://dx.doi.org/10.1124/jpet.108.148395] [PMID: 19188481]

[111]  Li, Q.; Wang, Z.; Xie, Y.; Hu, H. Antitumor activity and mechanism of costunolide and dehydrocostus lactone: Two natural sesquiterpene lactones from the Asteraceae family. *Biomed. Pharmacother.,* **2020**, *125*, 109955.
[http://dx.doi.org/10.1016/j.biopha.2020.109955] [PMID: 32014691]

[112]  Kamatou, G.P.P.; Viljoen, A.M.A. Review of the Application and Pharmacological Properties of α-Bisabolol and α-Bisabolol-Rich Oils. *J. Am. Oil Chem. Soc.,* **2010**, *87*, 1-7.
[http://dx.doi.org/10.1007/s11746-009-1483-3]

[113]  Chen, W.; Hou, J.; Yin, Y.; Jang, J.; Zheng, Z.; Fan, H.; Zou, G. alpha-Bisabolol induces dose- and time-dependent apoptosis in HepG2 cells *via* a Fas- and mitochondrial-related pathway, involves p53 and NFkappaB. *Biochem. Pharmacol.,* **2010**, *80*(2), 247-254.
[http://dx.doi.org/10.1016/j.bcp.2010.03.021] [PMID: 20346922]

[114]  Seki, T.; Kokuryo, T.; Yokoyama, Y.; Suzuki, H.; Itatsu, K.; Nakagawa, A.; Mizutani, T.; Miyake, T.; Uno, M.; Yamauchi, K.; Nagino, M. Antitumor effects of α-bisabolol against pancreatic cancer. *Cancer Sci.,* **2011**, *102*(12), 2199-2205.
[http://dx.doi.org/10.1111/j.1349-7006.2011.02082.x] [PMID: 21883695]

[115]  Zhong, Z.; Dang, Y.; Yuan, X.; Guo, W.; Li, Y.; Tan, W.; Cui, J.; Lu, J.; Zhang, Q.; Chen, X.; Wang, Y. Furanodiene, a natural product, inhibits breast cancer growth both *in vitro* and *in vivo*. *Cell. Physiol. Biochem.,* **2012**, *30*(3), 778-790.
[http://dx.doi.org/10.1159/000341457] [PMID: 22854281]

[116]  Xiao, Y.; Yang, F.Q.; Li, S.P.; Gao, J.L.; Hu, G.; Lao, S.C.; Conceição, E.L.; Fung, K.P.; Wangl, Y.T.; Lee, S.M. Furanodiene induces G2/M cell cycle arrest and apoptosis through MAPK signaling and

mitochondria-caspase pathway in human hepatocellular carcinoma cells. *Cancer Biol. Ther.,* **2007**, *6*(7), 1044-1050.
[http://dx.doi.org/10.4161/cbt.6.7.4317] [PMID: 17611410]

[117] Miao, R.; Wei, J.; Zhang, Q.; Sajja, V.; Yang, J.; Wang, Q. Redifferentiation of human hepatoma cells (SMMC-7721) induced by two new highly oxygenated bisabolane-type sesquiterpenes. *J. Biosci.,* **2008**, *33*(5), 723-730.
[http://dx.doi.org/10.1007/s12038-008-0092-x] [PMID: 19179760]

[118] Rasul, A.; Bao, R.; Malhi, M.; Zhao, B.; Tsuji, I.; Li, J.; Li, X. Induction of apoptosis by costunolide in bladder cancer cells is mediated through ROS generation and mitochondrial dysfunction. *Molecules,* **2013**, *18*(2), 1418-1433.
[http://dx.doi.org/10.3390/molecules18021418] [PMID: 23348995]

[119] Yang, Y.I.; Kim, J.H.; Lee, K.T.; Choi, J.H. Costunolide induces apoptosis in platinum-resistant human ovarian cancer cells by generating reactive oxygen species. *Gynecol. Oncol.,* **2011**, *123*(3), 588-596.
[http://dx.doi.org/10.1016/j.ygyno.2011.08.031] [PMID: 21945308]

[120] Hsu, J.L.; Pan, S.L.; Ho, Y.F.; Hwang, T.L.; Kung, F.L.; Guh, J.H. Costunolide induces apoptosis through nuclear calcium2+ overload and DNA damage response in human prostate cancer. *J. Urol.,* **2011**, *185*(5), 1967-1974.
[http://dx.doi.org/10.1016/j.juro.2010.12.091] [PMID: 21421237]

[121] Zhang, J.H.; Liu, W.J.; Luo, H.M. The research of progress of the medicinal plant terpenoids. *World Sci. Tech. Mod. Trad. Chinese Med. Materia Med.,* **2018**, *20*(3), 419-430.

[122] Chen, T.C.; Fonseca, C.O.D.; Schönthal, A.H. Preclinical development and clinical use of perillyl alcohol for chemoprevention and cancer therapy. *Am. J. Cancer Res.,* **2015**, *5*(5), 1580-1593.
[PMID: 26175929]

[123] Sakinah, S.A.; Handayani, S.T.; Hawariah, L.P. Zerumbone induced apoptosis in liver cancer cells *via* modulation of Bax/Bcl-2 ratio. *Cancer Cell Int.,* **2007**, *7*, 4.
[http://dx.doi.org/10.1186/1475-2867-7-4] [PMID: 17407577]

[124] Nwankwo, J.O. Anticancer Potentials of Phytochemicals from Some Indigenous Food and Medicinal Plants of West Africa. *Adv. Cancer Prev.,* **2018**, *3*(1), 124.
[http://dx.doi.org/10.4172/2472-0429.1000124]

[125] Lanzotti, V. Diterpenes for therapeutic use. *Nat. Prod,* **2013**, 3173-3191.

[126] Perveen, S. Introductory Chapter: Terpenes and Terpenoids. In: *Terpenes and Terpenoids - Recent Advances*; Perveen, S.; Al-Taweel, A. M., Eds.; IntechOpen: London, **2021**. https://www.inte chopen.com/chapters/77011
[http://dx.doi.org/10.5772/intechopen.98261]

[127] Drummond, G.J.; Grant, P.S.; Brimble, M.A. ent-Atisane diterpenoids: isolation, structure and bioactivity. *Nat. Prod. Rep.,* **2020**.
[http://dx.doi.org/10.1039/D0NP00039F] [PMID: 32716458]

[128] Roy, P.K.; Maarisit, W.; Roy, M.C.; Taira, J.; Ueda, K. Five new diterpenoids from an Okinawan soft coral, Cespitularia sp. *Mar. Drugs,* **2012**, *10*(12), 2741-2748.
[http://dx.doi.org/10.3390/md10122741] [PMID: 23201595]

[129] Ma, G.X.; Xu, X.D.; Cao, L.; Yuan, J.Q.; Yang, J.S.; Ma, L.Y. Cassane-type diterpenes from the seeds of Caesalpinia minax with their antineoplastic activity. *Planta Med.,* **2012**, *78*(12), 1363-1369.
[http://dx.doi.org/10.1055/s-0032-1314976] [PMID: 22753035]

[130] Wang, S.J.; Li, Y.X.; Bao, L.; Han, J.J.; Yang, X.L.; Li, H.R.; Wang, Y.Q.; Li, S.J.; Liu, H.W. Eryngiolide A, a cytotoxic macrocyclic diterpenoid with an unusual cyclododecane core skeleton produced by the edible mushroom Pleurotus eryngii. *Org. Lett.,* **2012**, *14*(14), 3672-3675.
[http://dx.doi.org/10.1021/ol301519m] [PMID: 22769974]

[131]  Xu, Y.; Lang, J.H.; Jiao, W.H.; Wang, R.P.; Peng, Y.; Song, S.J.; Zhang, B.H.; Lin, H.W. Formamido-diterpenes from the South China Sea sponge Acanthella cavernosa. *Mar. Drugs,* **2012,** *10*(7), 1445-1458.
[http://dx.doi.org/10.3390/md10071445] [PMID: 22851918]

[132]  Ma, G.X.; Xu, N.; Yuan, J.Q.; Wei, H.; Zheng, Q.X.; Sun, Z.C.; Yang, J.S.; Xu, X.D. Two new diterpenes, neocaesalpin MR and minaxin C, from Caesalpinia minax. *J. Asian Nat. Prod. Res.,* **2012,** *14*(12), 1156-1161.
[http://dx.doi.org/10.1080/10286020.2012.734504] [PMID: 23134417]

[133]  Nguyen, H.X.; Nguyen, M.T.T.; Nguyen, T.A.; Nguyen, N.Y.T.; Phan, D.A.T.; Thi, P.H.; Nguyen, T.H.P.; Dang, P.H.; Nguyen, N.T.; Ueda, J.Y.; Awale, S. Cleistanthane diterpenes from the seed of Caesalpinia sappan and their antiausterity activity against PANC-1 human pancreatic cancer cell line. *Fitoterapia,* **2013,** *91*, 148-153.
[http://dx.doi.org/10.1016/j.fitote.2013.08.018] [PMID: 24001712]

[134]  Abou-El-Wafa, G.S.; Shaaban, M.; Shaaban, K.A.; El-Naggar, M.E.; Maier, A.; Fiebig, H.H.; Laatsch, H. Pachydictyols B and C: new diterpenes from Dictyota dichotoma Hudson. *Mar. Drugs,* **2013,** *11*(9), 3109-3123.
[http://dx.doi.org/10.3390/md11093109] [PMID: 23975221]

[135]  Zheng, C.J.; Zhu, J.Y.; Yu, W.; Ma, X.Q.; Rahman, K.; Qin, L.P. Labdane-type diterpenoids from the fruits of Vitex trifolia. *J. Nat. Prod.,* **2013,** *76*(2), 287-291.
[http://dx.doi.org/10.1021/np300679x] [PMID: 23327905]

[136]  Tsai, T.C.; Wu, Y.J.; Su, J.H.; Lin, W.T.; Lin, Y.S. A new spatane diterpenoid from the cultured soft coral Sinularia leptoclados. *Mar. Drugs,* **2013,** *11*(1), 114-123.
[http://dx.doi.org/10.3390/md11010114] [PMID: 23306171]

[137]  Han, Y.; Di, X.X.; Li, H.Z.; Shen, T.; Ren, D.M.; Lou, H.X.; Wang, X.N. Podoimbricatin A, a cytotoxic diterpenoid with an unprecedented 6/6/5/6-fused tetracyclic ring system from the twigs and leaves of Podocarpus imbricatus. *Bioorg. Med. Chem. Lett.,* **2014,** *24*(15), 3326-3328.
[http://dx.doi.org/10.1016/j.bmcl.2014.05.100] [PMID: 24953598]

[138]  Al-Lihaibi, S.S.; Alarif, W.M.; Abdel-Lateff, A.; Ayyad, S.E.; Abdel-Naim, A.B.; El-Senduny, F.F.; Badria, F.A. Three new cembranoid-type diterpenes from Red Sea soft coral Sarcophyton glaucum: isolation and antiproliferative activity against HepG2 cells. *Eur. J. Med. Chem.,* **2014,** *81*, 314-322.
[http://dx.doi.org/10.1016/j.ejmech.2014.05.016] [PMID: 24852278]

[139]  Zhang, X.; Tan, Y.; Li, Y.; Jin, L.; Wei, N.; Wu, H.; Ma, G.; Zheng, Q.; Tian, Y.; Yang, J.; Zhang, J.; Xu, X. Aphanamixins A-F, acyclic diterpenoids from the stem bark of Aphanamixis polystachya. *Chem. Pharm. Bull. (Tokyo),* **2014,** *62*(5), 494-498.
[http://dx.doi.org/10.1248/cpb.c14-00056] [PMID: 24789934]

[140]  Lin, C.Z.; Zhao, Z.X.; Xie, S.M.; Mao, J.H.; Zhu, C.C.; Li, X.H.; Zeren-dawa, B.; Suolang-qimei, K.; Zhu, D.; Xiong, T.Q.; Wu, A.Z. Diterpenoid alkaloids and flavonoids from Delphinium trichophorum. *Phytochemistry,* **2014,** *97*, 88-95.
[http://dx.doi.org/10.1016/j.phytochem.2013.10.011] [PMID: 24256579]

[141]  Li, W.F.; Wang, J.; Zhang, J.J.; Song, X.; Ku, C.F.; Zou, J.; Li, J.X.; Rong, L.J.; Pan, L.T.; Zhang, H.J. Henrin A: a new anti-HIV ent-kaurane diterpene from Pteris henryi. *Int. J. Mol. Sci.,* **2015,** *16*(11), 27978-27987.
[http://dx.doi.org/10.3390/ijms161126071] [PMID: 26610490]

[142]  Nguyen, H.X.; Nguyen, N.T.; Dang, P.H.; Thi Ho, P.; Nguyen, M.T.T.; Van Can, M.; Dibwe, D.F.; Ueda, J.Y.; Awale, S. Cassane diterpenes from the seed kernels of Caesalpinia sappan. *Phytochemistry,* **2016,** *122*, 286-293.
[http://dx.doi.org/10.1016/j.phytochem.2015.12.018] [PMID: 26769396]

[143]  Kang, N.; Cao, S.J.; Zhou, Y.; He, H.; Tashiro, S.; Onodera, S.; Qiu, F.; Ikejima, T. Inhibition of caspase-9 by oridonin, a diterpenoid isolated from Rabdosia rubescens, augments apoptosis in human

laryngeal cancer cells. *Int. J. Oncol.,* **2015**, *47*(6), 2045-2056.
[http://dx.doi.org/10.3892/ijo.2015.3186] [PMID: 26648189]

[144]   Gu, Z.; Wang, X.; Qi, R.; Wei, L.; Huo, Y.; Ma, Y.; Shi, L.; Chang, Y.; Li, G.; Zhou, L. Oridonin induces apoptosis in uveal melanoma cells by upregulation of Bim and downregulation of Fatty Acid Synthase. *Biochem. Biophys. Res. Commun.,* **2015**, *457*(2), 187-193.
[http://dx.doi.org/10.1016/j.bbrc.2014.12.086] [PMID: 25545058]

[145]   Xu, B.; Shen, W.; Liu, X.; Zhang, T.; Ren, J.; Fan, Y.; Xu, J. Oridonin inhibits BxPC-3 cell growth through cell apoptosis. *Acta Biochim. Biophys. Sin. (Shanghai),* **2015**, *47*(3), 164-173.
[http://dx.doi.org/10.1093/abbs/gmu134] [PMID: 25651847]

[146]   Chang, F.R.; Huang, S.T.; Liaw, C.C.; Yen, M.H.; Hwang, T.L.; Chen, C.Y.; Hou, M.F.; Yuan, S.S.; Cheng, Y.B.; Wu, Y.C. Diterpenes from Grangea maderaspatana. *Phytochemistry,* **2016**, *131*, 124-129.
[http://dx.doi.org/10.1016/j.phytochem.2016.08.009] [PMID: 27567453]

[147]   Chen, W.; Su, H.; Feng, L.; Zheng, X. Andrographolide suppresses preadipocytes proliferation through glutathione antioxidant systems abrogation. *Life Sci.,* **2016**, *156*, 21-29.
[http://dx.doi.org/10.1016/j.lfs.2016.05.030] [PMID: 27221023]

[148]   Li, L.; Yue, G.G.; Lau, C.B.; Sun, H.; Fung, K.P.; Leung, P.C.; Han, Q.; Leung, P.S. Eriocalyxin B induces apoptosis and cell cycle arrest in pancreatic adenocarcinoma cells through caspase- and p53-dependent pathways. *Toxicol. Appl. Pharmacol.,* **2012**, *262*(1), 80-90.
[http://dx.doi.org/10.1016/j.taap.2012.04.021] [PMID: 22561874]

[149]   Munagala, R.; Aqil, F.; Jeyabalan, J.; Gupta, R.C. Tanshinone IIA inhibits viral oncogene expression leading to apoptosis and inhibition of cervical cancer. *Cancer Lett.,* **2015**, *356*(2 Pt B), 536-546.
[http://dx.doi.org/10.1016/j.canlet.2014.09.037] [PMID: 25304375]

[150]   Oliveira, A.; Beyer, G.; Chugh, R.; Skube, S.J.; Majumder, K.; Banerjee, S.; Sangwan, V.; Li, L.; Dawra, R.; Subramanian, S.; Saluja, A.; Dudeja, V. Triptolide abrogates growth of colon cancer and induces cell cycle arrest by inhibiting transcriptional activation of E2F. *Lab. Invest.,* **2015**, *95*(6), 648-659.
[http://dx.doi.org/10.1038/labinvest.2015.46] [PMID: 25893635]

[151]   Wang, L.; He, H.S.; Yu, H.L.; Zeng, Y.; Han, H.; He, N.; Liu, Z.G.; Wang, Z.Y.; Xu, S.J.; Xiong, M. Sclareol, a plant diterpene, exhibits potent antiproliferative effects *via* the induction of apoptosis and mitochondrial membrane potential loss in osteosarcoma cancer cells. *Mol. Med. Rep.,* **2015**, *11*(6), 4273-4278.
[http://dx.doi.org/10.3892/mmr.2015.3325] [PMID: 25672419]

[152]   Du, J.; Chen, C.; Sun, Y.; Zheng, L.; Wang, W. Ponicidin suppresses HT29 cell growth *via* the induction of G1 cell cycle arrest and apoptosis. *Mol. Med. Rep.,* **2015**, *12*(4), 5816-5820.
[http://dx.doi.org/10.3892/mmr.2015.4150] [PMID: 26239027]

[153]   Gao, Q.; Liu, H.; Yao, Y.; Geng, L.; Zhang, X.; Jiang, L.; Shi, B.; Yang, F. Carnosic acid induces autophagic cell death through inhibition of the Akt/mTOR pathway in human hepatoma cells. *J. Appl. Toxicol.,* **2015**, *35*(5), 485-492.
[http://dx.doi.org/10.1002/jat.3049] [PMID: 25178877]

[154]   Ma, Y.C.; Su, N.; Zhao, N.M.; Li, Q.Y.; Zhang, M.; Zhao, H.W.; Liu, H.M.; Qin, Y.H. [Jaridonin, a new diterpenoid from Isodon rubescens, induces cell cycle arrest in gastric cancer cells through activating ataxia telangiectasia mutated kinase]. *Zhonghua Zhong Liu Za Zhi,* **2016**, *38*(4), 258-262.
[PMID: 27087371]

[155]   Zhou, L.; Zuo, Z.; Chow, M.S. Danshen: an overview of its chemistry, pharmacology, pharmacokinetics, and clinical use. *J. Clin. Pharmacol.,* **2005**, *45*(12), 1345-1359.
[http://dx.doi.org/10.1177/0091270005282630] [PMID: 16291709]

[156]   Sung, H.J.; Choi, S.M.; Yoon, Y.; An, K.S. Tanshinone IIA, an ingredient of Sal*via* miltiorrhiza BUNGE, induces apoptosis in human leukemia cell lines through the activation of caspase-3. *Exp. Mol. Med.,* **1999**, *31*(4), 174-178.

[http://dx.doi.org/10.1038/emm.1999.28] [PMID: 10630370]

[157]   Wang, X.; Wei, Y.; Yuan, S.; Liu, G.; Lu, Y.; Zhang, J.; Wang, W. Potential anticancer activity of tanshinone IIA against human breast cancer. *Int. J. Cancer,* **2005**, *116*(5), 799-807.
[http://dx.doi.org/10.1002/ijc.20880] [PMID: 15849732]

[158]   Su, C.C.; Chen, G.W.; Kang, J.C.; Chan, M.H. Growth inhibition and apoptosis induction by tanshinone IIA in human colon adenocarcinoma cells. *Planta Med.,* **2008**, *74*(11), 1357-1362.
[http://dx.doi.org/10.1055/s-2008-1081299] [PMID: 18622903]

[159]   Su, C.C.; Lin, Y.H. Tanshinone IIA down-regulates the protein expression of ErbB-2 and up-regulates TNF-alpha in colon cancer cells *in vitro* and *in vivo. Int. J. Mol. Med.,* **2008**, *22*(6), 847-851.
[PMID: 19020785]

[160]   Won, S.H.; Lee, H.J.; Jeong, S.J.; Lee, H.J.; Lee, E.O.; Jung, D.B.; Shin, J.M.; Kwon, T.R.; Yun, S.M.; Lee, M.H.; Choi, S.H.; Lü, J.; Kim, S.H. Tanshinone IIA induces mitochondria dependent apoptosis in prostate cancer cells in association with an inhibition of phosphoinositide 3-kinase/AKT pathway. *Biol. Pharm. Bull.,* **2010**, *33*(11), 1828-1834.
[http://dx.doi.org/10.1248/bpb.33.1828] [PMID: 21048307]

[161]   Wang, J.; Wang, X.; Jiang, S.; Yuan, S.; Lin, P.; Zhang, J.; Lu, Y.; Wang, Q.; Xiong, Z.; Wu, Y.; Ren, J.; Yang, H. Growth inhibition and induction of apoptosis and differentiation of tanshinone IIA in human glioma cells. *J. Neurooncol.,* **2007**, *82*(1), 11-21.
[http://dx.doi.org/10.1007/s11060-006-9242-x] [PMID: 16955220]

[162]   Yuxian, X.; Feng, T.; Ren, L.; Zhengcai, L. Tanshinone II-A inhibits invasion and metastasis of human hepatocellular carcinoma cells *in vitro* and *in vivo. Tumori,* **2009**, *95*(6), 789-795.
[http://dx.doi.org/10.1177/030089160909500623] [PMID: 20210245]

[163]   Shan, Y.F.; Shen, X.; Xie, Y.K.; Chen, J.C.; Shi, H.Q.; Yu, Z.P.; Song, Q.T.; Zhou, M.T.; Zhang, Q.Y. Inhibitory effects of tanshinone II-A on invasion and metastasis of human colon carcinoma cells. *Acta Pharmacol. Sin.,* **2009**, *30*(11), 1537-1542.
[http://dx.doi.org/10.1038/aps.2009.139] [PMID: 19820721]

[164]   Liu, J.J.; Liu, W.D.; Yang, H.Z.; Zhang, Y.; Fang, Z.G.; Liu, P.Q.; Lin, D.J.; Xiao, R.Z.; Hu, Y.; Wang, C.Z.; Li, X.D.; He, Y.; Huang, R.W. Inactivation of PI3k/Akt signaling pathway and activation of caspase-3 are involved in tanshinone I-induced apoptosis in myeloid leukemia cells *in vitro. Ann. Hematol.,* **2010**, *89*(11), 1089-1097.
[http://dx.doi.org/10.1007/s00277-010-0996-z] [PMID: 20512574]

[165]   Lee, W.Y.; Liu, K.W.; Yeung, J.H. Reactive oxygen species-mediated kinase activation by dihydrotanshinone in tanshinones-induced apoptosis in HepG2 cells. *Cancer Lett.,* **2009**, *285*(1), 46-57.
[http://dx.doi.org/10.1016/j.canlet.2009.04.040] [PMID: 19467570]

[166]   Park, I.J.; Kim, M.J.; Park, O.J.; Park, M.G.; Choe, W.; Kang, I.; Kim, S.S.; Ha, J. Cryptotanshinone sensitizes DU145 prostate cancer cells to Fas(APO1/CD95)-mediated apoptosis through Bcl-2 and MAPK regulation. *Cancer Lett.,* **2010**, *298*(1), 88-98.
[http://dx.doi.org/10.1016/j.canlet.2010.06.006] [PMID: 20638780]

[167]   Wang, Y.; Lu, J.J.; He, L. Triptolide (TPL) Inhibits Global Transcription by Inducing Proteasome-Dependent Degradation of RNA Polymerase II (PolII). *PLoS One,* **2011**, *6*, 23993.
[http://dx.doi.org/10.1371/journal.pone.0023993]

[168]   McCallum, C.; Kwon, S.; Leavitt, P.; Shen, D.M.; Liu, W.; Gurnett, A. Triptolide binds covalently to a 90 kDa nuclear protein. Role of epoxides in binding and activity. *Immunobiology,* **2007**, *212*(7), 549-556.
[http://dx.doi.org/10.1016/j.imbio.2007.02.002] [PMID: 17678712]

[169]   Titov, D.V.; Gilman, B.; He, Q.L.; Bhat, S.; Low, W.K.; Dang, Y.; Smeaton, M.; Demain, A.L.; Miller, P.S.; Kugel, J.F.; Goodrich, J.A.; Liu, J.O. XPB, a subunit of TFIIH, is a target of the natural product triptolide. *Nat. Chem. Biol.,* **2011**, *7*(3), 182-188.

[http://dx.doi.org/10.1038/nchembio.522] [PMID: 21278739]

[170] Zhou, Z.L.; Luo, Z.G.; Yu, B.; Jiang, Y.; Chen, Y.; Feng, J.M.; Dai, M.; Tong, L.J.; Li, Z.; Li, Y.C.; Ding, J.; Miao, Z.H. Increased accumulation of hypoxia-inducible factor-1α with reduced transcriptional activity mediates the antitumor effect of triptolide. *Mol. Cancer,* **2010**, *9*, 268. [http://dx.doi.org/10.1186/1476-4598-9-268] [PMID: 20932347]

[171] Pan, D.J.; Li, Z.L.; Hu, C.Q.; Chen, K.; Chang, J.J.; Lee, K.H. The cytotoxic principles of Pseudolarix kaempferi: pseudolaric acid-A and -B and related derivatives. *Planta Med.,* **1990**, *56*(4), 383-385. [http://dx.doi.org/10.1055/s-2006-960989] [PMID: 2236294]

[172] Wong, V.K.; Chiu, P.; Chung, S.S.; Chow, L.M.; Zhao, Y.Z.; Yang, B.B.; Ko, B.C. Pseudolaric acid B, a novel microtubule-destabilizing agent that circumvents multidrug resistance phenotype and exhibits antitumor activity in vivo. *Clin. Cancer Res.,* **2005**, *11*(16), 6002-6011. [http://dx.doi.org/10.1158/1078-0432.CCR-05-0209] [PMID: 16115945]

[173] Anton Aparicio, L.M.; Pulido, E.G.; Gallego, G.A. Vinflunine: a new vision that may translate into antiangiogenic and antimetastatic activity. *Anticancer Drugs,* **2011**, *23*(1), 1-11. [http://dx.doi.org/10.1097/CAD.0b013e32834d237b] [PMID: 20938340]

[174] Jordan, M.A.; Wilson, L. Microtubules as a target for anticancer drugs. *Nat. Rev. Cancer,* **2004**, *4*(4), 253-265. [http://dx.doi.org/10.1038/nrc1317] [PMID: 15057285]

[175] Tan, W.F.; Zhang, X.W.; Li, M.H.; Yue, J.M.; Chen, Y.; Lin, L.P.; Ding, J. Pseudolarix acid B inhibits angiogenesis by antagonizing the vascular endothelial growth factor-mediated anti-apoptotic effect. *Eur. J. Pharmacol.,* **2004**, *499*(3), 219-228. [http://dx.doi.org/10.1016/j.ejphar.2004.07.063] [PMID: 15381043]

[176] Li, M.H.; Miao, Z.H.; Tan, W.F.; Yue, J.M.; Zhang, C.; Lin, L.P.; Zhang, X.W.; Ding, J. Pseudolaric acid B inhibits angiogenesis and reduces hypoxia-inducible factor 1alpha by promoting proteasome-mediated degradation. *Clin. Cancer Res.,* **2004**, *10*(24), 8266-8274. [http://dx.doi.org/10.1158/1078-0432.CCR-04-0951] [PMID: 15623602]

[177] a) Yu, J.H.; Wang, H.J.; Li, X.R.; Tashiro, S.; Onodera, S.; Ikejima, T. Protein tyrosine kinase, JNK, and ERK involvement in pseudolaric acid B-induced apoptosis of human breast cancer MCF-7 cells. *Acta Pharmacol. Sin.,* **2008**, *29*(9), 1069-1076. [http://dx.doi.org/10.1111/j.1745-7254.2008.00835.x] [PMID: 18718176] b) Bhatia, R.; Singh, R.K. Introductory Chapter: Protein Kinases as Promising Targets for Drug Design against Cancer.*Protein Kinases - Promising Targets for Anticancer Drug Research*; Singh, R.K., Ed.; IntechOpen: London, **2021**. [http://dx.doi.org/10.5772/intechopen.100315]

[178] a)Ji, L.; Liu, T.; Liu, J.; Chen, Y.; Wang, Z. Andrographolide inhibits human hepatoma-derived Hep3B cell growth through the activation of c-Jun N-terminal kinase. *Planta Med.,* **2007**, *73*(13), 1397-1401. [http://dx.doi.org/10.1055/s-2007-990230] [PMID: 17918040] b)Mehta, S.; Sharma, A.K.; Singh, R.K. Pharmacological activities and molecular mechanisms of pure and crude extract of Andrographis paniculata: An update. *Phytomedicine Plus,* **2021**, *1*(4)100085 [http://dx.doi.org/10.1016/j.phyplu.2021.100085] c)Mehta, S.; Sharma, A.K.; Singh, R.K. Therapeutic Journey of Andrographis paniculata (Burm.f.) Nees from Natural to Synthetic and Nanoformulations. *Mini Rev. Med. Chem.,* **2021**, *21*(12), 1556-1577. [http://dx.doi.org/10.2174/1389557521666210315162354] [PMID: 33719961] d)Mehta, S.; Sharma, A.K.; Singh, R.K. Ethnobotany, Pharmacological activities and Bioavailability studies of "King of Bitter" (Kalmegh): A Review (2010-2020). *Comb. Chem. High Throughput Screen,* **2022**, *25*(5), 788-807. [http://dx.doi.org/10.2174/1386207324666210310140611] [PMID: 33745423]

[179] Xia, Y.F.; Ye, B.Q.; Li, Y.D.; Wang, J.G.; He, X.J.; Lin, X.; Yao, X.; Ma, D.; Slungaard, A.; Hebbel, R.P.; Key, N.S.; Geng, J.G. Andrographolide attenuates inflammation by inhibition of NF-kappa B

activation through covalent modification of reduced cysteine 62 of p50. *J. Immunol.,* **2004**, *173*(6), 4207-4217.
[http://dx.doi.org/10.4049/jimmunol.173.6.4207] [PMID: 15356172]

[180]  Wang, L.J.; Zhou, X.; Wang, W.; Tang, F.; Qi, C.L.; Yang, X.; Wu, S.; Lin, Y.Q.; Wang, J.T.; Geng, J.G. Andrographolide inhibits oral squamous cell carcinogenesis through NF-κB inactivation. *J. Dent. Res.,* **2011**, *90*(10), 1246-1252.
[http://dx.doi.org/10.1177/0022034511418341] [PMID: 21841043]

[181]  Kuttan, G.; Pratheeshkumar, P.; Manu, K.A.; Kuttan, R. Inhibition of tumor progression by naturally occurring terpenoids. *Pharm. Biol.,* **2011**, *49*(10), 995-1007.
[http://dx.doi.org/10.3109/13880209.2011.559476] [PMID: 21936626]

[182]  Ikezoe, T.; Yang, Y.; Bandobashi, K.; Saito, T.; Takemoto, S.; Machida, H.; Togitani, K.; Koeffler, H.P.; Taguchi, H. Oridonin, a diterpenoid purified from Rabdosia rubescens, inhibits the proliferation of cells from lymphoid malignancies in association with blockade of the NF-kappa B signal pathways. *Mol. Cancer Ther.,* **2005**, *4*(4), 578-586.
[http://dx.doi.org/10.1158/1535-7163.MCT-04-0277] [PMID: 15827331]

[183]  Huang, J.; Wu, L.; Tashiro, S.; Onodera, S.; Ikejima, T. Reactive oxygen species mediate oridonin-induced HepG2 apoptosis through p53, MAPK, and mitochondrial signaling pathways. *J. Pharmacol. Sci.,* **2008**, *107*(4), 370-379.
[http://dx.doi.org/10.1254/jphs.08044FP] [PMID: 18719315]

[184]  Hu, H.Z.; Yang, Y.B.; Xu, X.D.; Shen, H.W.; Shu, Y.M.; Ren, Z.; Li, X.M.; Shen, H.M.; Zeng, H.T. Oridonin induces apoptosis *via* PI3K/Akt pathway in cervical carcinoma HeLa cell line. *Acta Pharmacol. Sin.,* **2007**, *28*(11), 1819-1826.
[http://dx.doi.org/10.1111/j.1745-7254.2007.00667.x] [PMID: 17959034]

[185]  Cheng, Y.; Qiu, F.; Ye, Y.C.; Guo, Z.M.; Tashiro, S.; Onodera, S.; Ikejima, T. Autophagy inhibits reactive oxygen species-mediated apoptosis *via* activating p38-nuclear factor-kappa B survival pathways in oridonin-treated murine fibrosarcoma L929 cells. *FEBS J.,* **2009**, *276*(5), 1291-1306.
[http://dx.doi.org/10.1111/j.1742-4658.2008.06864.x] [PMID: 19187231]

[186]  Zhang, Y.H.; Wu, Y.L.; Tashiro, S.; Onodera, S.; Ikejima, T. Reactive oxygen species contribute to oridonin-induced apoptosis and autophagy in human cervical carcinoma HeLa cells. *Acta Pharmacol. Sin.,* **2011**, *32*(10), 1266-1275.
[http://dx.doi.org/10.1038/aps.2011.92] [PMID: 21892202]

[187]  Islam, M.T.; Ali, E.S.; Uddin, S.J.; Shaw, S.; Islam, M.A.; Ahmed, M.I.; Chandra Shill, M.; Karmakar, U.K.; Yarla, N.S.; Khan, I.N.; Billah, M.M.; Pieczynska, M.D.; Zengin, G.; Malainer, C.; Nicoletti, F.; Gulei, D.; Berindan-Neagoe, I.; Apostolov, A.; Banach, M.; Yeung, A.W.K.; El-Demerdash, A.; Xiao, J.; Dey, P.; Yele, S.; Jóźwik, A.; Strzałkowska, N.; Marchewka, J.; Rengasamy, K.R.R.; Horbańczuk, J.; Kamal, M.A.; Mubarak, M.S.; Mishra, S.K.; Shilpi, J.A.; Atanasov, A.G. Phytol: A review of biomedical activities. *Food Chem. Toxicol.,* **2018**, *121*, 82-94.
[http://dx.doi.org/10.1016/j.fct.2018.08.032] [PMID: 30130593]

[188]  Deng, R.; Tang, J.; Xia, L.P.; Li, D.D.; Zhou, W.J.; Wang, L.L.; Feng, G.K.; Zeng, Y.X.; Gao, Y.H.; Zhu, X.F. ExcisaninA, a diterpenoid compound purified from Isodon MacrocalyxinD, induces tumor cells apoptosis and suppresses tumor growth through inhibition of PKB/AKT kinase activity and blockade of its signal pathway. *Mol. Cancer Ther.,* **2009**, *8*(4), 873-882.
[http://dx.doi.org/10.1158/1535-7163.MCT-08-1080] [PMID: 19372560]

[189]  Wani, M.C.; Taylor, H.L.; Wall, M.E.; Coggon, P.; McPhail, A.T. Plant antitumor agents. VI. The isolation and structure of taxol, a novel antileukemic and antitumor agent from Taxus brevifolia. *J. Am. Chem. Soc.,* **1971**, *93*(9), 2325-2327.
[http://dx.doi.org/10.1021/ja00738a045] [PMID: 5553076]

[190]  Ziaei, S.; Halaby, R. Immunosuppressive, anti-inflammatory and anti-cancer properties of triptolide: A mini review. *Avicenna J. Phytomed.,* **2016**, *6*(2), 149-164.
[PMID: 27222828]

[191]   Qiu, D.; Zhao, G.; Aoki, Y.; Shi, L.; Uyei, A.; Nazarian, S.; Ng, J.C.; Kao, P.N. Immunosuppressant PG490 (triptolide) inhibits T-cell interleukin-2 expression at the level of purine-box/nuclear factor of activated T-cells and NF-kappaB transcriptional activation. *J. Biol. Chem.,* **1999**, *274*(19), 13443-13450.
[http://dx.doi.org/10.1074/jbc.274.19.13443] [PMID: 10224109]

[192]   Westerheide, S.D.; Kawahara, T.L.; Orton, K.; Morimoto, R.I. Triptolide, an inhibitor of the human heat shock response that enhances stress-induced cell death. *J. Biol. Chem.,* **2006**, *281*(14), 9616-9622.
[http://dx.doi.org/10.1074/jbc.M512044200] [PMID: 16469748]

[193]   Chang, W.T.; Kang, J.J.; Lee, K.Y.; Wei, K.; Anderson, E.; Gotmare, S.; Ross, J.A.; Rosen, G.D. Triptolide and chemotherapy cooperate in tumor cell apoptosis. A role for the p53 pathway. *J. Biol. Chem.,* **2001**, *276*(3), 2221-2227.
[http://dx.doi.org/10.1074/jbc.M009713200] [PMID: 11053449]

[194]   Vispé, S.; DeVries, L.; Créancier, L.; Besse, J.; Bréand, S.; Hobson, D.J.; Svejstrup, J.Q.; Annereau, J.P.; Cussac, D.; Dumontet, C.; Guilbaud, N.; Barret, J.M.; Bailly, C. Triptolide is an inhibitor of RNA polymerase I and II-dependent transcription leading predominantly to down-regulation of short-lived mRNA. *Mol. Cancer Ther.,* **2009**, *8*(10), 2780-2790.
[http://dx.doi.org/10.1158/1535-7163.MCT-09-0549] [PMID: 19808979]

[195]   Hassan, S.B.; Gali-Muhtasib, H.; Göransson, H.; Larsson, R. Alpha terpineol: a potential anticancer agent which acts through suppressing NF-kappaB signalling. *Anticancer Res.,* **2010**, *30*(6), 1911-1919.
[PMID: 20651334]

[196]   Khaleel, C.; Tabanca, N.; Buchbauer, G. α-Terpineol, a natural monoterpene: A review of its biological properties. *Open Chem.,* **2018**, *16*, 349-361.
[http://dx.doi.org/10.1515/chem-2018-0040]

[197]   Yoshida, M.; Feng, W.; Saijo, N.; Ikekawa, T. Antitumor activity of daphnane-type diterpene gnidimacrin isolated from Stellera chamaejasme L. *Int. J. Cancer,* **1996**, *66*(2), 268-273.
[http://dx.doi.org/10.1002/(SICI)1097-0215(19960410)66:2<268::AID-IJC22>3.0.CO;2-7]   [PMID: 8603823]

[198]   Yoshida, M.; Matsui, Y.; Iizuka, A.; Ikarashi, Y. G2-phase arrest through p21(WAF1 / Cip1) induction and cdc2 repression by gnidimacrin in human hepatoma HLE cells. *Anticancer Res.,* **2009**, *29*(4), 1349-1354.
[PMID: 19414386]

[199]   a) Dimas, K.; Kokkinopoulos, D.; Demetzos, C.; Vaos, B.; Marselos, M.; Malamas, M.; Tzavaras, T. The effect of sclareol on growth and cell cycle progression of human leukemic cell lines. *Leuk. Res.,* **1999**, *23*(3), 217-234.
[http://dx.doi.org/10.1016/S0145-2126(98)00134-9] [PMID: 10071073] b) Hatziantoniou, S.; Dimas, K.; Georgopoulos, A.; Sotiriadou, N.; Demetzos, C. Cytotoxic and antitumor activity of liposome-incorporated sclareol against cancer cell lines and human colon cancer xenografts. *Pharmacol. Res.,* **2006**, *53*(1), 80-87.
[http://dx.doi.org/10.1016/j.phrs.2005.09.008] [PMID: 16253514]

[200]   Kingston, D.G. Taxol: the chemistry and structure-activity relationships of a novel anticancer agent. *Trends Biotechnol,* **1994**, *12*(6), 222-7.
[http://dx.doi.org/10.1016/0167-7799(94)90120-1] [PMID: 7765351]

[201]   Wu, Y.B.; Ni, Z.Y.; Shi, Q.W.; Dong, M.; Kiyota, H.; Gu, Y.C.; Cong, B. Constituents from Sal*via* species and their biological activities. *Chem. Rev.,* **2012**, *112*(11), 5967-6026.
[http://dx.doi.org/10.1021/cr200058f] [PMID: 22967178]

[202]   Cai, Y.; Zhang, W.; Chen, Z.; Shi, Z.; He, C.; Chen, M. Recent insights into the biological activities and drug delivery systems of tanshinones. *Int. J. Nanomedicine,* **2016**, *11*, 121-130.
[PMID: 26792989]

[203]   Lai, Z.; He, J.; Zhou, C. Tanshinones: An Update in the Medicinal Chemistry in Recent 5 Years. *Curr.*

*Med. Chem.,* **2020**, *27*, 1.
[PMID: 32436817]

[204]  a) Schafer, B. Taxol: Hoffnunggegen Krebs. *Chem. Unserer Zeit,* **2014**, *45*, 32-46.
[http://dx.doi.org/10.1002/ciuz.201100539] b) Weaver, B.A. How Taxol/paclitaxel kills cancer cells.
*Mol. Biol. Cell,* **2014**, *25*(18), 2677-2681.
[http://dx.doi.org/10.1091/mbc.e14-04-0916] [PMID: 25213191]

[205]  Liu, Y.; Wang, L.; Jung, J.H.; Zhang, S. Sesterterpenoids. *Nat. Prod. Rep.,* **2007**, *24*(6), 1401-1429.
[http://dx.doi.org/10.1039/b617259h] [PMID: 18033586]

[206]  Wang, L.; Yang, B.; Lin, X.P.; Zhou, X.F.; Liu, Y. Sesterterpenoids. *Nat. Prod. Rep.,* **2013**, *30*(3),
455-473.
[http://dx.doi.org/10.1039/c3np20089b] [PMID: 23385977]

[207]  Harborne, J.B. *Phytochemical methods.A guide to modern techniques of plant analysis,* 3$^{rd}$ ed;
Thompson Science: London, UK, **1998**, p. 1317.

[208]  Chudzik, M.; Korzonek-Szlacheta, I.; Król, W. Triterpenes as potentially cytotoxic compounds.
*Molecules,* **2015**, *20*(1), 1610-1625.
[http://dx.doi.org/10.3390/molecules20011610] [PMID: 25608043]

[209]  Connolly, J.D.; Hill, R.A. Triterpenoids. *Nat. Prod. Rep.,* **2001**, *18*(5), 560-578.
[http://dx.doi.org/10.1039/b104602k] [PMID: 11699886]

[210]  Cascão, R.; Fonseca, J.E.; Moita, L.F. Celastrol: A Spectrum of Treatment Opportunities in Chronic
Diseases. *Front. Med. (Lausanne),* **2017**, *4*, 69.
[http://dx.doi.org/10.3389/fmed.2017.00069] [PMID: 28664158]

[211]  Calixto, J.B.; Campos, M.M.; Otuki, M.F.; Santos, A.R. Anti-inflammatory compounds of plant
origin. Part II. modulation of pro-inflammatory cytokines, chemokines and adhesion molecules. *Planta
Med.,* **2004**, *70*(2), 93-103.
[http://dx.doi.org/10.1055/s-2004-815483] [PMID: 14994184]

[212]  Allison, A.C.; Cacabelos, R.; Lombardi, V.R.; Alvarez, X.A.; Vigo, C. Celastrol, a potent antioxidant
and anti-inflammatory drug, as a possible treatment for Alzheimer's disease. *Prog.
Neuropsychopharmacol. Biol. Psychiatry,* **2001**, *25*(7), 1341-1357.
[http://dx.doi.org/10.1016/S0278-5846(01)00192-0] [PMID: 11513350]

[213]  Seo, W.Y.; Ju, S.M.; Song, H.Y.; Goh, A.R.; Jun, J.G.; Kang, Y.H.; Choi, S.Y.; Park, J. Celastrol
suppresses IFN-gamma-induced ICAM-1 expression and subsequent monocyte adhesiveness *via* the
induction of heme oxygenase-1 in the HaCaT cells. *Biochem. Biophys. Res. Commun.,* **2010**, *398*(1),
140-145.
[http://dx.doi.org/10.1016/j.bbrc.2010.06.053] [PMID: 20599745]

[214]  Pang, X.; Yi, Z.; Zhang, J.; Lu, B.; Sung, B.; Qu, W.; Aggarwal, B.B.; Liu, M. Celastrol suppresses
angiogenesis-mediated tumor growth through inhibition of AKT/mammalian target of rapamycin
pathway. *Cancer Res.,* **2010**, *70*(5), 1951-1959.
[http://dx.doi.org/10.1158/0008-5472.CAN-09-3201] [PMID: 20160026]

[215]  Yang, H.; Chen, D.; Cui, Q.C.; Yuan, X.; Dou, Q.P. Celastrol, a triterpene extracted from the Chinese
"Thunder of God Vine," is a potent proteasome inhibitor and suppresses human prostate cancer growth
in nude mice. *Cancer Res.,* **2006**, *66*(9), 4758-4765.
[http://dx.doi.org/10.1158/0008-5472.CAN-05-4529] [PMID: 16651429]

[216]  Yang, H.; Dou, Q.P. Targeting apoptosis pathway with natural terpenoids: implications for treatment
of breast and prostate cancer. *Curr. Drug Targets,* **2010**, *11*(6), 733-744.
[http://dx.doi.org/10.2174/138945010791170842] [PMID: 20298150]

[217]  Hong, J.; Min, H.Y.; Xu, G.H.; Lee, J.G.; Lee, S.H.; Kim, Y.S.; Kang, S.S.; Lee, S.K. Growth
inhibition and G1 cell cycle arrest mediated by 25-methoxyhispidol A, a novel triterpenoid, isolated
from the fruit of *Poncirus trifoliata* in human hepatocellular carcinoma cells. *Planta Med.,* **2008**,

*74*(2), 151-155.
[http://dx.doi.org/10.1055/s-2008-1034286] [PMID: 18219600]

[218]   Yan, S.L.; Huang, C.Y.; Wu, S.T.; Yin, M.C. Oleanolic acid and ursolic acid induce apoptosis in four human liver cancer cell lines. *Toxicol.,* **2010**, *24*(3), 842-848.
[http://dx.doi.org/10.1016/j.tiv.2009.12.008] [PMID: 20005942]

[219]   Zhang, R.X.; Li, Y.; Tian, D.D.; Liu, Y.; Nian, W.; Zou, X.; Chen, Q.Z.; Zhou, L.Y.; Deng, Z.L.; He, B.C. Ursolic acid inhibits proliferation and induces apoptosis by inactivating Wnt/β-catenin signaling in human osteosarcoma cells. *Int. J. Oncol.,* **2016**, *49*(5), 1973-1982.
[http://dx.doi.org/10.3892/ijo.2016.3701] [PMID: 27665868]

[220]   Gai, W.T.; Yu, D.P.; Wang, X.S.; Wang, P.T. Anti-cancer effect of ursolic acid activates apoptosis through ROCK/PTEN mediated mitochondrial translocation of cofilin-1 in prostate cancer. *Oncol. Lett.,* **2016**, *12*(4), 2880-2885.
[http://dx.doi.org/10.3892/ol.2016.5015] [PMID: 27698874]

[221]   Lewinska, A.; Adamczyk-Grochala, J.; Kwasniewicz, E.; Deregowska, A.; Wnuk, M. Ursolic acid-mediated changes in glycolytic pathway promote cytotoxic autophagy and apoptosis in phenotypically different breast cancer cells. *Apoptosis,* **2017**, *22*(6), 800-815.
[http://dx.doi.org/10.1007/s10495-017-1353-7] [PMID: 28213701]

[222]   Li, T.; Chen, X.; Liu, Y.; Fan, L.; Lin, L.; Xu, Y.; Chen, S.; Shao, J. pH-Sensitive mesoporous silica nanoparticles anticancer prodrugs for sustained release of ursolic acid and the enhanced anti-cancer efficacy for hepatocellular carcinoma cancer. *Eur. J. Pharm. Sci.,* **2017**, *96*, 456-463.
[http://dx.doi.org/10.1016/j.ejps.2016.10.019] [PMID: 27771513]

[223]   Wang, S.; Meng, X.; Dong, Y. Ursolic acid nanoparticles inhibit cervical cancer growth *in vitro* and *in vivovia* apoptosis induction. *Int. J. Oncol.,* **2017**, *50*(4), 1330-1340.
[http://dx.doi.org/10.3892/ijo.2017.3890] [PMID: 28259944]

[224]   Salminen, A.; Lehtonen, M.; Paimela, T.; Kaarniranta, K. Celastrol: Molecular targets of Thunder God Vine. *Biochem. Biophys. Res. Commun.,* **2010**, *394*(3), 439-442.
[http://dx.doi.org/10.1016/j.bbrc.2010.03.050] [PMID: 20226165]

[225]   Chambliss, O.L.; Jones, C.M. Cucurbitacins: specific insect attractants in Cucurbitaceae. *Science,* **1966**, *153*(3742), 1392-1393.
[http://dx.doi.org/10.1126/science.153.3742.1392] [PMID: 17814391]

[226]   Zhang, M.; Zhang, H.; Sun, C.; Shan, X.; Yang, X.; Li-Ling, J.; Deng, Y. Targeted constitutive activation of signal transducer and activator of transcription 3 in human hepatocellular carcinoma cells by cucurbitacin B. *Cancer Chemother. Pharmacol.,* **2009**, *63*(4), 635-642.
[http://dx.doi.org/10.1007/s00280-008-0780-0] [PMID: 18521604]

[227]   Chan, K.T.; Meng, F.Y.; Li, Q.; Ho, C.Y.; Lam, T.S.; To, Y.; Lee, W.H.; Li, M.; Chu, K.H.; Toh, M. Cucurbitacin B induces apoptosis and S phase cell cycle arrest in BEL-7402 human hepatocellular carcinoma cells and is effective *via* oral administration. *Cancer Lett.,* **2010**, *294*(1), 118-124.
[http://dx.doi.org/10.1016/j.canlet.2010.01.029] [PMID: 20153103]

[228]   Lee, D.H.; Iwanski, G.B.; Thoennissen, N.H. Cucurbitacin: ancient compound shedding new light on cancer treatment. *ScientificWorldJournal,* **2010**, *10*, 413-418.
[http://dx.doi.org/10.1100/tsw.2010.44] [PMID: 20209387]

[229]   Li, Y.; Wang, R.; Ma, E.; Deng, Y.; Wang, X.; Xiao, J.; Jing, Y. The induction of G2/M cell-cycle arrest and apoptosis by cucurbitacin E is associated with increased phosphorylation of eIF2alpha in leukemia cells. *Anticancer Drugs,* **2010**, *21*(4), 389-400.
[http://dx.doi.org/10.1097/CAD.0b013e328336b383] [PMID: 20110807]

[230]   Alghasham, A.A. Cucurbitacins - a promising target for cancer therapy. *Int. J. Health Sci. (Qassim),* **2013**, *7*(1), 77-89.
[http://dx.doi.org/10.12816/0006025] [PMID: 23559908]

[231]  Pan, L.; Yong, Y.; Deng, Y.; Lantvit, D.D.; Ninh, T.N.; Chai, H.; Carcache de Blanco, E.J.; Soejarto, D.D.; Swanson, S.M.; Kinghorn, A.D. Isolation, structure elucidation, and biological evaluation of 16,23-epoxycucurbitacin constituents from Eleaocarpus chinensis. *J. Nat. Prod.,* **2012**, *75*(3), 444-452.
[http://dx.doi.org/10.1021/np200879p] [PMID: 22239601]

[232]  Hsu, H.S.; Huang, P.I.; Chang, Y.L.; Tzao, C.; Chen, Y.W.; Shih, H.C.; Hung, S.C.; Chen, Y.C.; Tseng, L.M.; Chiou, S.H. Cucurbitacin I inhibits tumorigenic ability and enhances radiochemosensitivity in nonsmall cell lung cancer-derived CD133-positive cells. *Cancer,* **2011**, *117*(13), 2970-2985.
[http://dx.doi.org/10.1002/cncr.25869] [PMID: 21225866]

[233]  Tang, J.Z.; Kong, X.J.; Banerjee, A.; Muniraj, N.; Pandey, V.; Steiner, M.; Perry, J.K.; Zhu, T.; Liu, D.X.; Lobie, P.E. STAT3alpha is oncogenic for endometrial carcinoma cells and mediates the oncogenic effects of autocrine human growth hormone. *Endocrinology,* **2010**, *151*(9), 4133-4145.
[http://dx.doi.org/10.1210/en.2010-0273] [PMID: 20668024]

[234]  Momma, K.; Masuzawa, Y.; Nakai, N.; Chujo, M.; Murakami, A.; Kioka, N.; Kiyama, Y.; Akita, T.; Nagao, M. Direct interaction of Cucurbitacin E isolated from Alsomitra macrocarpa to actin filament. *Cytotechnology,* **2008**, *56*(1), 33-39.
[http://dx.doi.org/10.1007/s10616-007-9100-5] [PMID: 19002839]

[235]  Yin, D.; Wakimoto, N.; Xing, H.; Lu, D.; Huynh, T.; Wang, X.; Black, K.L.; Koeffler, H.P. Cucurbitacin B markedly inhibits growth and rapidly affects the cytoskeleton in glioblastoma multiforme. *Int. J. Cancer,* **2008**, *123*(6), 1364-1375.
[http://dx.doi.org/10.1002/ijc.23648] [PMID: 18561312]

[236]  Lee, K.Y.; Lee, S.K. Ginsenoside-Rg1 positively regulates cyclin E-dependent kinase activity in human hepatoma SK-HEP-1 cells. *Biochem. Mol. Biol. Int.,* **1996**, *39*(3), 539-546.
[http://dx.doi.org/10.1080/15216549600201591] [PMID: 8828805]

[237]  Lee, K.Y.; Lee, Y.H.; Kim, S.I.; Park, J.H.; Lee, S.K. Ginsenoside-Rg5 suppresses cyclin E-dependent protein kinase activity *via* up-regulating p21Cip/WAF1 and down-regulating cyclin E in SK-HEP-1 cells. *Anticancer Res.,* **1997**, *17*(2A), 1067-1072.
[PMID: 9137450]

[238]  Lee, K.Y.; Park, J.A.; Chung, E.; Lee, Y.H.; Kim, S.I.; Lee, S.K. Ginsenoside-Rh2 blocks the cell cycle of SK-HEP-1 cells at the G1/S boundary by selectively inducing the protein expression of p27kip1. *Cancer Lett.,* **1996**, *110*(1-2), 193-200.
[http://dx.doi.org/10.1016/S0304-3835(96)04502-8] [PMID: 9018101]

[239]  Park, J.A.; Lee, K.Y.; Oh, Y.J.; Kim, K.W.; Lee, S.K. Activation of caspase-3 protease *via* a Bcl--insensitive pathway during the process of ginsenoside Rh2-induced apoptosis. *Cancer Lett.,* **1997**, *121*(1), 73-81.
[http://dx.doi.org/10.1016/S0304-3835(97)00333-9] [PMID: 9459177]

[240]  Ko, H.; Kim, Y.J.; Park, J.S.; Park, J.H.; Yang, H.O. Autophagy inhibition enhances apoptosis induced by ginsenoside Rk1 in hepatocellular carcinoma cells. *Biosci. Biotechnol. Biochem.,* **2009**, *73*(10), 2183-2189.
[http://dx.doi.org/10.1271/bbb.90250] [PMID: 19809182]

[241]  Huang, Z.R.; Lin, Y.K.; Fang, J.Y. Biological and pharmacological activities of squalene and related compounds: potential uses in cosmetic dermatology. *Molecules,* **2009**, *14*(1), 540-554.
[http://dx.doi.org/10.3390/molecules14010540] [PMID: 19169201]

[242]  Vazquez, L.H.; Palazon, J.; Navarro-Ocan, A. *The Pentacyclic Triterpenes α, β-amyrins: A Review of Sources and Biological Activities: Phytochemicals – A Global Perspective of Their Role in Nutrition and Health*; Venketeshwer Rao, IntechOpen, **2012**.

[243]  Mlala, S.; Oyedeji, A.O.; Gondwe, M.; Oyedeji, O.O. Ursolic Acid and Its Derivatives as Bioactive Agents. *Molecules,* **2019**, *24*(15), 2751.
[http://dx.doi.org/10.3390/molecules24152751] [PMID: 31362424]

[244] Tian, Z.; Liu, Y.M.; Chen, S.B.; Yang, J.S.; Xiao, P.G.; Wang, L.; Wu, E. Cytotoxicity of two triterpenoids from *Nigella glandulifera. Molecules,* **2006**, *11*(9), 693-699.
[http://dx.doi.org/10.3390/11090693] [PMID: 17971743]

[245] Weng, C.J.; Chau, C.F.; Hsieh, Y.S.; Yang, S.F.; Yen, G.C. Lucidenic acid inhibits PMA-induced invasion of human hepatoma cells through inactivating MAPK/ERK signal transduction pathway and reducing binding activities of NF-kappaB and AP-1. *Carcinogenesis,* **2008**, *29*(1), 147-156.
[http://dx.doi.org/10.1093/carcin/bgm261] [PMID: 18024477]

[246] Law, B.Y.; Wang, M.; Ma, D.L.; Al-Mousa, F.; Michelangeli, F.; Cheng, S.H.; Ng, M.H.; To, K.F.; Mok, A.Y.; Ko, R.Y.; Lam, S.K.; Chen, F.; Che, C.M.; Chiu, P.; Ko, B.C. Alisol B, a novel inhibitor of the sarcoplasmic/endoplasmic reticulum Ca(2+) ATPase pump, induces autophagy, endoplasmic reticulum stress, and apoptosis. *Mol. Cancer Ther.,* **2010**, *9*(3), 718-730.
[http://dx.doi.org/10.1158/1535-7163.MCT-09-0700] [PMID: 20197400]

[247] Huang, Y.T.; Huang, D.M.; Chueh, S.C.; Teng, C.M.; Guh, J.H. Alisol B acetate, a triterpene from Alismatis rhizoma, induces Bax nuclear translocation and apoptosis in human hormone-resistant prostate cancer PC-3 cells. *Cancer Lett.,* **2006**, *231*(2), 270-278.
[http://dx.doi.org/10.1016/j.canlet.2005.02.011] [PMID: 16399228]

[248] Giner, E.M.; Máñez, S.; Recio, M.C.; Giner, R.M.; Cerdá-Nicolás, M.; Ríos, J.L. *In vivo* studies on the anti-inflammatory activity of pachymic and dehydrotumulosic acids. *Planta Med.,* **2000**, *66*(3), 221-227.
[http://dx.doi.org/10.1055/s-2000-8563] [PMID: 10821046]

[249] Ling, H.; Zhang, Y.; Ng, K.Y.; Chew, E.H. Pachymic acid impairs breast cancer cell invasion by suppressing nuclear factor-κB-dependent matrix metalloproteinase-9 expression. *Breast Cancer Res. Treat.,* **2011**, *126*(3), 609-620.
[http://dx.doi.org/10.1007/s10549-010-0929-5] [PMID: 20521099]

[250] Ling, H.; Jia, X.; Zhang, Y.; Gapter, L.A.; Lim, Y.S.; Agarwal, R.; Ng, K.Y. Pachymic acid inhibits cell growth and modulates arachidonic acid metabolism in nonsmall cell lung cancer A549 cells. *Mol. Carcinog.,* **2010**, *49*(3), 271-282.
[http://dx.doi.org/10.1002/mc.20597] [PMID: 19918789]

[251] Gapter, L.; Wang, Z.; Glinski, J.; Ng, K.Y. Induction of apoptosis in prostate cancer cells by pachymic acid from Poria cocos. *Biochem. Biophys. Res. Commun.,* **2005**, *332*(4), 1153-1161.
[http://dx.doi.org/10.1016/j.bbrc.2005.05.044] [PMID: 15913545]

[252] Einbond, L.S.; Soffritti, M.; Esposti, D.D.; Park, T.; Cruz, E.; Su, T.; Wu, H.A.; Wang, X.; Zhang, Y.J.; Ham, J.; Goldberg, I.J.; Kronenberg, F.; Vladimirova, A. Actein activates stress- and statin-associated responses and is bioavailable in Sprague-Dawley rats. *Fundam. Clin. Pharmacol.,* **2009**, *23*(3), 311-321.
[http://dx.doi.org/10.1111/j.1472-8206.2009.00673.x] [PMID: 19527300]

[253] Li, M.; Wei, S.Y.; Xu, B.; Guo, W.; Liu, D.L.; Cui, J.R.; Yao, X.S. Pro-apoptotic and microtubule-disassembly effects of ardisiacrispin (A+B), triterpenoid saponins from Ardisia crenata on human hepatoma Bel-7402 cells. *J. Asian Nat. Prod. Res.,* **2008**, *10*(7-8), 739-746.
[http://dx.doi.org/10.1021/np700739t] [PMID: 18696326]

[254] Qi, H.; Wei, L.; Han, Y.; Zhang, Q.; Lau, A.S.; Rong, J. Proteomic characterization of the cellular response to chemopreventive triterpenoid astragaloside IV in human hepatocellular carcinoma cell line HepG2. *Int. J. Oncol.,* **2010**, *36*(3), 725-735.
[PMID: 20126993]

[255] Lee, Y.S.; Jin, D.Q.; Kwon, E.J.; Park, S.H.; Lee, E.S.; Jeong, T.C.; Nam, D.H.; Huh, K.; Kim, J.A. Asiatic acid, a triterpene, induces apoptosis through intracellular Ca$^{2+}$ release and enhanced expression of p53 in HepG2 human hepatoma cells. *Cancer Lett.,* **2002**, *186*(1), 83-91.
[http://dx.doi.org/10.1016/S0304-3835(02)00260-4] [PMID: 12183079]

[256] Eichenmüller, M.; von Schweinitz, D.; Kappler, R. Betulinic acid treatment promotes apoptosis in

hepatoblastoma cells. *Int. J. Oncol.*, **2009**, *35*(4), 873-879.
[PMID: 19724925]

[257] Tong, X.; Lin, S.; Fujii, M.; Hou, D.X. Molecular mechanisms of echinocystic acid-induced apoptosis in HepG2 cells. *Biochem. Biophys. Res. Commun.*, **2004**, *321*(3), 539-546.
[http://dx.doi.org/10.1016/j.bbrc.2004.07.004] [PMID: 15358141]

[258] Zhou, X.Y.; Fu, F.H.; Li, Z.; Dong, Q.J.; He, J.; Wang, C.H. Escin, a natural mixture of triterpene saponins, exhibits antitumor activity against hepatocellular carcinoma. *Planta Med.*, **2009**, *75*(15), 1580-1585.
[http://dx.doi.org/10.1055/s-0029-1185838] [PMID: 19579181]

[259] Yang, H.L. Ganoderic acid produced from submerged culture of Ganoderma lucidum induces cell cycle arrest and cytotoxicity in human hepatoma cell line BEL7402. *Biotechnol. Lett.*, **2005**, *27*(12), 835-838.
[http://dx.doi.org/10.1007/s10529-005-6191-y] [PMID: 16086244]

[260] Chang, U.M.; Li, C.H.; Lin, L.I.; Huang, C.P.; Kan, L.S.; Lin, S.B. Ganoderiol F, a ganoderma triterpene, induces senescence in hepatoma HepG2 cells. *Life Sci.*, **2006**, *79*(12), 1129-1139.
[http://dx.doi.org/10.1016/j.lfs.2006.03.027] [PMID: 16635496]

[261] Khanal, P.; Oh, W.K.; Thuong, P.T.; Cho, S.D.; Choi, H.S. 24-hydroxyursolic acid from the leaves of the Diospyros kaki (Persimmon) induces apoptosis by activation of AMP-activated protein kinase. *Planta Med.*, **2010**, *76*(7), 689-693.
[http://dx.doi.org/10.1055/s-0029-1240678] [PMID: 19960411]

[262] Thoppil, R.J.; Bishayee, A. Terpenoids as potential chemopreventive and therapeutic agents in liver cancer. *World J. Hepatol.*, **2011**, *3*(9), 228-249.
[http://dx.doi.org/10.4254/wjh.v3.i9.228] [PMID: 21969877]

[263] Neto, C.C. Ursolic acid and other pentacyclic triterpenoids: anticancer activities and occurrence in berries. In: *Berries and Cancer Prevention*; Springer: New York, **2011**.

[264] Ayeleso, T.B.; Matumba, M.G.; Mukwevho, E. Oleanolic Acid and Its Derivatives: Biological Activities and Therapeutic Potential in Chronic Diseases. *Molecules*, **2017**, *22*(11), 1915.
[http://dx.doi.org/10.3390/molecules22111915] [PMID: 29137205]

[265] Yan, X.J.; Gong, L.H.; Zheng, F.Y.; Cheng, K.J.; Chen, Z.S.; Shi, Z. Triterpenoids as reversal agents for anticancer drug resistance treatment. *Drug Discov. Today*, **2014**, *19*(4), 482-488.
[http://dx.doi.org/10.1016/j.drudis.2013.07.018] [PMID: 23954181]

[266] Youn, S.H.; Lee, J.S.; Lee, M.S.; Cha, E.Y.; Thuong, P.T.; Kim, J.R.; Chang, E.S. Anticancer properties of pomolic acid-induced AMP-activated protein kinase activation in MCF7 human breast cancer cells. *Biol. Pharm. Bull.*, **2012**, *35*(1), 105-110.
[http://dx.doi.org/10.1248/bpb.35.105] [PMID: 22223345]

[267] Bishayee, A.; Ahmed, S.; Brankov, N.; Perloff, M. Triterpenoids as potential agents for the chemoprevention and therapy of breast cancer. *Front. Biosci.*, **2011**, *16*(3), 980-996.
[http://dx.doi.org/10.2741/3730] [PMID: 21196213]

[268] Mu, X.; Shi, W.; Sun, L.; Li, H.; Jiang, Z.; Zhang, L. Pristimerin, a triterpenoid, inhibits tumor angiogenesis by targeting VEGFR2 activation. *Molecules*, **2012**, *17*(6), 6854-6868.
[http://dx.doi.org/10.3390/molecules17066854] [PMID: 22669041]

[269] Swain, S.S.; Rout, K.K.; Chand, P.K. Production of triterpenoid anti-cancer compound taraxerol in Agrobacterium-transformed root cultures of butterfly pea (Clitoria ternatea L.). *Appl. Biochem. Biotechnol.*, **2012**, *168*(3), 487-503.
[http://dx.doi.org/10.1007/s12010-012-9791-8] [PMID: 22843061]

[270] Kim, S.E.; Lee, Y.H.; Park, J.H.; Lee, S.K. Ginsenoside-Rs3, a new diol-type ginseng saponin, selectively elevates protein levels of p53 and p21WAF1 leading to induction of apoptosis in SK-HE-1 cells. *Anticancer Res.*, **1999**, *19*(1A), 487-491.

[PMID: 10226587]

[271] Wang, Q.F.; Chen, J.C.; Hsieh, S.J.; Cheng, C.C.; Hsu, S.L. Regulation of Bcl-2 family molecules and activation of caspase cascade involved in gypenosides-induced apoptosis in human hepatoma cells. *Cancer Lett.,* **2002**, *183*(2), 169-178.
[http://dx.doi.org/10.1016/S0304-3835(01)00828-X] [PMID: 12065092]

[272] Oh, S.H.; Lee, B.H. A ginseng saponin metabolite-induced apoptosis in HepG2 cells involves a mitochondria-mediated pathway and its downstream caspase-8 activation and Bid cleavage. *Toxicol. Appl. Pharmacol.,* **2004**, *194*(3), 221-229.
[http://dx.doi.org/10.1016/j.taap.2003.09.011] [PMID: 14761678]

[273] Ming, Y.L.; Song, G.; Chen, L.H.; Zheng, Z.Z.; Chen, Z.Y.; Ouyang, G.L.; Tong, Q.X. Anti-proliferation and apoptosis induced by a novel intestinal metabolite of ginseng saponin in human hepatocellular carcinoma cells. *Cell Biol. Int.,* **2007**, *31*(10), 1265-1273.
[http://dx.doi.org/10.1016/j.cellbi.2007.05.005] [PMID: 17587608]

[274] Liu, J.J.; Nilsson, A.; Oredsson, S.; Badmaev, V.; Duan, R.D. Keto- and acetyl-keto-boswellic acids inhibit proliferation and induce apoptosis in Hep G2 cells *via* a caspase-8 dependent pathway. *Int. J. Mol. Med.,* **2002**, *10*(4), 501-505.
[http://dx.doi.org/10.3892/ijmm.10.4.501] [PMID: 12239601]

[275] Weng, C.J.; Chau, C.F.; Chen, K.D.; Chen, D.H.; Yen, G.C. The anti-invasive effect of lucidenic acids isolated from a new Ganoderma lucidum strain. *Mol. Nutr. Food Res.,* **2007**, *51*(12), 1472-1477.
[http://dx.doi.org/10.1002/mnfr.200700155] [PMID: 17979098]

[276] Zhang, L.; Zhang, Y.; Zhang, L.; Yang, X.; Lv, Z. Lupeol, a dietary triterpene, inhibited growth, and induced apoptosis through down-regulation of DR3 in SMMC7721 cells. *Cancer Invest.,* **2009**, *27*(2), 163-170.
[http://dx.doi.org/10.1080/07357900802210745] [PMID: 19235588]

[277] Zhang, Z.; Wang, S.; Qiu, H.; Duan, C.; Ding, K.; Wang, Z. Waltonitone induces human hepatocellular carcinoma cells apoptosis *in vitro* and *in vivo*. *Cancer Lett.,* **2009**, *286*(2), 223-231.
[http://dx.doi.org/10.1016/j.canlet.2009.05.023] [PMID: 19539424]

[278] Wang, Y.; Zhang, D.; Ye, W.; Yin, Z.; Fung, K.P.; Zhao, S.; Yao, X. Triterpenoid saponins from Androsace umbellata and their anti-proliferative activities in human hepatoma cells. *Planta Med.,* **2008**, *74*(10), 1280-1284.
[http://dx.doi.org/10.1055/s-2008-1081291] [PMID: 18622900]

[279] Moghaddam, M.G.; Ahmad, F.B.H. Biological Activity of Betulinic Acid: A Review. *Pharmacol. Pharm.,* **2012**, *3*, 119-123.
[http://dx.doi.org/10.4236/pp.2012.32018]

[280] Hordyjewska, A.; Ostapiuk, A.; Horecka, A. Betulin and betulinic acid: triterpenoids derivatives with a powerful biological potential. *Phytochem. Rev.,* **2019**, *18*, 929-951.
[http://dx.doi.org/10.1007/s11101-019-09623-1]

[281] Garg, S.; Kaul, S.C.; Wadhwa, R. Cucurbitacin B and cancer intervention: Chemistry, biology and mechanisms (Review). *Int. J. Oncol.,* **2018**, *52*(1), 19-37. [Review].
[PMID: 29138804]

[282] Mahavir, H.G.; Prasad, G.J. Role of Pentacyclic Triterpenoids in Chemoprevention and Anticancer Treatment: An Overview on Targets and Underling Mechanisms. *J. Pharmacopuncture,* **2019**, *22*(2), 055-067.

[283] Saeidnia, S.; Manayi, A.; Gohari, A.R. The Story of Beta-sitosterol- A Review. *European J. Med. Plants,* **2014**, *4*(5), 590-609.
[http://dx.doi.org/10.9734/EJMP/2014/7764]

[284] Kaur, N.; Chaudhary, J.; Jain, A. Stigmasterol: A Comprehensive review. *Int. J. Pharm. Sci. Res.,* **2011**, *2*(9), 2259-2265.

[285]  Huang, M.; Lu, J.J.; Huang, M.Q.; Bao, J.L.; Chen, X.P.; Wang, Y.T. Terpenoids: natural products for cancer therapy. *Expert Opin. Investig. Drugs,* **2012**, *21*(12), 1801-1818.
[http://dx.doi.org/10.1517/13543784.2012.727395] [PMID: 23092199]

[286]  Tapiero, H.; Townsend, D.M.; Tew, K.D. The role of carotenoids in the prevention of human pathologies. *Biomed. Pharmacother.,* **2004**, *58*(2), 100-110.
[http://dx.doi.org/10.1016/j.biopha.2003.12.006] [PMID: 14992791]

[287]  Das, S.K.; Hashimoto, T.; Kanazawa, K. Growth inhibition of human hepatic carcinoma HepG2 cells by fucoxanthin is associated with down-regulation of cyclin D. *Biochim. Biophys. Acta,* **2008**, *1780*(4), 743-749.
[http://dx.doi.org/10.1016/j.bbagen.2008.01.003] [PMID: 18230364]

[288]  Liu, C.L.; Huang, Y.S.; Hosokawa, M.; Miyashita, K.; Hu, M.L. Inhibition of proliferation of a hepatoma cell line by fucoxanthin in relation to cell cycle arrest and enhanced gap junctional intercellular communication. *Chem. Biol. Interact.,* **2009**, *182*(2-3), 165-172.
[http://dx.doi.org/10.1016/j.cbi.2009.08.017] [PMID: 19737546]

[289]  Huang, C.S.; Fan, Y.E.; Lin, C.Y.; Hu, M.L. Lycopene inhibits matrix metalloproteinase-9 expression and down-regulates the binding activity of nuclear factor-kappa B and stimulatory protein-1. *J. Nutr. Biochem.,* **2007**, *18*(7), 449-456.
[http://dx.doi.org/10.1016/j.jnutbio.2006.08.007] [PMID: 17049831]

[290]  Park, Y.O.; Hwang, E.S.; Moon, T.W. The effect of lycopene on cell growth and oxidative DNA damage of Hep3B human hepatoma cells. *Biofactors,* **2005**, *23*(3), 129-139.
[http://dx.doi.org/10.1002/biof.5520230302] [PMID: 16410635]

[291]  Hwang, E.S.; Lee, H.J. Inhibitory effects of lycopene on the adhesion, invasion, and migration of SK-Hep1 human hepatoma cells. *Exp. Biol. Med. (Maywood),* **2006**, *231*(3), 322-327.
[http://dx.doi.org/10.1177/153537020623100313] [PMID: 16514180]

[292]  Elgass, S.; Cooper, A.; Chopra, M. Lycopene inhibits angiogenesis in human umbilical vein endothelial cells and rat aortic rings. *Br. J. Nutr.,* **2012**, *108*(3), 431-439.
[http://dx.doi.org/10.1017/S0007114511005800] [PMID: 22142444]

[293]  Huang, C.S.; Chuang, C.H.; Lo, T.F.; Hu, M.L. Anti-angiogenic effects of lycopene through immunomodualtion of cytokine secretion in human peripheral blood mononuclear cells. *J. Nutr. Biochem.,* **2013**, *24*(2), 428-434.
[http://dx.doi.org/10.1016/j.jnutbio.2012.01.003] [PMID: 22704783]

[294]  Chen, M.L.; Lin, Y.H.; Yang, C.M.; Hu, M.L. Lycopene inhibits angiogenesis both *in vitro* and *in vivo* by inhibiting MMP-2/uPA system through VEGFR2-mediated PI3K-Akt and ERK/p38 signaling pathways. *Mol. Nutr. Food Res.,* **2012**, *56*(6), 889-899.
[http://dx.doi.org/10.1002/mnfr.201100683] [PMID: 22707264]

[295]  Uppala, P.T.; Dissmore, T.; Lau, B.H.; Andacht, T.; Rajaram, S. Selective inhibition of cell proliferation by lycopene in MCF-7 breast cancer cells *in vitro*: a proteomic analysis. *Phytother. Res.,* **2013**, *27*(4), 595-601.
[http://dx.doi.org/10.1002/ptr.4764] [PMID: 22718574]

[296]  Wójcik, M.; Bobowiec, R.; Martelli, F. Effect of carotenoids on *in vitro* proliferation and differentiation of oval cells during neoplastic and non-neoplastic liver injuries in rats. *J. Physiol. Pharmacol.,* **2008**, *59*(2) Suppl. 2, 203-213.
[PMID: 18812639]

[297]  Cui, Y.; Lu, Z.; Bai, L.; Shi, Z.; Zhao, W.E.; Zhao, B. beta-Carotene induces apoptosis and up-regulates peroxisome proliferator-activated receptor gamma expression and reactive oxygen species production in MCF-7 cancer cells. *Eur. J. Cancer,* **2007**, *43*(17), 2590-2601.
[http://dx.doi.org/10.1016/j.ejca.2007.08.015] [PMID: 17911009]

[298]  Eid, S.Y.; El-Readi, M.Z.; Wink, M. Carotenoids reverse multidrug resistance in cancer cells by

interfering with ABC-transporters. *Phytomedicine,* **2012**, *19*(11), 977-987.
[http://dx.doi.org/10.1016/j.phymed.2012.05.010] [PMID: 22770743]

[299]  Gyémánt, N.; Tanaka, M.; Molnár, P.; Deli, J.; Mándoky, L.; Molnár, J. Reversal of multidrug resistance of cancer cells *in vitro*: modification of drug resistance by selected carotenoids. *Anticancer Res.,* **2006**, *26*(1A), 367-374.
[PMID: 16475720]

[300]  Kim, Y.; Seo, J.H.; Kim, H. β-Carotene and lutein inhibit hydrogen peroxide-induced activation of NF-κB and IL-8 expression in gastric epithelial AGS cells. *J. Nutr. Sci. Vitaminol. (Tokyo),* **2011**, *57*(3), 216-223.
[http://dx.doi.org/10.3177/jnsv.57.216] [PMID: 21908944]

[301]  Nepali, K.; Bande, M.S.; Dhar, K.L. Antitussive effects of azepino[2,1-b]quinazolones. *Med. Chem. Res.,* **2012**, *21*, 1271-1277.
[http://dx.doi.org/10.1007/s00044-011-9641-1]

[302]  Popoola, M.O.K.; Elbagory, A.M.; Ameer, F. Marrubiin. *Molecules,* **2013**, *18*(8), 9049-9060.
[http://dx.doi.org/10.3390/molecules18089049] [PMID: 23899837]

[303]  Ding, C.; Tian, Q.; Li, J.; Jiao, M.; Song, S.; Wang, Y.; Miao, Z.; Zhang, A. Structural Modification of Natural Product Tanshinone I Leading to Discovery of Novel Nitrogen-Enriched Derivatives with Enhanced Anticancer Profile and Improved Drug-like Properties. *J. Med. Chem.,* **2018**, *61*(3), 760-776.
[http://dx.doi.org/10.1021/acs.jmedchem.7b01259] [PMID: 29294282]

[304]  Das, B.; Chowdhury, C.; Kumar, D.; Sen, R.; Roy, R.; Das, P.; Chatterjee, M. Synthesis, cytotoxicity, and structure-activity relationship (SAR) studies of andrographolide analogues as anti-cancer agent. *Bioorg. Med. Chem. Lett.,* **2010**, *20*(23), 6947-6950.
[http://dx.doi.org/10.1016/j.bmcl.2010.09.126] [PMID: 20974534]

[305]  Yogeeswari, P.; Sriram, D. Betulinic acid and its derivatives: a review on their biological properties. *Curr. Med. Chem.,* **2005**, *12*(6), 657-666.
[http://dx.doi.org/10.2174/0929867053202214] [PMID: 15790304]

[306]  Zhang, B. Artemisinin-derived dimers as potential anticancer agents: Current developments, action mechanisms, and structure-activity relationships. *Arch Pharm (Weinheim),* **2020**, *353*(2), e1900240.
[http://dx.doi.org/10.1002/ardp.201900240] [PMID: 31797422]

# CHAPTER 3

# Recent Advances in Synthesis and the Anticancer Activity of Benzothiazole Hybrids as Anticancer Agents

**Rajesh Kumar**[1,*], **Monika Sharma**[1], **Sarita Sharma**[2] and **Rajesh K. Singh**[1,*]

[1] *Department of Pharmaceutical Chemistry, Shivalik College of Pharmacy, Nangal Distt. Rupnagar, 140126, Punjab, India*

[2] *Mount Carmel Sr.Sec. School, Rakkar Colony Distt. Una, 174303, Himachal Pradesh, India*

**Abstract:** Cancer is known as a silent killer that wreaks havoc on our immune systems. Cancer is the leading cause of death in the majority of cases. Resistance to anticancer drugs is becoming more agile, which encourages researchers to develop more effective cancer therapies. Heterocyclic compounds have long been important in advanced medicinal chemistry. Among the various heterocyclic scaffolds, benzothiazole (BT) is one of the most privileged moieties with a diverse range of biological activities such as anticancer, antidiabetic, anti-inflammatory, antiviral, antifungal, and so on. A large number of novel benzothiazole derivatives have been synthesized. Some of the mechanisms used by BT to treat cancer include tyrosine-kinase inhibitors, topoisomerase II inhibitors, CYP450 enzyme inhibitors, Abl kinase inhibitors, tubulin polymerase inhibitors, and HSP90 inhibitors. In this chapter, we will discuss various benzothiazole-hybrid compounds that optimise potency as well as anticancer activity in a concise manner. The goal of this chapter is to highlight recent research on benzothiazole scaffolds and their anticancer activity against various biological targets. The chapter will also provide updates on benzothiazole-containing drugs that are currently in clinical trials as well as those that have recently been granted patents.

**Keywords:** Anticancer activity, Benzothiazole, Bio targets, Heterocyclic scaffold, Structure-activity relationship (SAR), Synthesis.

## INTRODUCTION

Cancer is a life-threatening disease that transforms normal cells into infected cells, affecting our immune system. Various chemotherapeutic agents are used to treat various kinds of cancer. Conventional chemotherapeutic agents have higher toxicity in normal cells than in cancer cells, and they have low tolerability. As a

---

* **Corresponding author Rajesh Kumar and Rajesh Kumar:** Department of Pharmaceutical Chemistry, Shivalik College of Pharmacy, Nangal Distt. Rupnagar, 140126, Punjab, India; E-mails: rajeshduvedi@gmail.com, rksingh244@gmail.com

result, multi-targeted cytotoxic agents are used to overcome the limitations of the traditional treatment strategy due to their higher specificity towards abnormal cells and non-toxicity to normal cells. These agents have a wider therapeutic window and are more tolerable [1 - 3]. Recently, heterocyclic chemistry has exploded in popularity, and medicinal chemists are more interested than ever. More than 85% of drugs are derived from heterocyclic compounds. The primary reason for their wide applicability is that they function as biomimetics (having a structure similar to DNA base pairs). They also showed excellent pharmacological activity against a wide range of diseases [4 - 7]. The benzothiazole (BT) scaffold has a prominent position amongst all the heterocyclic compounds and exhibits a broad spectrum of pharmacological activities [8, 9]. Benzothiazole and its derivatives are abundant in nature and can be found in *Asparagus racemosus*, mango, roasted peanuts, soya bean milk, concentrated sterile milk, and other foods. Moreover, it can also be obtained by the isolation of boiled potatoes, green tea, and styrax. Some derivatives of benzothiazole have also been collected from fungi (*Aspergillus clavatus*), marine fish (*Cyprinodon variegates*), and also from culture extracts of Micrococcus sp. obtained by the fermentation process. It can also be manufactured on a large scale [10]. Benzothiazole is a bicyclic ring system formed by the conjugation of a benzene ring and a heterocyclic thiazole ring. Thiazole is a 5-membered ring system having hetero-atoms such as N and S and is mainly responsible for various pharmacological activities. Because of the ease of synthesis and the excellent biological profile of benzothiazole and its derivatives, there has been a surge in interest in the design and development of novel benzothiazole analogs. They have the potential to be used as chemotherapeutic agents and can also aid in the treatment of resistance to various anticancer drugs [11].

## BENZOTHIAZOLE CHEMISTRY AND NOMENCLATURE

In 1887, thiazole was first discussed by Hantzsch and Waber. Afterward, the structure of thiazole was confirmed in 1889. The numbering in the thiazole ring starts with the heteroatom S (sulfur). The fusion of the benzene ring at the 4, 5-position of the thiazole ring constitutes the core nucleus, 1, 3-benzothiazole, which is denoted as BT. Similar to thiazole, the sulphur atom in the benzothiazole scaffold is given higher priority [12].

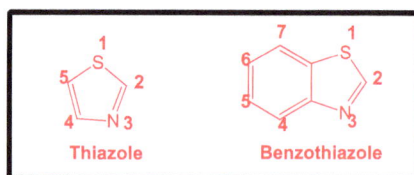

**Fig. (1).** Numbering and nomenclature of given heterocyclic compounds.

The IUPAC name of benzothiazole is 1, 3-benzothiazole or benzo[*d*]thiazole. The other names are benzosulfonazole, and 1-thia-3-azaindene. The tautomerism in benzothiazole-2-thiol is shown in Fig. (**2**).

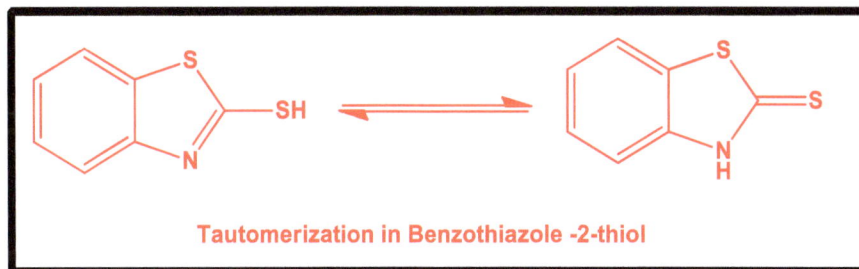

**Tautomerization in Benzothiazole -2-thiol**

**Fig. (2).** Tautomerization in the nucleus of benzothiazole-2-thiol.

Benzothiazole is a yellow, slightly viscous liquid having a boiling point of 227-228 °C and a melting point of 2 °C. The molecular formula of benzothiazole is $C_7H_5NS$, and its weight is 135.19 g/mol. It exhibits slight solubility in water and high solublility in ether. The $^1$H-NMR spectra provide a variety of signals such as 7.46, 7.51, 7.94, 8.14, 8.971 ppm [9].

## SYNTHETIC METHODOLOGY

In 1887, A. W. Hofmann was the first researcher who synthesized 2-substituted benzothiazoles due to their wide range of biological activities and their simple synthetic mechanism of cyclization [13]. Conventional methodologies for the synthesis of benzothiazole derivatives include condensation reactions of 2-aminothiophenols with substituted nitriles, aldehydes, carboxylic acids, acyl chlorides, or esters. But some limitations were observed in these traditional synthetic methods, such as in the preparation of readily oxidizable 2-aminothiophenols [14]. Moreover, microwave irradiation was used to prepare BT analogues by the reactions of *o*-aminothiophenol with chlorocinnamaldehydes, dibenzyl disulfides with *o*-aminothiophenol, reduction of *o, o'*-dinitrodiphenyl disulfide, and the reaction of S-aryl thiobenzoate with arylhaloamines, from 1, 2, 3-benzodithiazole-2-oxides, radical cyclization of benzyne intermediates, and Grignard reactions of aryl isothiocyanates [15]. A huge number of catalysts, namely, $ZrOCl_2.8H_2O$ [16], TMSCl [17], PCC [18], nano-CeO2 [19], cyanide [20], boron trifluoride etherate [21], mesoporous CdS nanospheres [22], silica-supported nano-copper (II) oxide [23], can be used as catalysts to prepare BT derivatives.

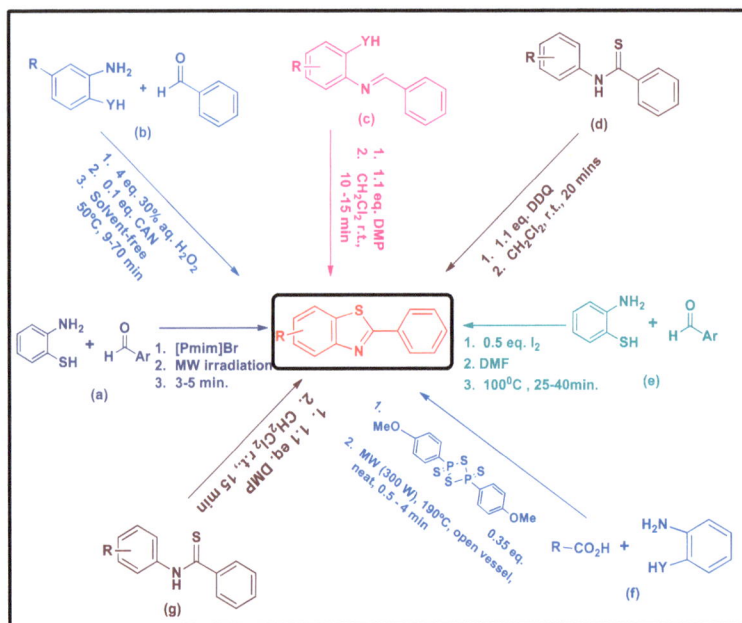

**Scheme. (1).** The conventional methods used for the synthesis of benzothiazole by using different catalysts (before 2010) [24 - 30].

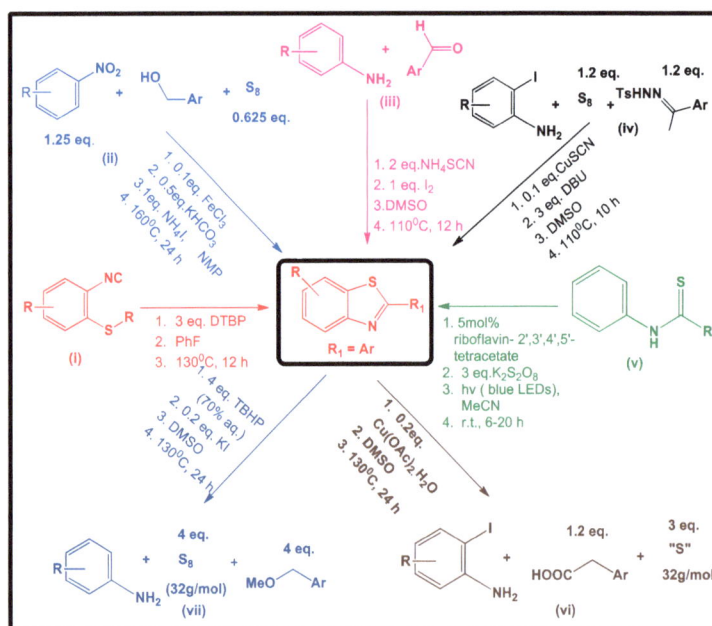

**Scheme. (2).** Various synthetic strategies are used to synthesize novel series of benzothiazole-containing compounds from 2011 to 2021 [31 - 37].

A few years ago, rapid progress occurred in the field of nanotechnology that fulfilled all the principles of green chemistry. Various nanocatalysts have been used for synthesizing BT analogs because they offer several merits over conventional strategies, including a fast synthetic route, excellent yield of the product with high selectivity, easy recovery, and recyclability. Moreover, their nanostructures help in the delivery of drugs specifically to the target site [38].

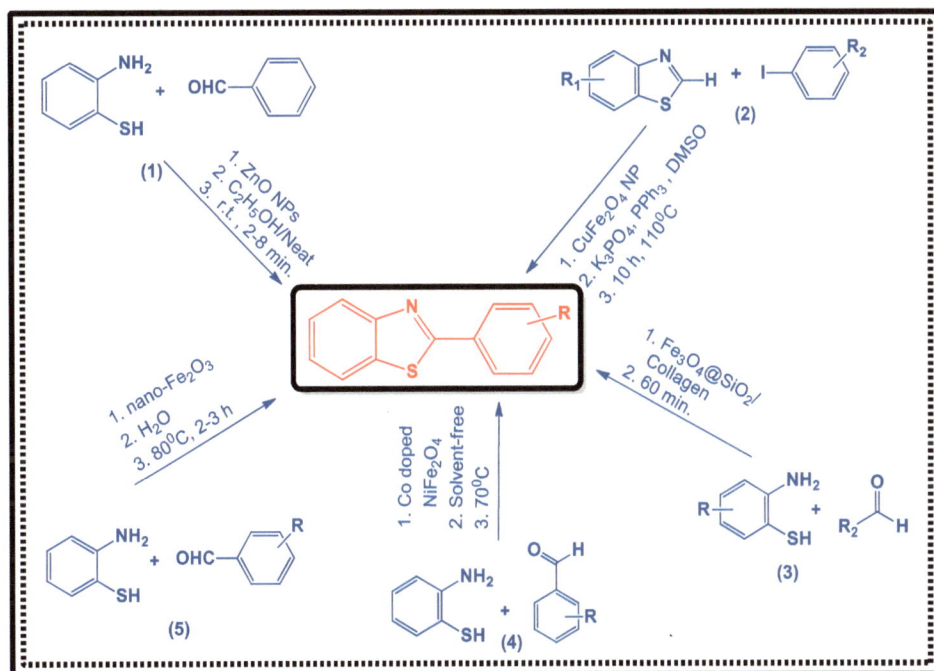

**Scheme. (3).** The advanced methodology for the synthesis of benzothiazole derivatives by employing nanocatalysts [39 - 43].

## BIOLOGICAL ACTIVITIES

The popularity of benzothiazole scaffolds is due to their enormous biological activities. The most important pharmacological activities include anticancer, antimicrobial, fungicidal, anticonvulsant, anti-inflammatory, anti-tubercular, antioxidant, *etc*. BT and its analogs have been explored as selective fatty acid amide hydrolase inhibitors, stearoyl co-enzyme A δ-9 desaturase inhibitors, anti-histamine specific to $H_2$ receptor, and $LTD_4$ receptor antagonists. It has also been used for the treatment of neurodegenerative disorders like Alzheimer's disease. Furthermore, any substitution on the benzothiazole scaffold affects the selectivity towards the target site, potency as well as biological activity. So, the nature and position of substitution are very crucial for the specific activity of a compound.

The benzothiazole nucleus is the basic unit in a variety of chemotherapeutic agents, which makes it the prominent nucleus for the synthesis and generation of various drugs, as shown in Fig. (**3**).

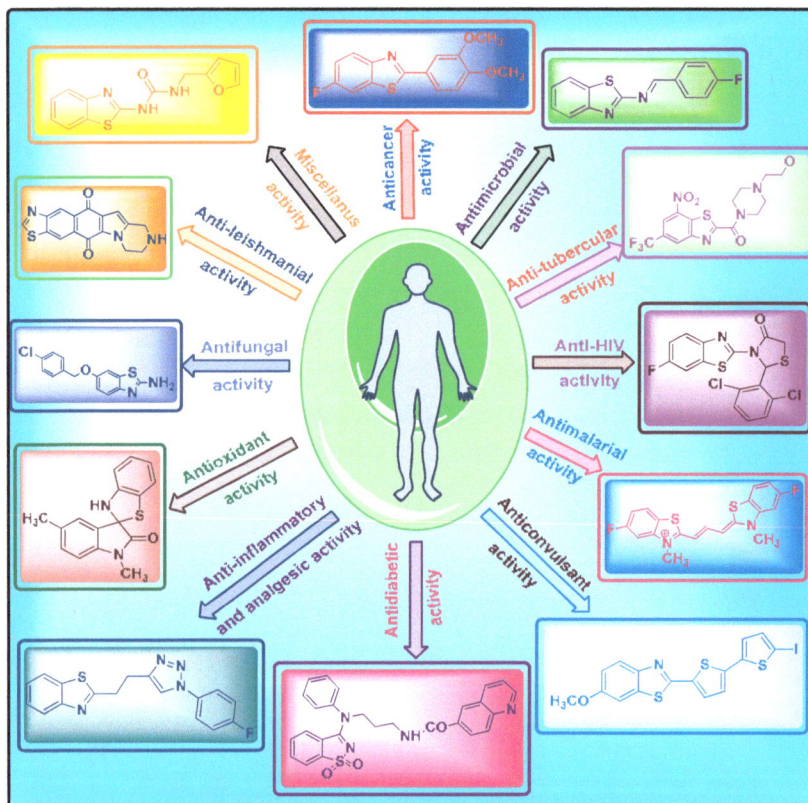

**Fig. (3).** Benzothiazole as a lead compound.

## Benzothiazole and its Derivatives as Anticancer Agents

A huge number of chemotherapeutic agents are already available on the market. But it becomes ineffective due to the quick resistance response of malignant cells toward antitumor drugs. As a result, the number of deaths increased all across the world. It encourages the medicinal chemist to identify a new lead compound that can show high selectivity, potency and have fewer chances of developing resistance. BT is chosen as one of the famous scaffolds that exhibit excellent anticancer activity. In conventional cancer therapy, therapies attack both normal and cancer cells, resulting in a broad spectrum of side effects. However, targeted drugs (such as EGFR tyrosine kinase inhibitors) attack cancer cells rather than normal cells, resulting in a better safety profile, less body damage, and more patient comfort [44, 45].

## Antimitotic Agent

Benzothiazole analogues are used to inhibit the abnormal growth of cancer cells *via* various mechanisms. Tubulin polymerase is one of the key target enzymes that is used to inhibit the abnormal proliferation of the cell. Microtubule-targeting agents (MTA) are the most widely used for cancer therapy. Microtubules are formed by the polymerization of α-and β-subunits of tubulin (the real part of a protein), and they are an essential component of the cytoskeleton and have been found in all eukaryotic cells. It has played a pivotal role in cell division, motility, cell shape maintenance, and transport of proteins and vesicles. It also helps in the separation of chromosomes during the mitosis cell cycle [46].

Antitubulin agents are one of the essential targets in the cancer war. Antimitotic drugs can stop the mitosis cell cycle. Vinca alkaloids and taxanes have been used for a long time due to their good cytotoxic activity. Vinca alkaloids (vincristine, vinblastine) inhibit the tubulin polymerization process, resulting in microtubule stabilization. Conversely, taxoid acts by inhibiting microtubule depolymerization. As MTA perturbs the function of mitotic spindles, it causes metaphase arrest [47, 48]. The mechanism by which antimitotic agents inhibit the tubulin polymerization process is depicted in Fig. (**4**).

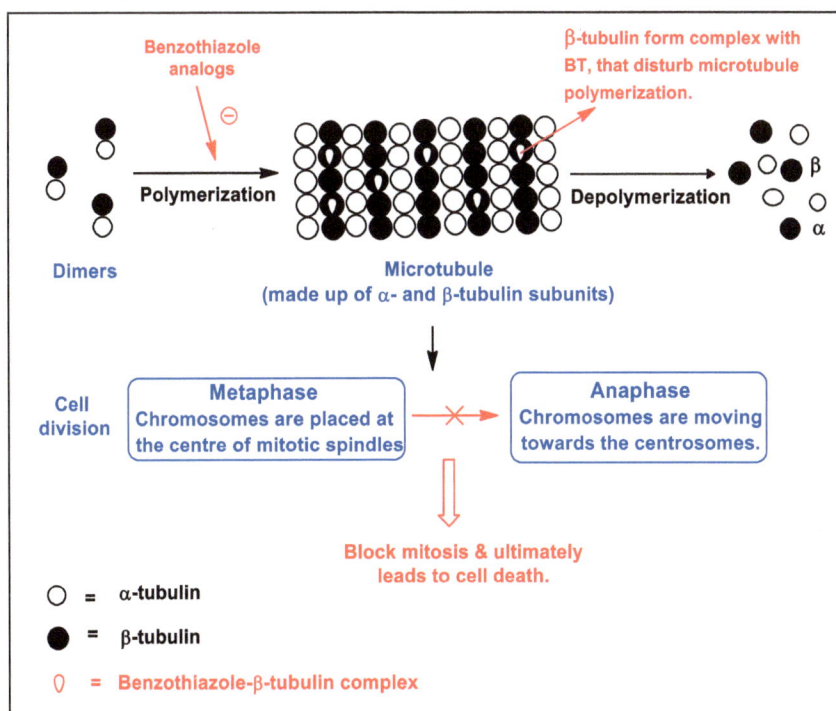

**Fig. (4).** Mechanism of action of benzothiazole-containing compounds as anti-mitotic agents [47].

Besides vinca alkaloids and taxanes, combretastatin A-4 (CA-4) is also a natural compound that exerts good anti-tumor action. It is a member of the stilbenes and was isolated from the bark of *Combretum caffrum* and *Combretum leprosum* species [49]. Because of its high cytotoxicity toward infected cells, it is used in the design of hybrid compounds.

In 2012, Kamal *et al.* synthesized enormous analogues of hybrid combretastatin–amidobenzothiazole compounds. Further, their anticancer activity has been evaluated against several human cancers (lung, leukemia, colon, melanoma, ovarian, renal, prostate, and breast cancer) at the National Cancer Institute (USA). Compound **1** (Fig. **5**) displayed good anti-proliferative activity against all the above cell lines with a $GI_{50}$ value of 0.019–11 μM. The *cis*-configuration of the olefinic bond has been playing a pivotal role in binding to the colchicine-binding site. The tubulin polymerization process has been inhibited by arresting the mitotic cell cycle at the $G_2/M$ phase. It further activates the caspase-3 enzyme, resulting in apoptotic cell death. Docking studies revealed that compound **1** is directly attached to the β-tubulin subunit onto the colchicine binding site (PDB code: 3E22) and results in extensive hydrophobic contacts of Lys 254 with the binding pocket of the chain [50].

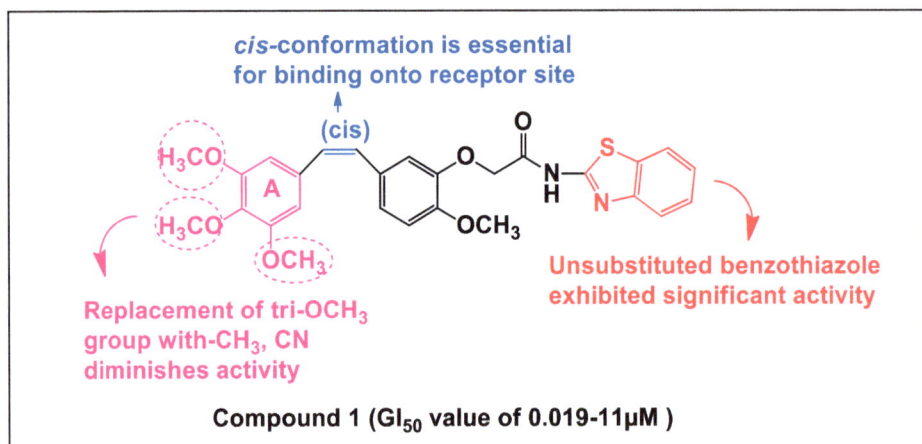

**Fig. (5).** Combretastatin bearing 2-amidobenzothiazole acts as an inhibitor of tubulin polymerase enzyme.

Furthermore, the innovative analogues of colchicine (structural similarities to CA-4) containing benzothiazole compounds have been incorporated into the study by Subba Rao *et al.* Colchicine is a natural alkaloid obtained from *Colchicum autumnale* and has demonstrated remarkable cytotoxicity against several cancer cell lines. It is a privileged structure and is present in a large number of anticancer drugs, such as 5F-203 and its Phortress prodrug. The rationale behind these hybrid analogues is to enhance their antiproliferative effect. Compounds **2** and **3** (Fig. **6**) showed excellent inhibitory activity towards the lung cancer cell line (A549) due to their high binding affinity for the β-tubulin subunit of a microtubule. It further perturbed microtubule assembly, polymerization, and finally cell division at metaphase. The *cis*-configuration of the olefinic bond has been retained by substituting the olefin bond with a tetrazole or triazole ring. It maintains the conformation geometry that is required for interacting with the colchicine-binding site [51].

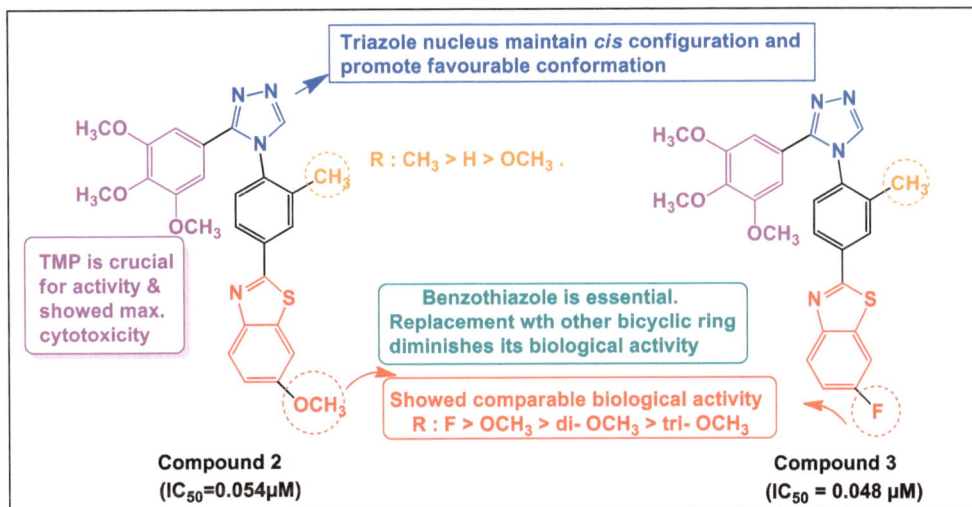

**Fig. (6).** Colchicine derivatives fused with benzothiazole moiety reported good cytotoxicity towards the lung cancer cell line (A549).

The *cis*-restricted benzothiazole analogues clubbed with mimics of combretastatin A-4 were synthesized by Ashraf *et al.* in 2016. Compounds **4** and **5** (Fig. **7**) are most commonly used because of their high potency and relatively easy synthetic route. They displayed excellent cytotoxicity against various cancer cell lines such as human ovarian, murine lymphocytic leukemia, and colon cancer cell lines. The pyridine nucleus has been inserted in place of the olefin bonds to restrict the *cis* conformation. These compounds mainly act by disturbing microtubule assembly, which arrests the mitotic cell division at the G$_2$/M phase. Docking studies also revealed that these analogues had a high affinity for various amino acid residues in the β-tubulin subunit [52].

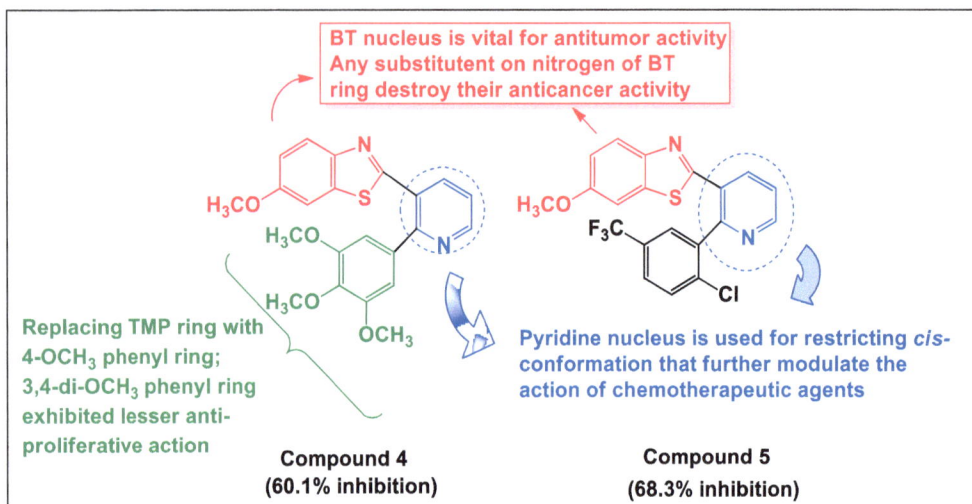

**Fig. (7).** *Cis*-restricted benzothiazole analogs act as a mitotic inhibitor.

A series of 2-aminobenzothiazole derivatives were fused with 2-anilinonicotinyl and were analyzed against several cancer cell lines for their cytotoxic effects. Out of numerous derivatives, only one compound (Compound **6**) (Fig. **8**) possesses more inhibitory activity in the treatment of cervical cancer. On the other hand, the remaining derivatives showed moderate cytotoxicity in human leukaemia HL-60 cells with $IC_{50}$ values ranging from 0.08 to 0.7 µM [53].

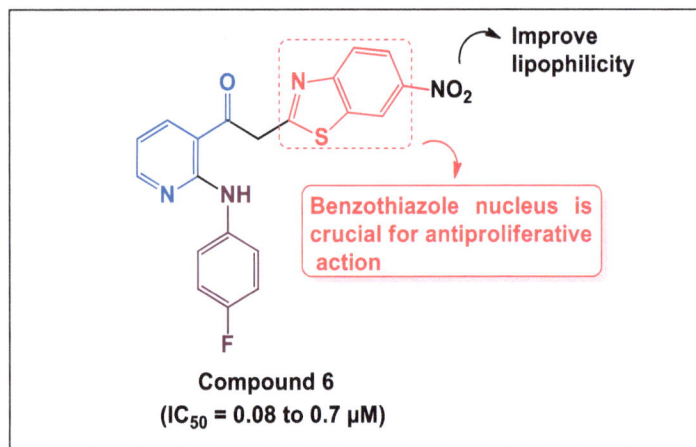

**Fig. (8).** Benzothiazole bearing 2-anilinonicotinyl analogs as anti-tubulin inhibitors.

In 2017, the numbers of 2-anilinopyridinyl-BT Schiff's bases were synthesized by Shaik *et al*. Moreover, their antiproliferative activity has been investigated against

A549, MCF7, and DU145 cell lines by the SRB assay. Compound **7** (Fig. **9**) exhibited good activity against all these cell lines, with $GI_{50}$ values of 17.0 µM, 12.0 µM, and 3.8 µM, respectively. The SAR study revealed that the presence of trimethoxy groups on the benzothiazole moiety and substituents at the 4th position of the aryl ring of the 2-anilinopyridinyl moiety, showed significant cytotoxicity. However, the effect of fluoro and chloro substituents on the benzothiazole nucleus was reported to have good cytotoxicity. A docking study was carried out; compound **7** binds at the interface of α and β chains of tubulin heterodimer (PDB code: 3E22) and is formed by several amino acid residues such as Asn101, Thr179, Ala180, Val181, Asn249, Ala250, Leu252, Arg253, Lys254, Leu255, Lys352, Thr353, *etc.*, surrounding the binding pocket [54].

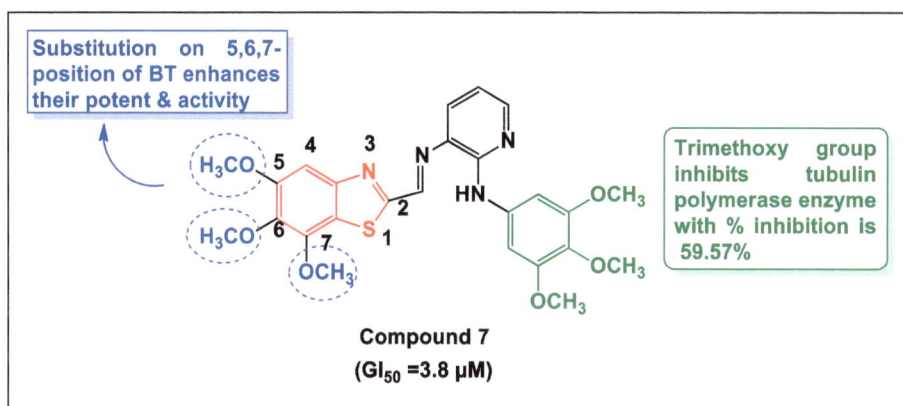

**Fig. (9).** Benzothiazole having 2-anilinopyridinyl Schiff's bases depicted maximum cytotoxicity and inhibitor of the mitosis cell cycle.

In 2018, a new class of hybrid pyrazole-benzothiazole derivatives was designed and prepared. Pyrazole-containing nitrogen heteroatoms are more abundant in natural as well as synthetic products and have excellent biological activity. Firstly, the Vilsmeyer-Haack reaction was used to synthesize pyrazole. Then it was fused with the benzothiazole motif by linkage of hydrazine or hydrazide *via* the formation of an imine bond in compounds **8** and **9**. Moreover, the exploration of their cytotoxic potential was estimated by utilizing an Allium assay. The design of hybrid molecules is an effective methodology to synthesize more active compounds. Likewise, pyrazole–benzothiazole hybrids were incorporated in their research work to enhance cytotoxicity against various cancer cells. Finally, the hydrazide linkage between pyrazole and benzothiazole was found to be more active than the hydrazine linkage (Fig. **10**) [55].

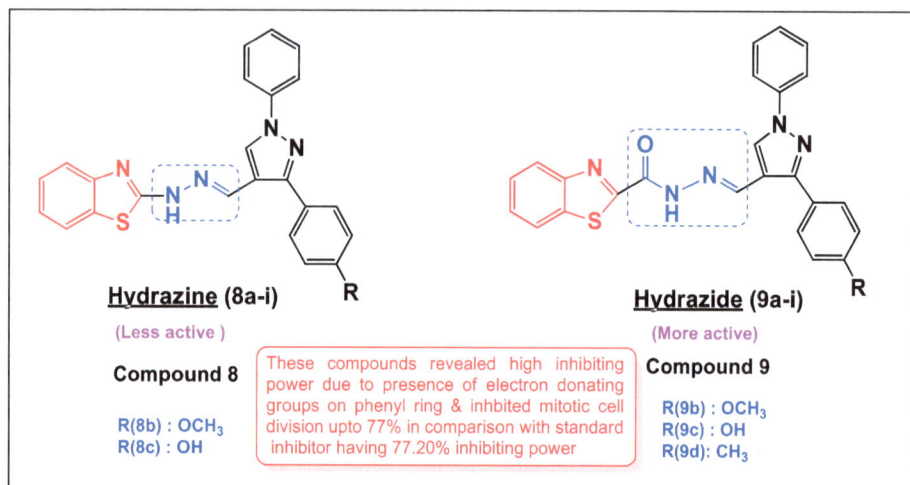

**Fig. (10).** Benzothiazole conjugated with pyrazole through two different linkages –hydrazine and hydrazide act as antimitotic agents.

Song *et al.* synthesized enormous analogues of tertiary amide-BT in 2020. Among all the reported compounds, only compound **10** (Fig. **11**) exerted excellent inhibition against HCT-116 cells, SGC-7901 cells, Mac-803 cells, and PC-3 cells. It is a potent inhibitor of the tubulin polymerase enzyme. It mainly acts by binding to the colchicine binding site of β-tubulin with an $IC_{50}$ value of 1.9 μM. It is typically obtained by opening the β-lactam ring and then optimizing a structure by substituting the BT moiety [56].

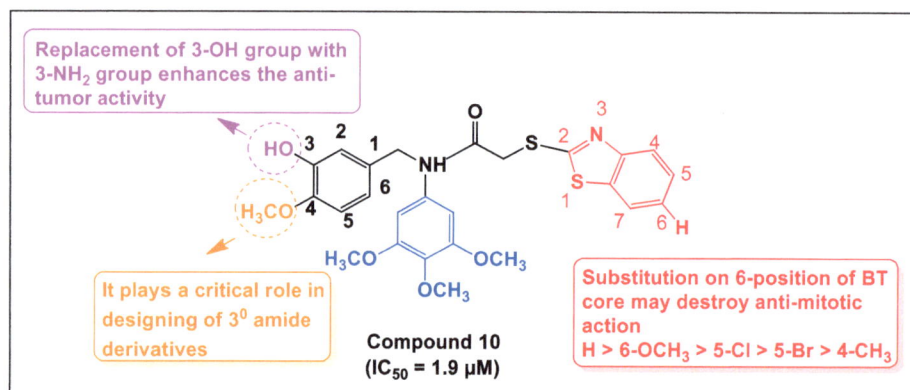

**Fig. (11).** Tertiary amide benzothiazole conjugates act as effective antiproliferative agents.

## A Tyrosine Kinase Inhibitor

TK is a protein kinase enzyme; it is one of the oldest enzymes that regulate cell growth [57, 58]. enzyme has been sub-divided into 2 major categories. First, receptor tyrosine kinases (RTKs) are present on the surface of the cell. The second type is non-receptor tyrosine kinase (NRTKs), which are found in the cell's cytoplasm [59].The induction and progression of a malignant tumour are mainly due to disturbances in the function of the tyrosine kinase enzyme. The tyrosine kinase is one of the major targets for cancer treatment [60].

## Epidermal Growth Factor Receptor (EGFR) Inhibitors

The first RTK enzyme, EGFR (Epidermal Growth Factor Receptor), regulates cell growth, differentiation, and survival [61].The second most popular kinase target for cancer therapy is HER2-TK. Its function is to control the growth of epithelial cells. Overactivation of HER2 leads to the production of aggressive metastatic breast cancer [62]. The third one is the thymidylate synthase enzyme whose activity is dependent on folate and it is the key enzyme utilized in the pathway of de novo biosynthesis of TMP. This enzyme is also crucial for cell growth. TS inhibition causes a deficiency of thymidylate, DNA damage, and activation of apoptosis [63]. The mode of action of anti-EGFR agents is depicted in Fig. (**12**).

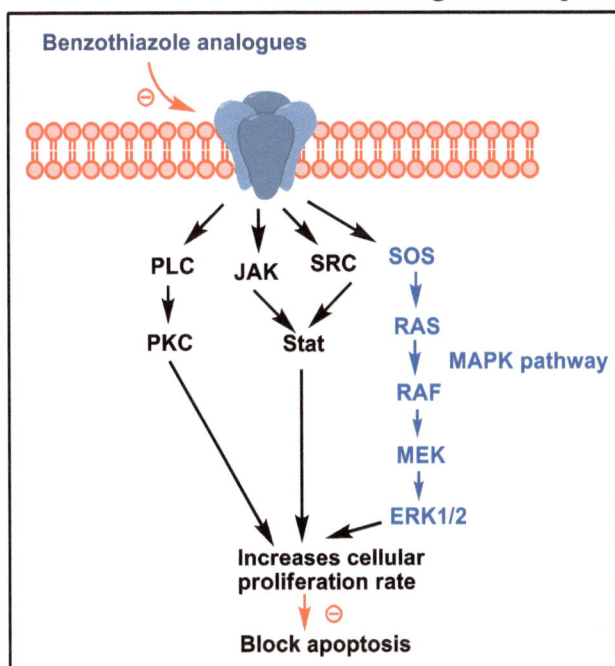

**Fig. (12).** Blockage of signal cascade pathway for combating cancer and acting as anti-EGFR agents [6].

Benzothiazole analogues work by perturbing the mutated therapeutic mechanism that is responsible for the production of cancer cells. The innovative derivatives of 2-phenyl-1 and 3-benzothiazole were designed and prepared. Afterward, all the compounds were explored for their anti-breast cancer activity. A few compounds showed moderate to good cytotoxicity to the MCF-7 breast cell line. It acts by competing with the ATP-binding site. SAR showed that any substitution in the benzothiazole motif affects the antiproliferative activity. Compounds **11** and **12** (with mono-substituted halogen) act as excellent cancer cell growth inhibitors in compounds **11**, **12**, and **13** (Fig. **13**). In contrast, di-substituted halogens on the BT moiety at positions 5, 6, and 7 significantly reduce their antiproliferative activity, as seen in compound 13 [64].

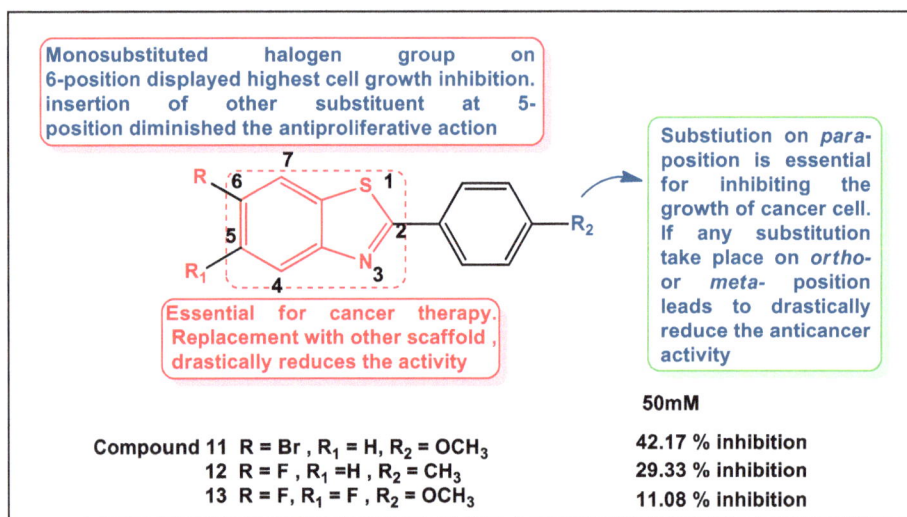

**Fig. (13).** Substituted 2-phenyl benzothiazole analogs as EGFR-TK inhibitor.

In 2012, Noolvi *et al.* reported that the 2-amino benzothiazole nucleus acts as a potent anti-EGFR agent. He reported that when the quinazoline core was replaced with the benzothiazole core, there was better inhibition of the binding site of the EGFR-TK enzyme. Based on the SAR study, the benzothiazole scaffold is essential for anticancer activity. But when the substituted aniline motif is attached to the benzothiazole core at position 2, it improves their hydrophobicity. The more lipophilic nature of antitumor agents at the binding site also enhances their potency and efficacy. Compound **14** (Fig. **14**) inhibited the HOP-92 (non-small cell lung) tumour cell line better, with $GI_{50}$ values of 7.18 to 10.8 μM [65].

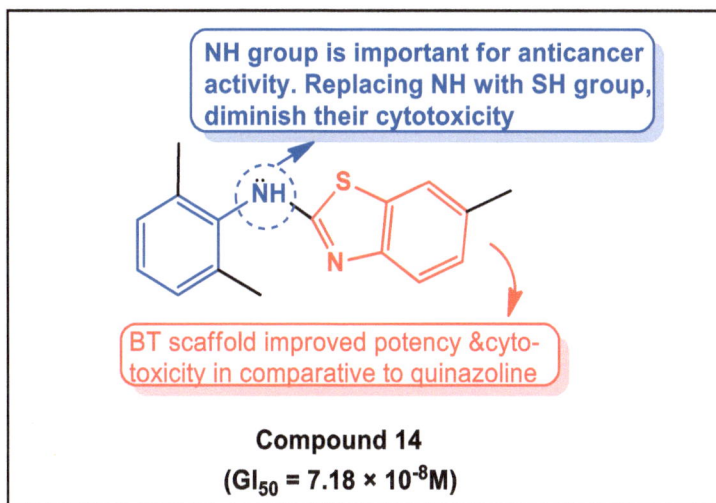

**Fig. (14).** 2-Aminobenzothiazole derivatives exerted more potent and cytotoxic EGFR inhibitors.

Gaber *et al*. (2014) synthesized 19 hybrid analogues of benzothiazole attached to different heterocyclic compounds. Afterward, screening was done by exploring these compounds against 60 subpanels of cancer cell lines. The most potent compounds were chosen. Those selectively and competitively inhibited ATP binding sites present in the EGFR domain at 10 µM concentrations. Compound **15** has demonstrated high potency, higher growth inhibition and also acts as a broad-spectrum anticancer agent. In compound **15** (Fig. **15**), the 2,5-dioxopyrrolidine motif was introduced to enhance the affinity towards the receptor of EGFR-TK [66].

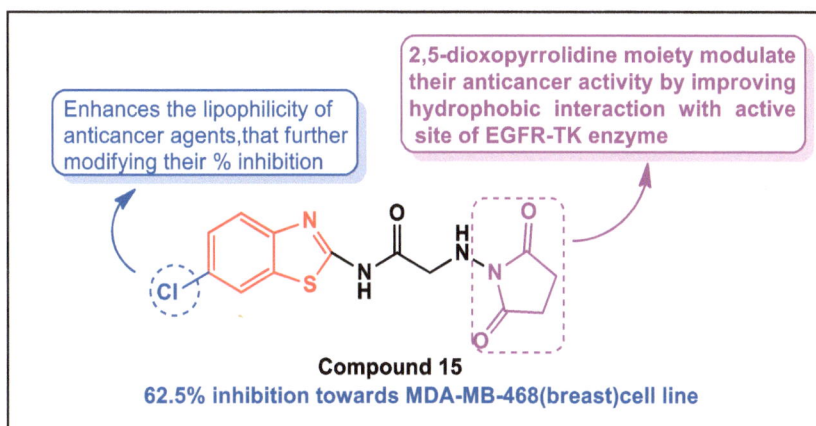

**Fig. (15).** Benzothiazole bearing pyrrolidine behaves like an anti-EGFR agent.

Moreover, Labib *et al.* (2018) synthesized various derivatives of benzothiazole-containing compounds. The evaluation of these compounds was done to identify their EGFR inhibition potential. Compound **16** (Fig. **16**) has shown better cytotoxicity against the human hepatic adenocarcinoma (HepG2) cell line. It was found to have an $IC_{50}$ value of 0.027-0.033 µM in comparison with the reference drug 5-FU ($IC_{50}$ = 0.038 µM). The compound **16** has high potency and also exerted good inhibition (47.28%). On the one hand, activation of caspase-3 and caspase-9 causes apoptosis, but this compound inhibits caspases more effectively in the $G_0$-$G_1$ phase [67].

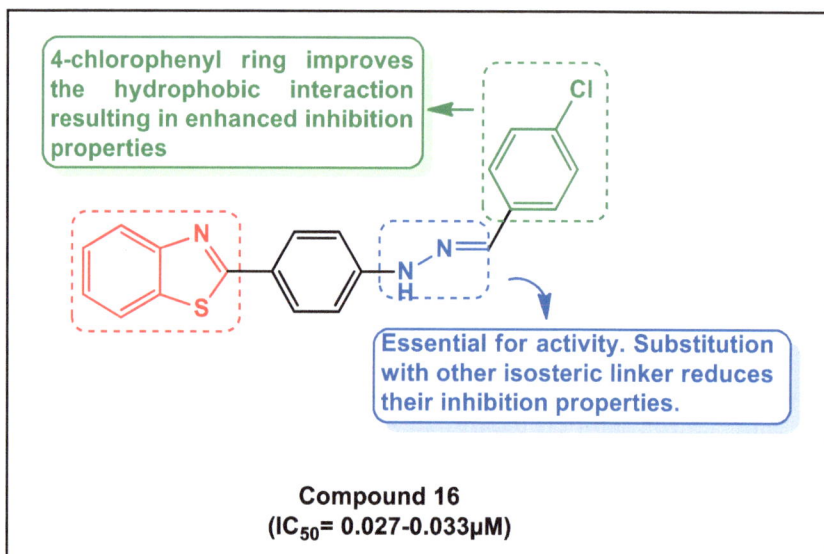

**Compound 16**
**($IC_{50}$= 0.027-0.033µM)**

**Fig. (16).** Benzothiazole conjugated with azole–hydrazone analogs exerted moderate inhibition against EGFR.

In addition, a number of novel benzothiazole-containing compounds were investigated. All essential groups with higher cytotoxicity against cancer cells were chosen. It is then combined in a single structure to produce compounds with higher cytotoxicity and lower resistance to anticancer agents. Abdellatif created and synthesized a number of BT nucleus derivatives with pyrimidine moieties. Only compound **17** (Fig. **17**) demonstrated moderate to good activity among all designed compounds. The phenyl ring at C-4 of the pyrimidine core was replaced with a chromone core, which modulated its activity. These benzothiazole derivatives compete for binding on the catalytic site of TK with ATP. The hydrophobic region II of EGFR and HER2 and the benzo-nucleus of BT have formed hydrophobic interactions. Similarly, the phenyl or chromone moiety on the pyrimidine nucleus participates in hydrophobic interactions [68].

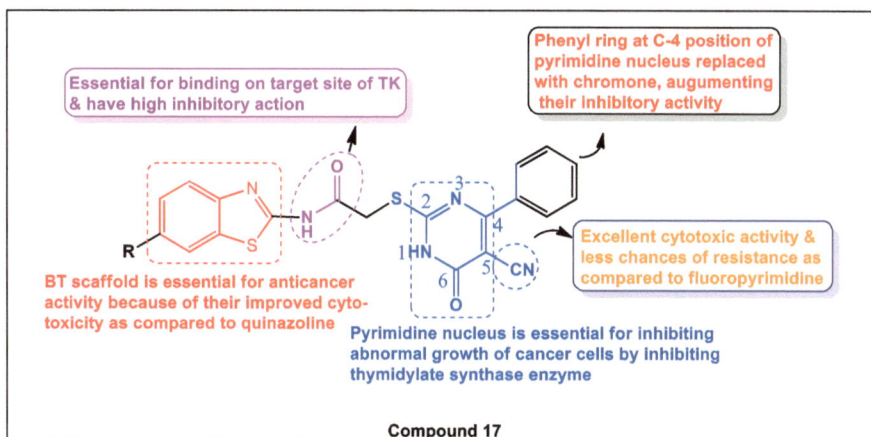

**Fig. (17).** Benzothiazole fused with pyrimidine ring and exhibited high cytotoxicity towards tumor cells.

The researchers created and synthesized a novel benzothiazole-containing hydrazone hybrid compound. After testing their anticancer activity *in vitro*, only two derivatives were chosen from a large number of compounds. These designed compounds have high potency and activity against 5 different cancer cell lines, including hepatocellular carcinoma (HepG2), colorectal carcinoma (HCT-116), mammary gland cancer (MCF-7), prostate cancer (PC-3), and epithelioid carcinoma (HeLa). Compounds **18a** and **18b** (Fig. **18**) inhibited EGFR excellently, with $IC_{50}$ values of 24.58 nM and 30.42 nM, respectively. In comparison to the standard lapatinib drug, the inhibition rate was 50.7–73.1% [69].

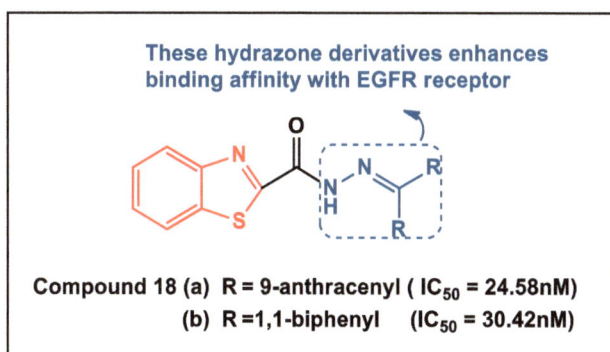

**Fig. (18).** Hybrid derivatives of a benzothiazole-hydrazone act against EGFR with more potency.

## A Bcr-Abl Kinase Inhibitor

c-Abl is a type of NRTK (non-receptor tyrosine kinase). It is a gene that regulates cellular processes such as cell division, adhesion, differentiation, and stress response. The reverse translocation between chromosomes 9, (Abelson kinase) gene and 22 Bcr (Breakpoint-cluster region) genes interferes with the function of the Abl gene (a proto-oncogene). The fusion of these two genes results in the formation of a chimeric bcr-abl gene. It is responsible for the uncontrolled cell growth that leads to the onset and progression of cancer [70]. The formation of the Philadelphia (Ph) chromosome is a sign of chronic myelogenous leukaemia (CML). Chronic myeloid leukaemia is a type of leukaemia that affects hematopoietic stem cells.

The Bcr-Abl kinase has been identified as a novel target, and its inhibition is required for CML treatment. Imatinib (STI-571) is a high-potency first-generation inhibitor of the Bcr-Abl gene that was approved by the FDA in 2001 for the treatment of CML. Patients with advanced CML are resistant to imatinib due to a point mutation in the bcr-abl gene. Second-generation drugs (dasatinib and nilotinib) were designed to address the issue of imatinib resistance. However, these drugs have no effect on the Abl-mutated gene. As a result, the researchers in this field generated a 3rd generation drug-like ponatinib by exploiting the action of the abl-T315I mutated kinase. However, these drugs have no effect on the Abl-mutated gene. As a result, the researchers in this field developed a 3rd generation drug-like ponatinib by exploiting the action of the abl-T315I mutated kinase. Nocodazole, which was developed a few years ago, inhibits both wild type and T315I mutant Abl [71]. The mechanisms of inhibition of the Abl-kinase enzyme for cancer therapy are as follows [72] (Fig. **19**).

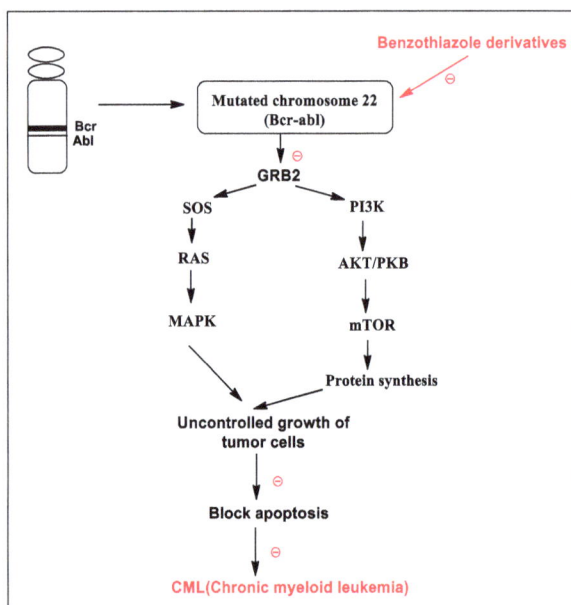

**Fig. (19).** Mechanism of action of Bcr-abl kinase inhibitor for cancer therapy.

*N*-methylpicolinamide is an imperative motif that is present in almost all potent anticancer agents with desirable physicochemical properties. Incorporation of *N*-methyl picolinamide at position 6 of the BT nucleus enhances their efficacy at the cellular and enzymatic level. The various drugs are used for the treatment of CML (1st, 2nd, and 3rd generation). But resistance to these drugs (like imatinib) fascinated the researchers, who developed a more effective, highly potent drug for CML treatment. Some of these molecules are in a stage of clinical development or pre-clinical studies. For instance, HS-438, **19** (Fig. **20**) and HS-543, **20** (Fig. **21**), these molecules displayed good inhibitory action on the $Abl^{T315I}$ *mutant* with an $IC_{50}$ value of 0.064 nM and 0.015 nM, respectively [73].

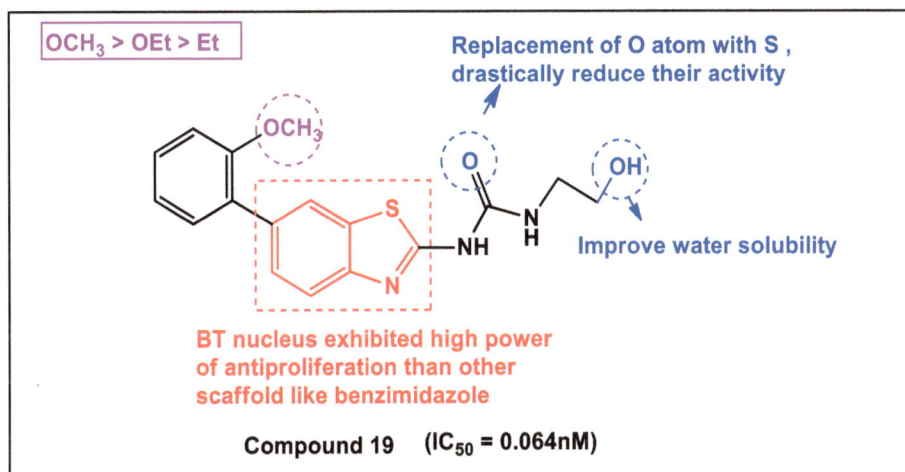

**Fig. (20).** Benzothiazole hybrid compound HS-438 as a potent inhibitor of Abl kinase enzyme.

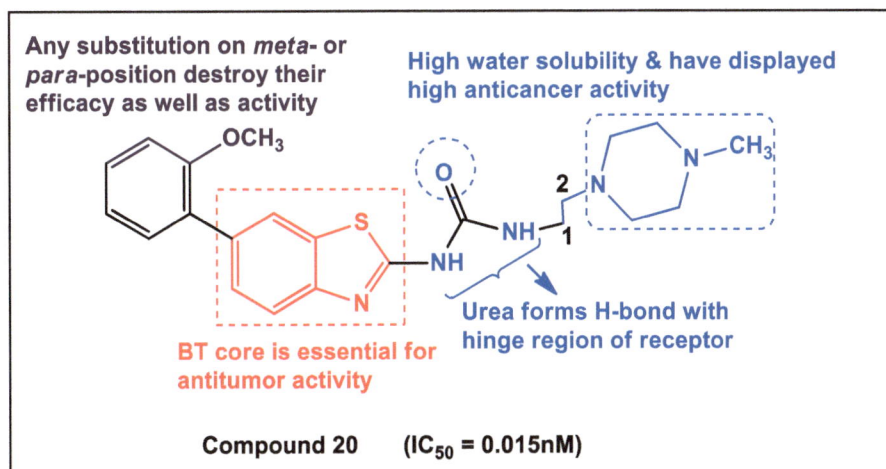

**Fig. (21).** HS-543 depicted excellent cytotoxicity towards mutant ABL-T315I kinase enzyme.

In 2015, El-Damasy *et al.* designed seventeen analogues of benzothiazole conjugated with picolinamide, and after screening, only eight were selected. Of the eight, only compound **21** (Fig. **22**) has more potency and has shown the best ABL kinase inhibition. In-*vitro* studies showed that compound **21** was found to have an $IC_{50}$ of 18.2 nM and 39.9 nM against both native and mutated *T315I Abl*. On the other hand, *in-vivo* studies showed 89.8% inhibition against K-562 leukaemia cells at 10 µM concentration. SAR studies demonstrated that the addition of a polar hydrophilic motif at the terminal of the side-chain improved the selectivity of the compound towards K-562. It has been demonstrated that the formation of H-bonds by the ether bridge, urea, and the nitrogen terminal of piperazine improves binding affinity at the receptor site [74].

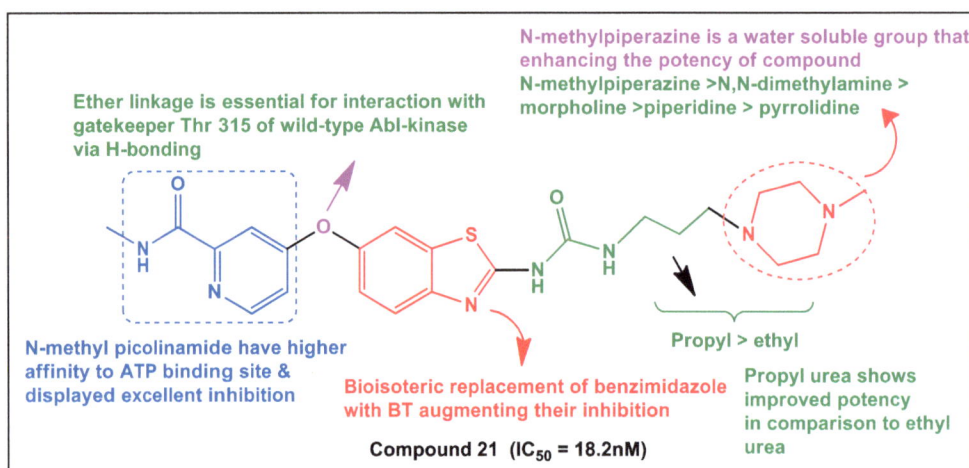

**Fig. (22).** Benzothiazole-picolinamide derivatives exerted excellent inhibition towards Abl kinase.

## PI3K/AKT/mTOR Enzyme Inhibitors

These enzymes are involved in a variety of cellular and metabolic processes, including cell proliferation, survival, metabolism, metastasis, and angiogenesis [75]. Tumorigenesis is caused by overactivation of the PI3k/AKT/mTOR signaling pathway caused by point mutations in PI3K genes or repression of tumour suppressor enzyme phosphatase and PTEN (tensin gene) [76]. Deregulation of these enzymes is responsible for the development of cancers such as ovarian, breast, and endometrial cancer [77]. To combat cancer, this signalling pathway is disrupted. Several inhibitors of these enzymes (alone or in combination) are currently in clinical trials [78]. The mechanism by which benzothiazole analogs interrupt the therapeutic signaling pathway of carcinogenesis is depicted below (Fig. **23**) [79, 80].

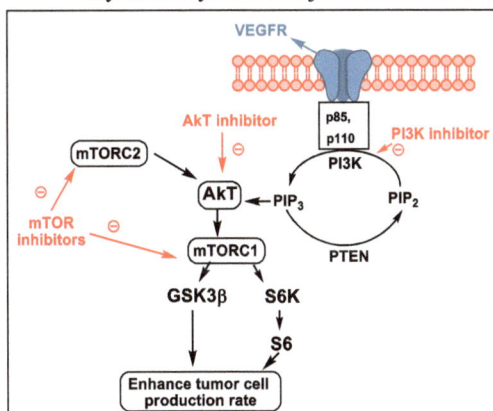

**Fig. (23).** Multiple target chemotherapeutic agents act as PI3K/AkT/mTOR inhibitors.

Li *et al.* designed novel hybrid compounds in 2014 by fusing a benzothiazole scaffold with a 2-substituted-3-sulfonylaminobenzamide ring. For cancer therapy, these were tested *in vitro* against MCF-7, A-549, HCT-116, and U-87MG cancer cell lines. It was also identified as a novel approach for cancer treatment by inhibiting the PI3K/AKT/mTOR signal transduction pathway. The SAR revealed that substituting a benzamide moiety for a substituted pyridine nucleus can more effectively disrupt the PI3K/AKT/mTOR mechanism with high cytotoxicity. Compounds **22** and **23** (Fig. **24**) demonstrated enhanced cytotoxicity against the aforementioned cancer cell lines, with $IC_{50}$ values of 1.95, 0.50, 1.70, and 4.75 µM, respectively [81].

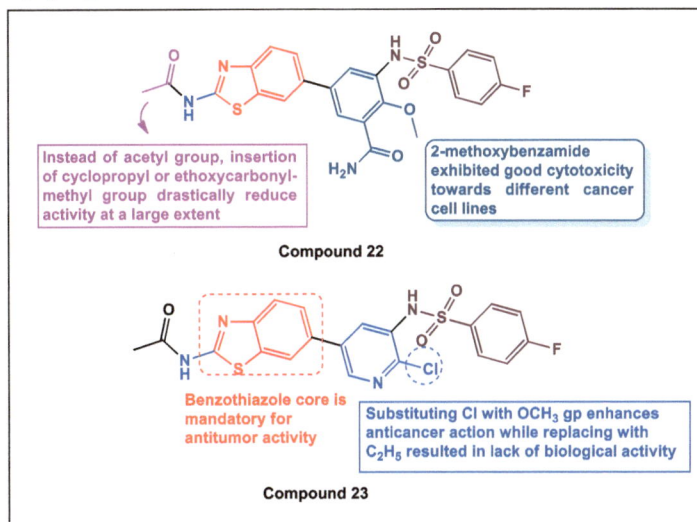

**Fig. (24).** Hybrid derivatives of benzothiazole –substituted 3-sulfonylamino compounds exhibited better ability to combat cancer.

Furthermore, by modifying compound **23** at the C-2 position of the benzothiazole nucleus, Xie *et al.* created a new series of compounds. These compounds were more effective at inhibiting the therapeutic mechanism of a kinase that causes cancer. The cytotoxicity of these benzothiazole analogues was investigated *in vitro* using a variety of cell lines including A-549, U87MG, HCT116, and MCF-7. Moreover, the activity of these compounds is compared to BEZ235 (a dual inhibitor of PI3K and mTOR). It was also investigated *in vivo* using the mouse homograft (S180) model. Compound **24** (Fig. **25**) demonstrated excellent cytoto xicity by inhibiting the PI3K and mTOR signal transduction pathways. The $IC_{50}$ value of compound **24** ranged from 0.17–0.45 μM in comparison with BEZ235 ($IC_{50}$ = 0.29–1.41 μM). A docking study also provides evidence that this compound more potently inhibits mTORC1 and PI3K enzymes [82].

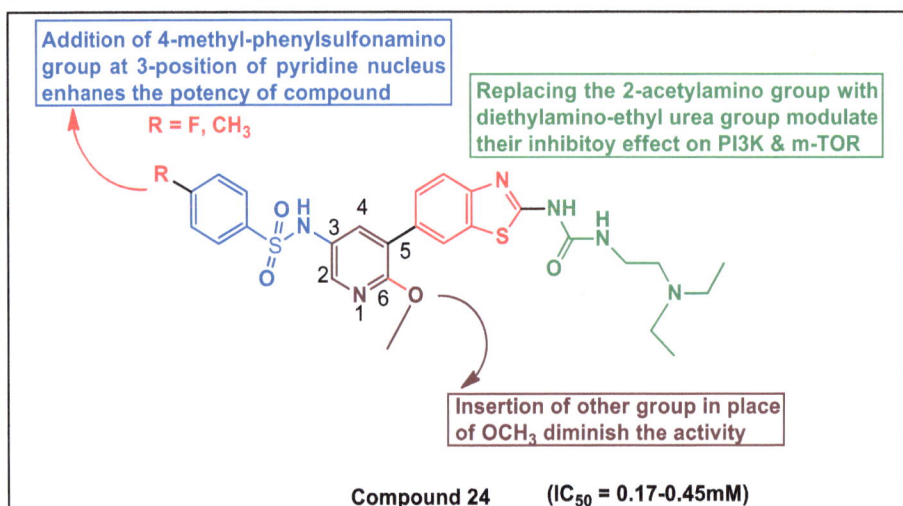

**Fig. (25).** Innovative series of benzothiazole analogs act as dual PI3K and mTOR inhibitors.

The novel benzothiazole-bearing derivatives were synthesized to fight against resistance. Hybrid benzothiazole-propylimidazole analogues were prepared and investigated for their antiproliferative action. Based on the docking study, it was concluded that compound **25** (Fig. **26**) bearing the side chain at C-2 of BT interacts with Lys 883 on the target receptor. The methoxy group present on the pyridine ring interacts with the Tyr867 residue of amino acids. The nitrogen of benzothiazole and the NH of amidic linkage form hydrogen bonds by binding with the Val amino acid residue located on the target site. Compound **25** acts as a selective inhibitor of PI3K [83].

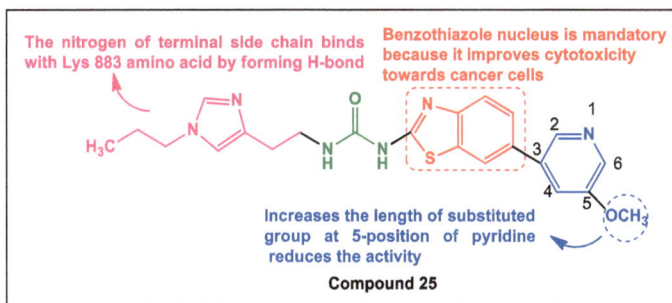

**Fig. (26).** Benzothiazole-propylimidazole hybrid derivatives act as selective PI3K inhibitors.

Several inhibitors of the PI3K/mTOR pathway are in various stages of clinical trials. For instance, BEZ255, BGT226, and GSK2126458 exhibited good potency *in vitro* and *in-vivo*.

## Inhibitors of the Braf Enzyme

*Braf* is a gene that is present in humans and encodes proteins. In normal cells, *RAF* has three kinds of protein, notably *A-RAF, B-RAF,* and *C-RAF,* whose stimulation is performed by phosphorylation. The mutated *Braf*$^{V600}$enzyme leads to an uncontrollable proliferation of cancer cells [84]. These inhibitors are recognised as a key target for melanoma treatment by blocking the expression of the mutated *Braf* gene. The kinase activity is augmented in tumour cells (10 times greater) than in normal cells due to the production of Braf-V600E protein, resulting in hyperactivation of the MAPK pathway. It promotes cancer cell proliferation. Fig. (**27**) represents the mechanism that inhibits the function of the mutated *Braf*$^{V600}$gene [85, 86].

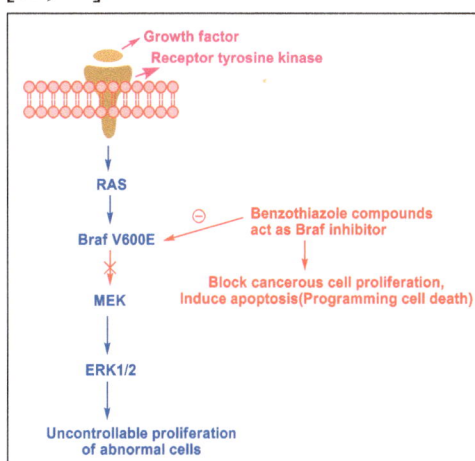

**Fig. (27).** Braf inhibitor is a novel target for preventing carcinogenesis.

The benzothiazole analogues bearing pyrrole ring-containing compounds were synthesized by Kamal *et al.* in 2013. The cytotoxic potential was investigated for all designed compounds, specifically in the MDA-MB-231 and MCF-7 cell lines. Compound **27** showed remarkable cytotoxicity against the MCF-7 breast cell line at a concentration of 4 µM, with $GI_{50} = 0.92$ µM, equal to the etoposide standard drug. Compounds **26** and **27** (Fig. **28**) were demonstrated as good inhibitors of the mitosis cell cycle at $G_2/M$ phase (*i.e.*, 48%), compared to etoposide (67%). The same molecule alleviates the oncogenic expression of Ras and simultaneously causes a downstream effect on molecules such as MEK1, ERK1/2, MAPK, and VEGF. According to the SAR study, the pyrrole is a well-known scaffold due to its excellent antineoplastic activity. So, the replacement of pyrrole with other heterocyclic rings reduces their remarkable activity [87].

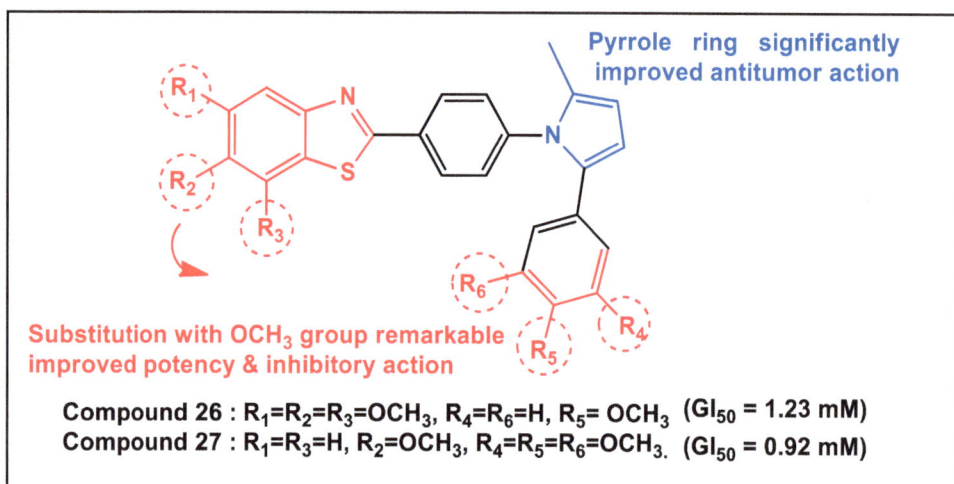

Compound 26 : $R_1=R_2=R_3=OCH_3$, $R_4=R_6=H$, $R_5=OCH_3$ $(GI_{50} = 1.23$ mM)
Compound 27 : $R_1=R_3=H$, $R_2=OCH_3$, $R_4=R_5=R_6=OCH_3$. $(GI_{50} = 0.92$ mM)

**Fig. (28).** Potential hybrid derivatives of benzothiazole possess pyrrole nucleus and exhibited remarkable cytotoxicity.

Song *et al.* developed a new class of benzothiazole derivatives with amide and urea motifs. These hybrid analogues were tested against various cancer cell lines, including NUGC-3 (gastric), MDA-MB-231 (breast), and human SK-Hep-1 (liver). These derivatives interfere with the binding of growth factors to receptor surfaces as well as the inhibiting signalling pathway that aids in undifferentiated cell proliferation. Among all the designed compounds, only compound **28** (Fig. **29**) displayed excellent inhibition with high potency. The $GI_{50}$ value of this compound was found to be 0.10 to 0.18 µg/ml in comparison with Adriamycin [88].

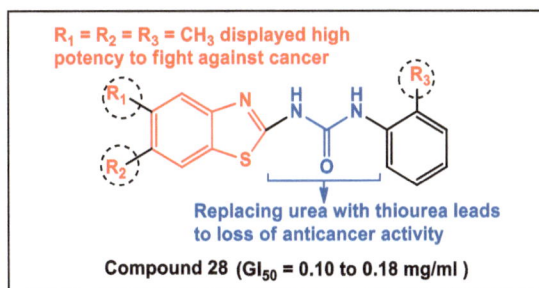

**Fig. (29).** Benzothiazole having amide and urea motifs exhibited remarkable cytotoxicity.

The hybrid benzothiazole-pyridyl amide urea analogues were synthesized by El-dasamy *et al.* in 2016. Their inhibitory effects on BRAF-V600E and c-Raf genes were examined to determine their chemoprotective potential. The screening of all discovered analogues was performed at a 10 µM concentration against various cancer cell lines. The highly hydrophobic nature of compound **29** (Fig. **30**) is demonstrated as an excellent inhibitor. This compound was shown to have an $IC_{50}$ value of 0.301–1.67 µM when a comparative study was done against standard sorafenib ($IC_{50}$ = 1.26–5.46 µM). Compound **30** was also effective in inhibiting the BRAF-V600E mutated gene by 67.6% and the *C-Raf* by 98.6%.

Compound **30** has an $IC_{50}$ value of 0.095 and 0.015 µM, respectively, in comparison to sorafenib (a standard drug), which has an $IC_{50}$ value of 0.038 µM and 0.006 µM. The urea linker was found to be essential for enhancing anticancer activity in the SAR study. Disubstituted derivatives are preferred over monosubstituted derivatives because they increase the potency of the compound by increasing lipophilicity [89].

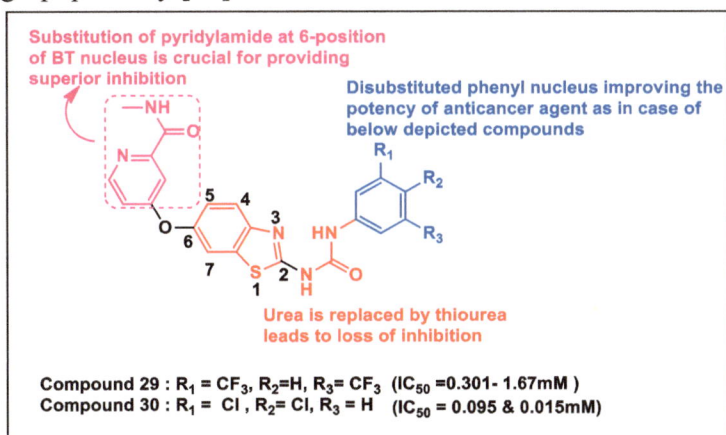

**Fig. (30).** BT clubbed with pyridyl amide and urea motifs exhibited maximum inhibition to Braf mutated gene.

**TAK-632,** a potential benzothiazole derivative (Compound **31**) Fig. (**31**) is a broad-spectrum anticancer agent that has been used to treat a variety of tumours. It effectively inhibited the mutated BRAF-V600E gene. According to in-vitro studies, it inhibits BRAFWT with an $IC_{50}$ of 8.3 nM and c-Raf with an $IC_{50}$ of 1.4 nM. Testing on nude rats was done in *in vivo* studies. They exhibited dose-dependent cytotoxicity against mutated genes, with a dose ranging from 3.9 to 24.1 mg/kg. Docking studies revealed that nitrogen from BT is involved in hydrogen bonding with the hinge region on the receptor's active site. The trifluoromethylphenyl motif, on the other hand, is buried in the receptor's lipophilic pocket [90].

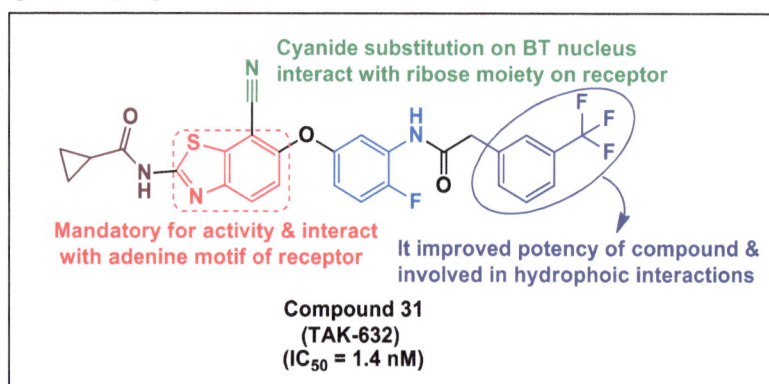

**Fig. (31).** Promising potential benzothiazole derivatives have a broad spectrum of anticancer activity.

## HDAC Inhibitor

Histones are proteins composed of small molecules of amino acids like lysine and arginine (both positively charged). It strengthens the chromosomes and aids in the regulation of gene expression. HDAC has recently been approved for the treatment of a variety of cancers, including solid tumours and hematological tumours. Disruptions in the maintained level of histone acetyltransferase (HAT) and histone deacetylase (HDAC) cause a variety of metabolic diseases and disorders [91]. Histone acetylation is a critical step in the regulation of gene expression. HDAC inhibitors work by preventing histone protein acetylation, thereby interfering with transcription. It is required for the transcription of a gene, cell differentiation, apoptosis, and carcinogenesis. This novel target has become more popular in the treatment of cancer [92]. HDAC inhibitors work by hyperacetylation of nucleosomal histones in cells, leading to aberrant gene expression. It further stops the proliferation of cancer cells and causes apoptosis, resulting in cell death. Fig. (**32**) depicts the mechanism of HDAC and its inhibition [93].

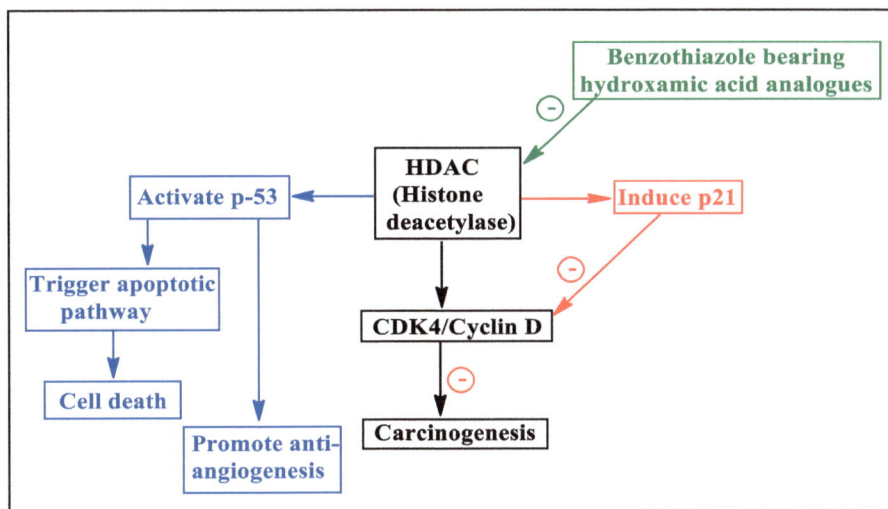

**Fig. (32).** Mode of action of a chemotherapeutic agent by inhibiting the function of HDAC enzyme.

Benzothiazole-bearing hydroxamic acids act as the most potent histone deacetylase inhibitors and so act as good antitumor agents. The benzothiazole moiety in compound **32(c),** (Fig. **33**), is linked to hydroxamic functional groups *via* a 6C-bridge linker. It displayed good inhibitory activity against HDAC3. It also exhibited potent cytotoxicity against chosen cancer cell lines at 1 µg/ml. The $IC_{50}$ values were 0.90 µM, 4.10 µM, 2.32 µM, 0.96 µM, and 1.10 µM, respectively, in SW620, MCF-7, PC3, AsPC-1, and NCI-H460 cell lines as compared to SAHA. Furthermore, compound **32(b)** inhibited HDAC8 *in vitro* due to its high affinity, but its activity was diminished *in vivo* due to methyl group oxidation in the liver [94 - 96].

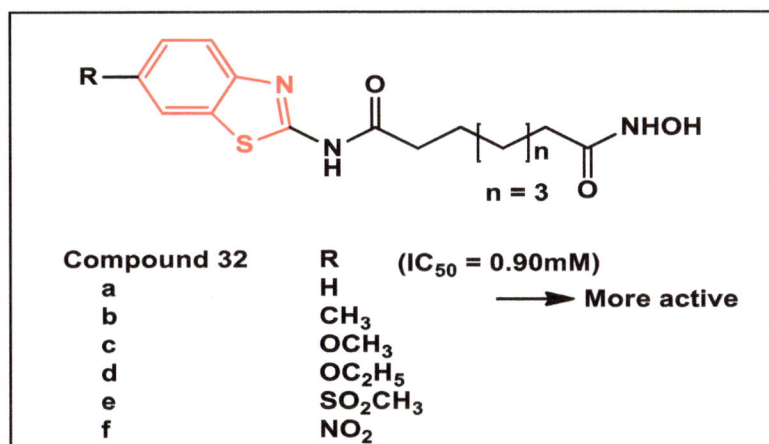

**Fig. (33).** Benzothiazole conjugated hydroxamic acid as HDAC inhibitor.

The efficacy of HDAC inhibitors was investigated, and they demonstrated greater cytotoxicity against hematological malignancies than solid tumours. Many research projects have been undertaken to develop various combination therapies. HDAC inhibitors, for example, are combined with other chemotherapeutic agents to avoid the aforementioned issue. However, in most cases, combination therapy results in undesirable drug-drug interactions as well as an abnormal PK profile [97]. Furthermore, one of the most effective approaches is to design and synthesize multi-targeted drugs by combining the pharmacophores of classical histone deacetylase inhibitors with other highly effective chemotherapeutic drugs. The phase I clinical trial for these multi-targeted HDAC/EGFR/HER2 inhibitors has been completed. It had higher cytotoxicity against solid tumours (NCT01384799). A few of them are still being studied in clinical trials [98].

A wide range of inhibition targets has been shown to improve therapeutic efficacy. It also ignores the issue of drug resistance. However, because of the numerous mechanisms involved in carcinogenesis, designing these compounds remains difficult. As a result, selecting a target is difficult [99].

**DNA-topoisomerase Inhibitor**

Topoisomerases (Top) are ubiquitous enzymes tasked with resolving topological issues. These issues primarily arise during DNA metabolism processes such as transcription, recombination, replication, and chromosome partitioning during cell division. Topoisomerases are essential for the survival of all organisms, from unicellular bacteria to humans, because they play this critical role. Topoisomerase is one of the most effective targets, and inhibiting it results in the generation of potential anticancer agents. Top I and Top II are the two main topoisomerase enzymes that play critical roles in cancer treatment. Overactivation of the topoisomerase I enzyme causes carcinogenesis. Top I inhibitors work by directly binding an inhibitor to the surface of a functional enzyme. (b) interact with DNA and alter its structure, preventing the Top enzyme from recognizing it. These inhibitors (campotethecin) convert the functional enzyme into a DNA-cleaving agent and are therefore referred to as "poisons." It severs a single strand of DNA helix, causing apoptosis and further impeding the carcinogenesis process. The top I poison cytotoxicity is restricted to the mitotic cell cycle's S-phase [100, 101]. Topoisomerase II antagonists, on the other hand, bind to the surface of the Top II enzyme, causing the enzyme's function to be altered. It resulted in the production of a cellular toxin that causes DNA breaks in both strands. It also has an impact on cellular activities such as replication, transcription, chromosome separation, and so on.

The whole catalytic cycle of topoisomerase II requires $Mg^{2+}$ and ATP. These agents are abundant in nature (*e.g.*, podophyllotoxin derivatives). These substances are abundant in nature (*e.g.*, podophyllotoxin derivatives). These benzothiazole hybrid analogues cut both strands of DNA at the same time, programming cell death. The stability of the complex was used to assess its cytotoxicity. There are numerous topoisomerase II inhibitors on the market. However, the demand for safer, more specific, and economically *via*ble drugs is still in its early stages [102]. Fig. (**34**) depicts a schematic diagram of the possible mechanism of DNA topoisomerase [103].

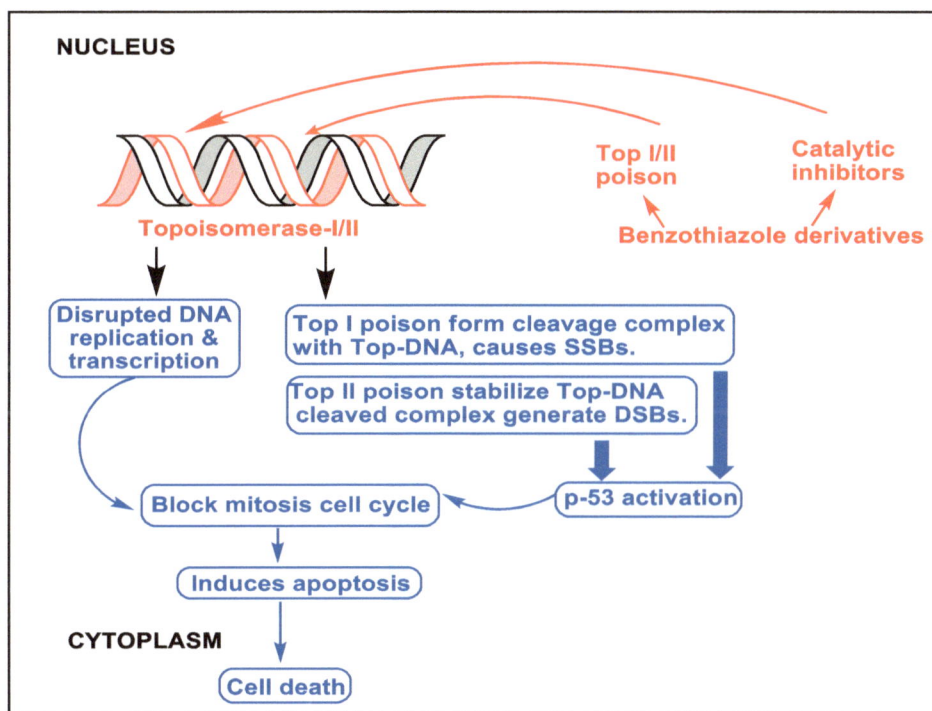

**Fig. (34).** Mechanism of DNA topoisomerase inhibitors for blocking pathway of tumorigenesis.

To avoid a variety of resistance issues, novel derivatives of hybrid compounds were developed. The rationale for using these moieties is that their active pharmacophores enhance antitumor activity. Etoposide, a natural derivative of podophyllotoxin, is widely used in the treatment of cancers such as lung cancer, testicular cancer, and leukemia (both lymphocytic as well as non-lymphocytic). Aside from their advantages, some shortcomings of these derivatives compel medical scientists to develop a better chemotherapeutic agent. Various reagents, including zirconium tetrachloride and NaI, were used to fuse the benzothiazole scaffold with the podophyllotoxin moiety. This synthetic method was chosen because of its ability to use zirconium salts to address issues such as slower reaction rates, longer reaction times, and toxicity.

These hybrid analogues were screened and chosen derivatives elicited excellent chemo-preventive properties at a lower dose. Further, their cytotoxic potential was analyzed against selected human cancerous lines. Compound **33** (Fig. **35**) depicted better inhibition towards Colo205, Hop-62, HT1080, and DWD, having IC$_{50}$ values of 7.0 µM, 15.2 µM, 9.5 µM and 5.2 µM, respectively, in comparison to reference drugs (adriamycin and podophyllotoxin).

Compound **34** (Fig. **35**) demonstrated similar antitumor activity with increased potency. It elicited more effective responses to colo205 and DWD, whose IC$_{50}$ values are 2.3 µM and 2.7 µM, respectively, when compared to reference drugs such as adriamycin (5.1 µM) and podophyllotoxin (5.0 µM). The inhibitory effect of the DNA-topoisomerase II enzyme increases as the inhibitor concentration increases from 10, 50, 100, 200 µM, and so on. According to SAR studies, benzothiazole and podophyllotoxin analogues linked by an aryl amino linker (phenyl or substituted phenylamino group) at the 2-position of BT and the 4-position of podophyllotoxin analogue have improved activity. These hybrid compounds effectively inhibited carcinogenesis by inhibiting the DNA-topoisomerase II enzyme [104].

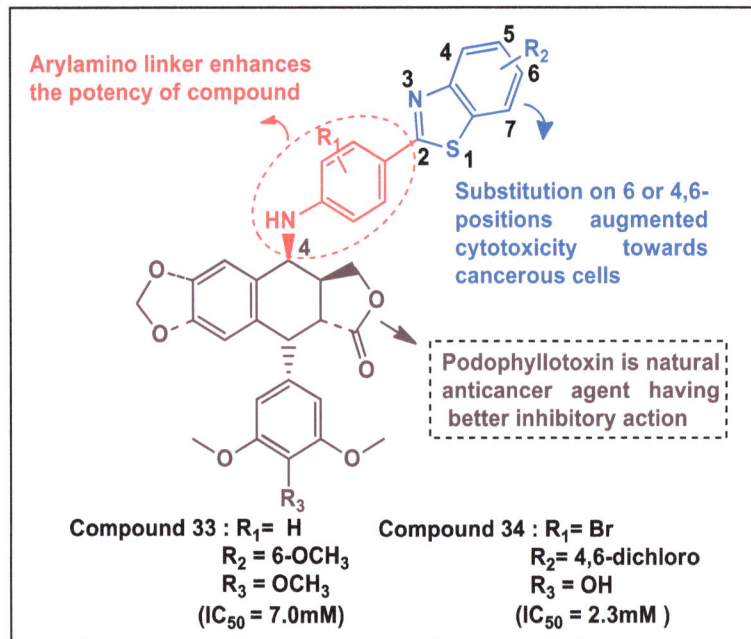

**Fig. (35).** Benzothiazole core clubbed with podophyllotoxin having excellent cytotoxicity towards selected human tumors.

Furthermore, the two active chemo-preventive agents have been conjugated to improve the compound's selectivity, specificity, and potency. Without the use of a catalyst, novel hybrid pyrazole-benzothiazole-β-naphthol derivatives were synthesized. The heterocyclic pyrazole nucleus is nitrogen-rich and plays an important role in cancer treatment. Benzothiazole analogues have a high affinity for DNA binding *via* the groove binding mode. The β-naphthol nucleus has anti-breast activity and is also used in the treatment of breast carcinoma as an estrogen receptor modulator. By acting as DNA intercalating agents, naphthalene analogues (amonafides) demonstrated excellent antitumor activity. Following screening, only a few analogues of these hybrid compounds inhibited the cervical (HeLa) cell line significantly. The cytotoxicity of these analogues was investigated against A549 (lung cancer), HeLa (cervical cancer), MCF-7 (breast cancer), and HEK-293 (human embryonic kidney cells). Compounds **35a, 35b, and 35c** (Fig. **36**) showed more dominant cytotoxicity towards cervical cancer cell lines than other cell lines, with $IC_{50}$ values of 5.20, 5.54, and 4.63 µM, respectively. SAR revealed that replacing $OCH_3$ and methyl groups on the benzothiazole nucleus reduces activity by seven times. The substitution of an electron-withdrawing group on the phenyl ring of 1, 3-biphenylpyrazole, on the other hand, increases its cytotoxicity when compared to electron-donating groups. Compound **35b and 35c** exhibited chemoprotective activity by either impeding the cell cycle at a specific stage, activating the apoptosis process, or both. They demonstrated cell accumulation of 19.9% and 25.3% at the $G_{2/}M$-phase at a concentration of 2.5 µM [105].

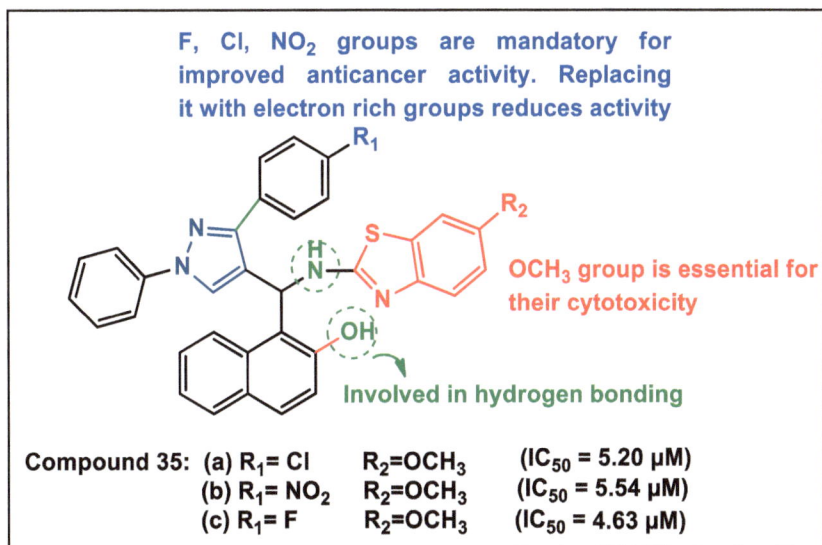

**Fig. (36).** Pyrazole-benzothiazole-β-naphthol hybrid derivatives exhibited considerable cytotoxicity towards the cervical cancerous line.

The continuous search for new compounds resulted in the development of hybrid naphthalimide-benzothiazole analogs. The evaluation of their cytotoxicity was carried out on a variety of carcinoma cells such as HT-29 (colon), A549 (lung), and MCF-7 (breast cancer). Amongst all the derivatives, only compounds **36** and **37** (Fig. **37**) demonstrated high cytotoxicity towards tumour cell lines. In comparison to the reference drug amonafide (5.459 and 7.762 µM), it had an $IC_{50}$ of 3.715 and 3.467 µM for colon cancer cell lines and an $IC_{50}$ of 4.074 and 3.890 µM for lung cancer cell lines. These compounds were identified as the most potent DNA-topoisomerase II inhibitors, and they work by intercalating both strands of DNA [106].

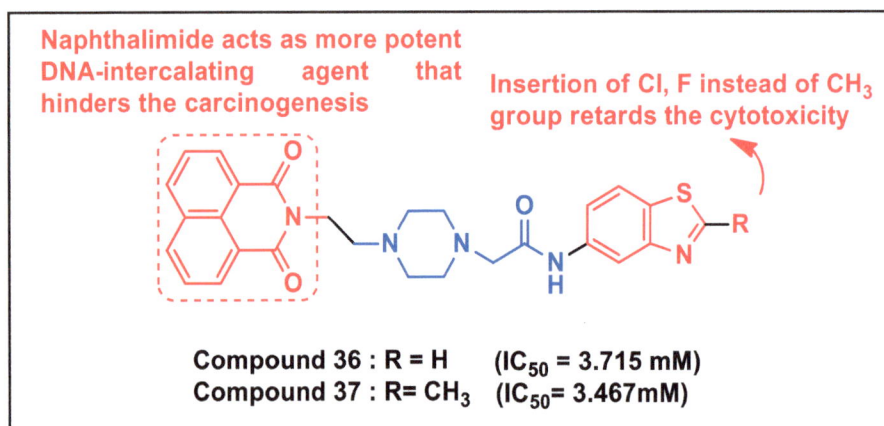

**Fig. (37).** Benzothiazole motif conjugated with naphthalimide acts as good DNA-intercalating agents.

In 2020, Tokalo *et al.* synthesized a new series of hybrid derivatives in which the β-carboline (natural origin) moiety was fused with the benzothiazole nucleus (synthetic origin) through carboxamide linkage. Out of thirty synthesized derivatives, only two compounds act as excellent DNA-intercalating agents. After screening, the compound's inhibitory effect was analyzed in adherent cell lines [A549 and NCI-H460 (lung), HCT-116 (colon)] and suspension cell lines [MOLT-4 (acute lymphoblastic leukemia), HL-60 (acute myeloblastic leukemia)]. Compounds **38** and **39** (Fig. **38**) displayed good cytotoxicity towards the lung cancer cell line (A549) with an $IC_{50}$ value of 1.46 and 1.81 µM. The SAR study revealed three sites for improving cytotoxic potential: C-1 of β-carboline, C-4, and position 6 of the benzothiazole nucleus. Molecular docking studies evidenced that these compounds are bound to the active site of the DNA-Top II complex. They stabilize this complex by interactions with base pairs of deoxyribose nucleic acid (DNA) and amino acid residues. Aside from that, various assays demonstrated their intercalating properties and excellent topoisomerase II inhibition [107].

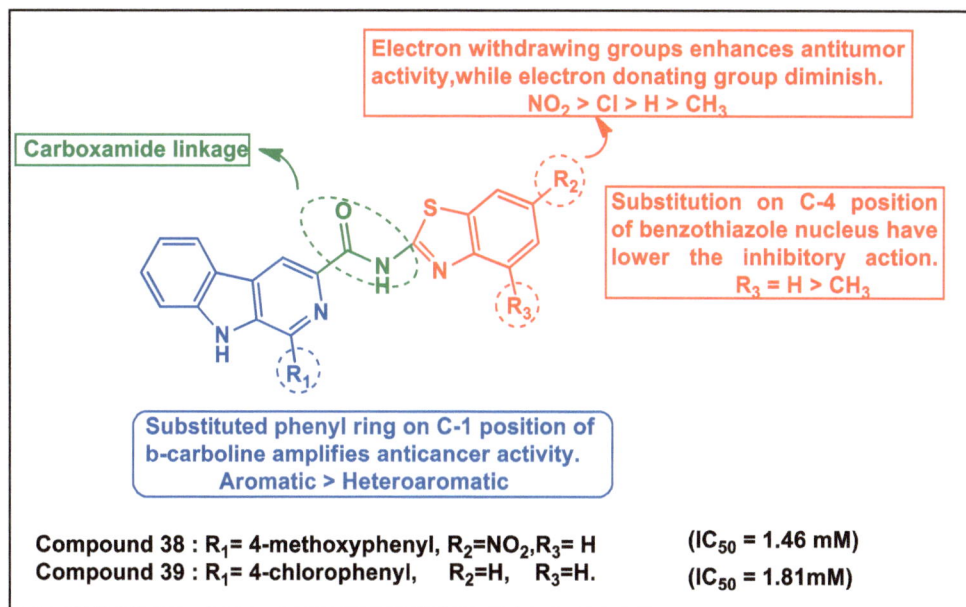

**Electron withdrawing groups enhances antitumor activity,while electron donating group diminish.**
$NO_2 > Cl > H > CH_3$

**Carboxamide linkage**

**Substitution on C-4 position of benzothiazole nucleus have lower the inhibitory action.**
$R_3 = H > CH_3$

**Substituted phenyl ring on C-1 position of b-carboline amplifies anticancer activity.**
**Aromatic > Heteroaromatic**

**Compound 38 : R₁= 4-methoxyphenyl, R₂=NO₂,R₃= H**          **(IC₅₀ = 1.46 mM)**
**Compound 39 : R₁= 4-chlorophenyl,     R₂=H,   R₃=H.**          **(IC₅₀ = 1.81mM)**

**Fig. (38).** BT motif adjoined with β-carboline *via* carboxamide linkage represented remarkable cytotoxicity.

## Aurora Kinase Inhibitors

Cell kinase is an important enzyme that regulates cell growth, division, and survival, among other things. Overexpression of these enzymes will serve as a pathway for the formation of abnormal cells. As a result, kinase inhibitors play an important role in the development of effective chemotherapeutic agents. Aurora kinase is one of the newer targets for cancer treatment among the various kinase inhibitors. It belongs to the Aurora A, B, and C subtypes of the serine/threonine kinase family. Aurora A is localized on arms of chromosomes or centrosomes during the G2/M phase. Aurora B acts as a chromosome passenger protein. All these aurora kinase enzymes regulate chromosome arrangements as well as monitor the mitotic spindle formation during the chromosomes separation. The aberrant Aurora-A causes apoptosis, while the interrupted function of Aurora B acts as an inhibitor of the cytokinesis process [108 - 110]. The mechanism of aurora kinase inhibitors is depicted in Fig. (**39**).

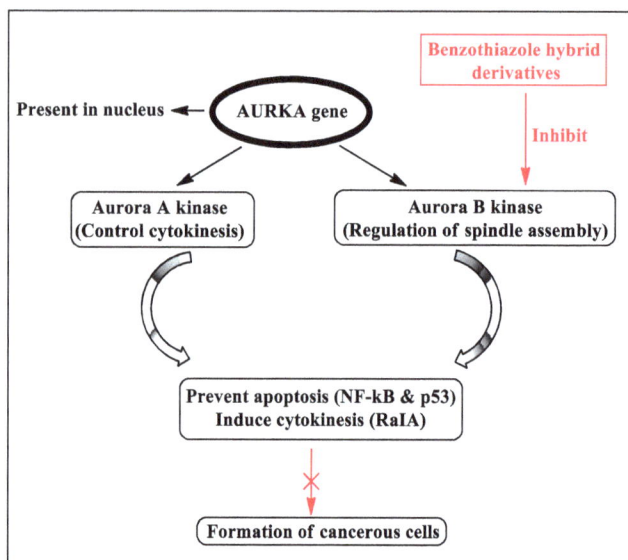

**Fig. (39).** Mechanism that targets Aurora kinase for cancer treatment.

In 2017, Lee *et al.* incorporated a new class of amidobenzothiazole analogues by bioisosteric replacement with an amidobenzoxazole scaffold. They enhanced their hydrophobicity, which resulted in enhanced potency as well as inhibition properties. Compounds **40** and **41** (Fig. **40**) exerted excellent inhibition towards the cervical cancer cell line (HeLa), with $IC_{50}$ values of 0.12 µM and 0.09 µM, respectively. These analogues act as selective inhibitors of Aurora-B kinase because of their higher affinity towards the ATP binding site present on the surface of the enzyme. These benzothiazole-bearing compounds stop the histone protein (H3) phosphorylation at Ser10 amino acid residues and also cause cell death by arresting cell division at the $G_2$/M phase [111].

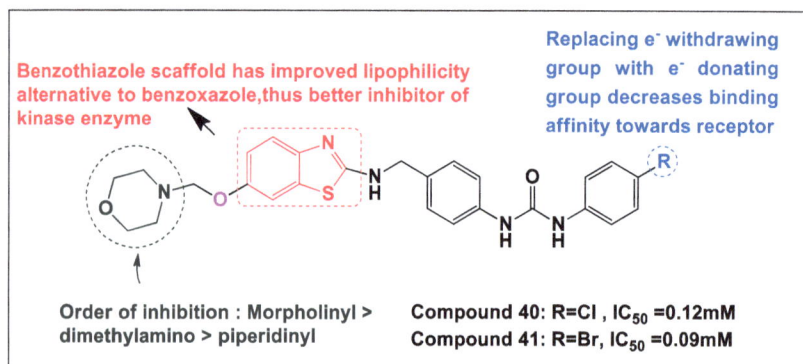

**Fig. (40).** Amidobenzothiazole compounds act as a potent inhibitor of the Aurora B kinase enzyme.

Moreover, Stefan *et al.* designed and synthesized a series of compounds in which the benzothiazole scaffold was conjugated with di-heteroaryl ether. Compound **42** (Fig. **41**) acts as a dual inhibitor of Aurora-A and B kinase. Besides this, it also showed a good $EC_{50}/IC_{50}$ ratio with cellular $EC_{50}$ values ranging from 60 to 800 nM and enzymatic $IC_{50}$ values of less than 100 nM. The discovery of a new antineoplastic agent is a necessary need for time. So, the researchers tried to design a combination therapy in which aurora kinase inhibitors were coupled with other antitumor drugs—to design an effective drug treatment and prevent the resistance issues [112, 113].

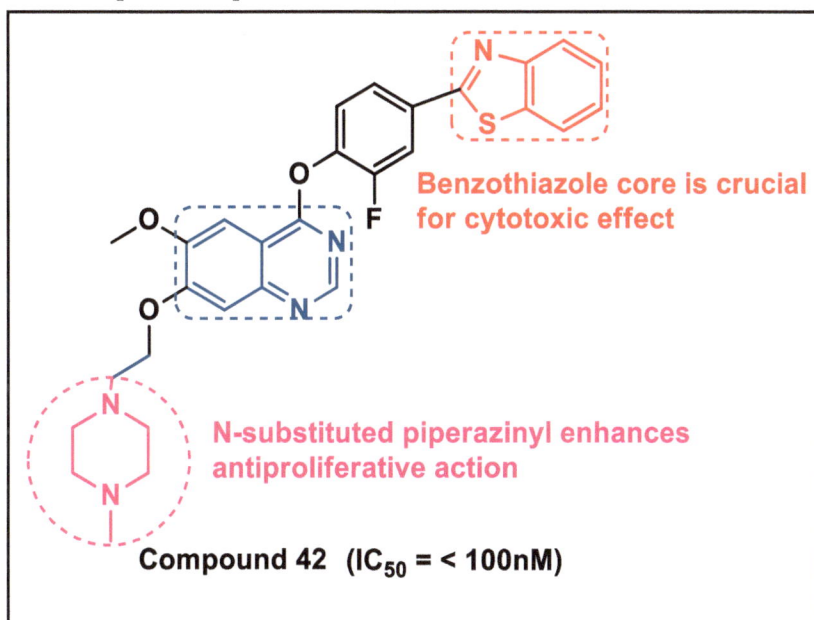

**Fig. (41).** Benzothiazole containing di-heteroaryl ether showed good inhibition on Aurora –A and B kinase enzymes.

The uninterrupted efforts of medical scientists designed and prepared another innovative series of compounds in which the benzothiazole nucleus was adjoined with dicarboxamide. Further, their inhibitory effect was evaluated against selected human carcinoma cells. Compounds **43, 44,** and **45** (Fig. **42**) exerted better cytotoxicity against A-549 (lung cancer) and DU-145 (prostate cancer) cell lines. Out of these three derivatives, compound **44** demonstrated good *in vitro* inhibitory action, possessing $IC_{50}$ values of 1.52 and 1.68 µM towards lung and prostate cancer cells against doxorubicin ($IC_{50}$ value of 1.71 µM) as a positive control. In the *in-vivo* study, compound **46** exerted good % inhibitions (61% and 38%) on Aurora-A and B kinase. According to the SAR study, when electron-rich groups were present with nitrogen (electron-deficient), it exhibited good cytotoxicity [114].

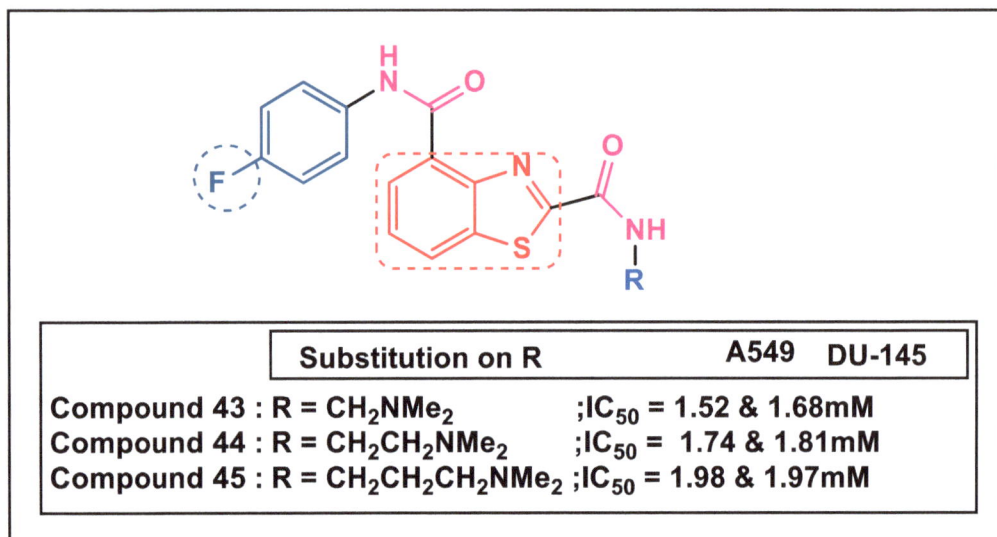

| Substitution on R | A549   DU-145 |
|---|---|
| Compound 43 : R = $CH_2NMe_2$ | ;$IC_{50}$ = 1.52 & 1.68mM |
| Compound 44 : R = $CH_2CH_2NMe_2$ | ;$IC_{50}$ = 1.74 & 1.81mM |
| Compound 45 : R = $CH_2CH_2CH_2NMe_2$ | ;$IC_{50}$ = 1.98 & 1.97mM |

**Fig. (42).** Hybrid benzothiazole possessing dicarboxamide exhibited better cytotoxicity against lung and prostate tumor cell lines.

## Inhibitor of Monoacylglycerol Lipase

A monoacylglycerol lipase enzyme is a type of serine hydrolase enzyme. It helps in the conversion of monoacylglycerol into its unsaturated fats. The molecular size of this protein is 33 kDa and it is composed of a larger number of amino acid residues (*i.e.*, 303). This enzyme is mainly present in different organs of humans, like the brain and kidney, the heart, adipose tissues, adrenal glands, *etc.* [115]. In cancer cells, the overactivation of monoacylglycerol lipase, in turn, exacerbates the various types of cancer, such as colon cancer, breast cancer, *etc*. It primarily augmented the metabolism that produced oncogenic mediators (those fascinating by the generation of free fatty acids). Their inhibitors, on the other hand, change the role of MAGL in cancerous cells, preventing cell migration, invasiveness, and proliferation. Notably, it was determined that monoacyl glycerol lipase aggravates cancer [116]. Inhibitors, on the other hand, are excellent chemoprotective agents. The two major enzymes responsible for prostaglandin degradation are monoacylglycerol lipase (MAGL) and unsaturated fatty acid amide hydrolase (FAAH) (PG-Gs). The best trigger for cancer therapy is advancement in this field. The mode of action of monoacylglycerol lipase inhibitors in cancer treatment is depicted in Fig. (**43**) [117].

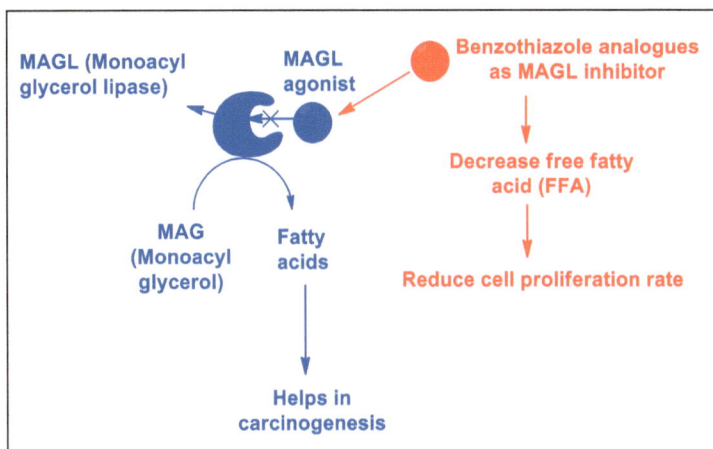

**Fig. (43).** Mechanism of MAGL inhibitor act as excellent antineoplastic agents.

Afzal *et al.* designed a series of novel benzothiazole derivatives. They primarily function as chemopreventive agents by interfering with the MAGL enzyme's function. In a cancerous cell, a high level of the monoacylglycerol lipase enzyme increased fatty acid formation. As a result, these benzothiazole analogues reduce the level of free fatty acids, which inhibits the formation of cancer cells. Only three of the thirty analogues are used because of their high cytotoxicity. Compound **46** (Fig. **44**) has a bromine substitution and is a highly potent MAGL inhibitor with an $IC_{50}$ value of 6.5 nM. Compounds **47** and **48** (Fig. **44**) inhibited the hMAGL enzyme in the same way.

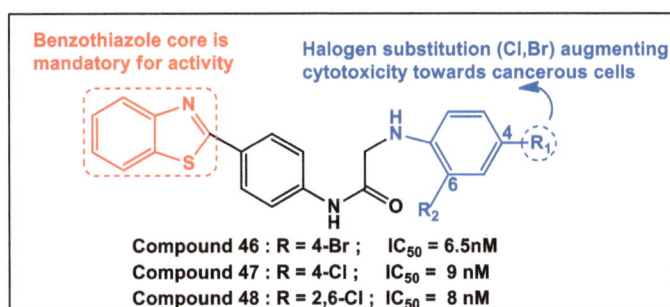

Compound 46 : R = 4-Br ;   $IC_{50}$ = 6.5nM
Compound 47 : R = 4-Cl ;    $IC_{50}$ = 9 nM
Compound 48 : R = 2,6-Cl ; $IC_{50}$ = 8 nM

**Fig. (44).** Benzothiazole nucleus conjugated with acetamide acts as a potent inhibitor of hMAGL enzyme.

These compounds have shown an $IC_{50}$ value of 9 nM and 8 nM on selected breast cancer cell lines (MCF-7 and MDA-MD-468), respectively, in comparison with the CAY10499 reference drug ($IC_{50}$ = 424 nM). The SAR study concluded that substituting an electron-donating group on the phenyl ring of an aniline derivative for an electron-withdrawing group reduces the cytotoxic potential of synthesized benzothiazole analogues [118].

## Inhibitors of the NEDD8 Activating Enzyme

Overstimulation of NEDD8 (Neural Precursor Cell-Expressed Developmentally Downregulated Protein 8) plays a significant role in tumour growth. It is a small protein-like ubiquitin molecule. The action of the enzyme was aberrant with the help of NEDD8 enzyme inhibitors. Inhibiting this activating pathway is one of the most effective ways to treat a wide range of tumours, including lung cancer, colon cancer, and the formation of osteosarcoma cells. In the Neddylation process, conjugation is mainly carried out between NEDD8 protein and substrate protein that further regulates the various cellular activities [119]. UBC12 is another protein that is involved in the degradation process. The disruption of the function of UBC12 suppresses cancer cell proliferation.

The UPS (Ubiquitin proteasome system) enzymes are classified into three types: E1 (Ubiquitin activator), E2 (Ubiquitin-conjugating), and E3 (Ubiquitin ligases). During the Neddylation cascade, the E1 enzyme (NAE) activates the NEDD8 protein, which then conjugates with the E2 (UBC12) enzyme. Finally, NEDD8 forms a conjugate complex with the cullin protein, which stimulates the cullin-RING ubiquitin E3 ligase (CRL) [120]. A combination strategy in which NEDD8 inhibitors are combined with DNA intercalating drugs is also used [121]. The schematic diagram depicts the mechanism of action of NEDD8 activating enzyme inhibitors, which is discussed in Fig. (45) [122].

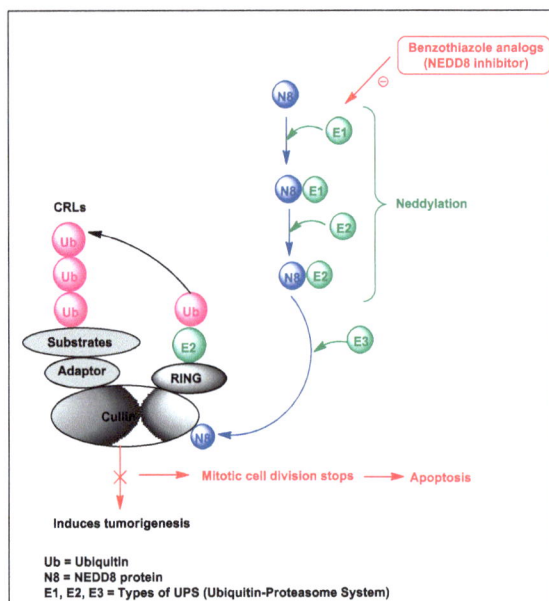

**Fig. (45).** Various steps in the generation of cancer cells are disrupted by NAE inhibitor (NEDD8 inhibitor) [122].

Researchers have worked tirelessly to develop novel benzothiazole derivatives that inhibit NAE non-covalently (NEDD8 activated enzyme). Ma *et al.* reported the anticancer properties of these novel non-sulfamide analogues of benzothiazole in 2017. As an alternative to standard MLN4924, the potential cytotoxicity of selected compounds was assessed against HCT116 (colon cancer) and U-2OS cell lines. Only compound **49** was more active and potent against the HCT116 (colon) cell line than it was against the U-2OS cell line (osteosarcoma cells). High potency is due to the presence of a 3-hydroxyphenyl group having an $IC_{50}$ value of 0.51 µM towards the HCT116 cell line analyzed by the MIT assay. Based on its mode of action, compound **49** (Fig. 46) was recognized as a new inhibitor of NAE (*i.e.*, NEDD8 activating enzyme) that aberrantly functions the function of NEDD8 protein and ultimately increases the level of UBC12 protein [126]. So, finally, it was concluded that the benzothiazole scaffold could act as the most promising lead compound for further development [123].

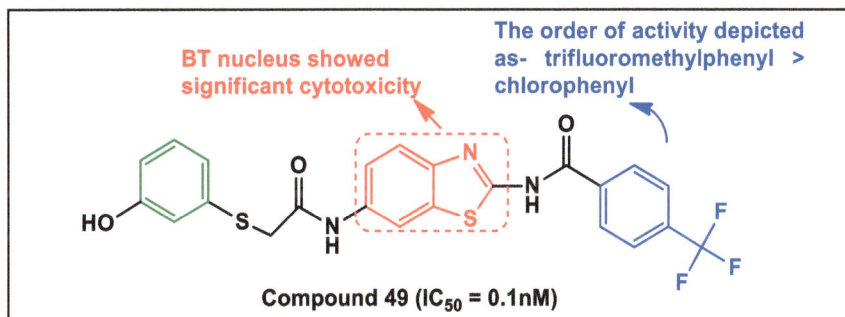

**Fig. (46).** Non-sulfamide analogs of benzothiazole displayed potent inhibitors of NEDD8 activating enzyme.

## Inhibitors of Heat Shock Protein 90

Heat shock protein is a chaperone that assists in the folding and refolding of proteins. Folding is done to stabilize new proteins, whereas unfolding is done to exclude proteins that have been damaged by cell stress. It can be divided into several classes based on molecular size. HSP 90 is one of the most important HSPs in the development of malignant tumours. It has a molecular weight of 90 kDa, as its name suggests. Furthermore, Her2, Akt, Raf1, CDK4/6, Src, telomerase, and survivin are Hsp90-dependent and ATP-dependent client proteins. These client proteins are related to cancer hallmarks, which aided in the discovery of the HSP 90 inhibitor for cancer therapy [124]. HSP90 inhibitors were designed using a variety of methods. The first method involves targeting the N-terminus of the ATP binding site of HSP. When it reaches the clinical trial stage, however, it produces a heat shock response (HSR), which causes cytostatic activity. The second method is to design an HSP inhibitor by targeting the C-terminus. This is a successful strategy because it does not cause HSR induction.

This approach was very successful, but it had a few drawbacks, such as the lack of a well-designed ligand-binding site in the protein's C-terminus. The third method is to prevent interaction between the client and the HSP protein [125]. These inhibitors selectively kill cancer cells while causing no or minimal side effects.

Novobiocin (an inhibitor of the DNA gyrase B enzyme) was chosen as a lead compound in the ongoing search for anticancer agents. Because both DNA gyrase B and heat shock protein 90 have similar structures as well as the Bergerat fold in the region of the ATP binding site, designing and developing selective inhibitors is fascinating. Furthermore, Novobiocin has been optimised to produce the first C-terminal HSP90 inhibitor with good antineoplastic properties and no heat shock response. Furthermore, their synthesis and cytotoxic properties against selected breast cancer lines were evaluated. Compound **50** (Fig. **47**) was known to exhibit better cytotoxicity at lower concentrations, with $EC_{50}$ values of 0.86 µM and 7.03 µM, respectively, against selected breast cancer lines SkBr3 and MCF-7. It makes a significant contribution to the SKBr3 breast cancer line [126].

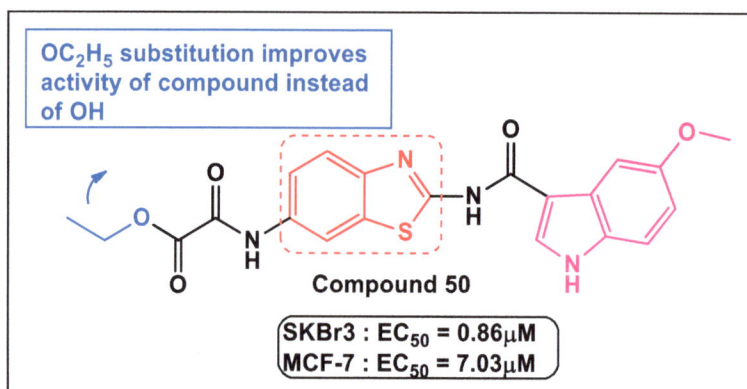

**Fig. (47).** Substituted benzothiazole analogs act as a potent inhibitor of Hsp 90 at the C-terminal.

## RECENTLY DEVELOPED BENZOTHIAZOLE ANALOGS AS AN ANTICANCER AGENT

BT-guanidino-propanoic acid conjugated compounds were synthesized and evaluated for antiproliferative activity against the human cancer cell line, HeLa. Compound **51** potently inhibited HeLa cells with an $IC_{50}$ of 1.8 µM, which was close to the value of the positive control, doxorubicin. As the SAR study reveals, the substitution of the -OH, -COOH, and $-SO_2NH_2$ groups at position 6 of the BT ring played an important role in the activity. The activity was found in the order of OH>COOH > $SO_2NH_2$ [127]. Afterward, 2-arylbenzothiazole analogues were synthesized and recognized as potent anticancer agents. Compound **52** displayed good cytotoxic activity against MCF-7 ($IC_{50}$ = 9.26 µM) and HeLa ($IC_{50}$ = 15.21

µM) cell lines as compared to cisplatin (reference drug) [$IC_{50}$ = 10 µM and 18 µM] by MTT assay. According to SAR studies, the electronegative fluorine atom in the *para*-position of the benzene ring increased the cytotoxic activity. The electron releasing group (2-Me, 2-OH, 2-OH-3-OMe) found in benzothiazole derivatives reduced anticancer efficacy. The cytotoxicity of benzothiazole derivatives has been increased by substituting heteroaryl groups at the 2-position [128].

Further, piperazine-benzothiazole analogues have been synthesized and evaluated for their *in vitro* cytotoxicity against Dalton's lymphoma ascites (DLA) cells by a cell *via*bility assay. Compound **53** showed potent cytotoxicity against the DLA ($IC_{50}$ = 22.6 µM) cell line. The SAR study was carried out by a bromo-group on phenyl rings and has shown promising antiproliferative efficacy [129]. Gabr and his coworker designed and synthesized benzothiazole Schiff bases as an antitumor agent. Compound **54** showed good activity against HeLa and COS-7 cell lines with $IC_{50}$ values of 2.41 µM and 4.31 µM, respectively, as compared to the reference drug of doxorubicin. The SAR study revealed that the presence of a 2-(4-hydroxy-2-methoxybenzylidene) hydrazino moiety at the $2^{nd}$ position of the benzothiazole ring enhanced the activity against HeLa and COS-7 cell lines. However, the replacement of the 4-hydroxy substituent in compound **54** with 4-methoxy resulted in decreased activity. Furthermore, changing the positions of the hydroxyl and methoxy substituents on the benzylidene moiety led to decreased activity. Docking studies revealed that the benzothiazole ring was isosteric with the adenine portion of ATP and could mimic the ATP competitive binding regions of EGFR-TK (PDB code: 1M17) [130].

Another novel benzothiazole analogue has been synthesized and tested for cytotoxicity against the MCF-7 cell line using the SRB assay with cisplatin as the reference drug. All synthesized derivatives were accompanied by the high production of hydrogen peroxide, nitric oxide, and other free radicals, causing tumour cell death as monitored by a reduction in the synthesis of protein and nucleic acids. Compound **55** showed good cytotoxic activity against the MCF-7 ($IC_{50}$ = 5.15 µM) cell line [131].

In recent years, Lad and his colleagues designed and synthesized methylsulfonyl benzothiazole (MSBT) derivatives as anticancer agents. All synthesized derivatives were examined for anticancer activity against HeLa and MCF-7 cancer cell lines by the SRB assay. Compound **56** displayed significant anti-proliferative activity against the HeLa ($GI_{50}$ = 0.1 µM) cell line. The cell proliferation rate was less than the benzothiazole moiety containing 4-nitrophenyl, diethyl, and tertiary butyl sulfonamide groups at the 4-position and an ethoxy group at the 5-position [132]. Innovative derivatives of 2-(4-aminophenyl) benzothiazole were designed and synthesized by Lei *et al*. The antitumor activity of these analogues has been evaluated against human U251 and rat C6 glioma cell lines by using the MTT assay. Compound **57** exhibited significant activity against human U251 and rat C6 glioma cells with $IC_{50}$ values of 3.5 μM and 4 μM, respectively. These derivatives demonstrated the reduction of tumour volume by 12% and showed remarkable inhibition of abnormal cell growth [133].

Abdelgawad and his co-worker designed and synthesized benzothiazole-substituted pyrazole derivatives as antiproliferative agents. All synthesized compounds were tested for their antiproliferative activity against MCF-7 and A549 cell lines using the MTT assay. Compound **58** showed good activity against MCF-7 and A549 cell lines with $IC_{50}$ values of 12.30 μM and 15.12 μM, respectively, as compared to doxorubicin as a reference drug. However, the docking study revealed that the most active compound **58** had been investigated for the three hydrogen binding interactions with His90, Arg513, and Tyr 356 residue within the binding site of the COX-2 enzyme (PDB: ID 1CX2) [134]. A series of 2-imidazolinyl substituted benzo[b]thieno-2-carboxamides with a benzothiazole subunit were synthesized and tested for anti-proliferative activity against a panel of human cancer cell lines *in vitro*. Compound **59** displayed good activity against SW620, HepG2, CFPAC-1, HeLa, and WI-38 cell lines with $IC_{50}$ values of 7.05 μM, 14.17 μM, 5.04 μM, 1.16 μM, and 4.24 μM, respectively, as compared to the reference drug 5-fluorouracil [135].

A series of 2-aminobenzothiazole derivatives have been synthesized and screened for their anti-hepatocellular carcinoma properties using the diethylnitrosamine (DEN) induced hepatocellular carcinoma rat model. Compound **60** displayed excellent activity against hepatocellular carcinoma ($IC_{50}$ = 60.32 μM) cell lines. Further, this compound combats the oxidative damage of hepatic cells due to the development of hepatocellular carcinoma induced by a chemical carcinogen, DEN. The docking study contains the compound **60**, which was shown to have different interactions (hydrophobic, Vander Waal, dispersion, hydrogen bonding, and other electrostatic interactions) between amino acids of the protein and the ligand binding of receptor Chk 1 (PDB entry: 1ZYS) and VEGFR-2 (PDB entry: 2QU5) [136]. Mono and binuclear Pt (II) and Pd (II) complexes with 2,20-dithiobis-(benzothiazole) derivatives were synthesized and tested for antitumor activity against two human tumour cell lines, MCF-7 and HepG2, using the MTT assay. Complex **61** exhibited more potent activity against MCF-7 and HepG2 cell lines with $IC_{50}$ values of 20.2 μM and 4.0 μM, respectively, as compared to cisplatin as a reference drug [137].

Eshkil and his coworker designed and synthesized benzothiazole thiourea derivatives as anticancer agents. All synthesized derivatives were evaluated for their cytotoxic activity against five different human and animal cancer cell lines, *viz.* MCF-7, HeLa, HT-29, K-562, and Neuro-2a by using the MTT assay. Compound **62** displayed good cytotoxic activity against all these above cell lines with $IC_{50}$ values of 6.72 µM, 4.97 µM, 3.90 µM, 40.5 µM, and 22.7 µM, respectively, as compared to the cisplatin reference drug [138]. By using the MTT method, new benzothiazole-pyrazole hybrids were synthesized and evaluated for their anticancer activity against A549, MCF7, and Hep3B cell lines. Compound **63** showed good cytotoxic activity against A549 (S.I = 5.27 µM), MCF7 (S.I = 0.15 µM) and Hep3B (S.I = 0.45 µM) cell lines with $IC_{50}$ values of 6.99 µM, 231.66 µM, and 81.49 µM, respectively. A SAR study revealed that the acyl moiety at the C3 position in benzothiazole/pyrazole hybrids leads to diminished anticancer activity and poor selectivity towards cancer *versus* the normal cell line. However, substituting C3 of the pyrazolone/benzoxazole hybrid with *p*-nitro or *p*-chloro benzaldehyde groups showed greater inhibitory activity towards COX-2 than coxib and was also active against A549 and MCF7 cell lines [139].

A series of novel bis-benzothiazole derivatives were designed and synthesized as anticancer agents. Compound **64** showed the highest antiproliferative activities on U937, HL60, and HeLa cells with $IC_{50}$ values of 6.76 µM, 7.21 µM, and 8.67 µM, respectively, as compared to 5-FU and the Hoechst 33258 standard drug [140]. The benzothiazole derivatives clubbed with metal-ligand and their anti-tumor activity were evaluated by thermal denaturation. It displayed strong DNA interaction at a concentration of 104 M-1. The cytotoxicity of compound **65** was measured *in vitro* against MCF-7 and MDA-MB-231 (human breast carcinoma cell lines) and DSF (human skin fibroblasts) lines. Compound **65** exhibited good inhibition, having an $IC_{50}$ value of 20 µM against MCF-7, an alternative to the cisplatin drug that acts as a positive control. The inhibitory action was revealed by causing an alteration in the structure of DNA [141]. Moreover, another class of benzothiazole-berberine hybrid derivatives were synthesized, and their tumour inhibitory properties were determined by testing of suitably chosen tumour cell lines. Compound **66** has been shown to have remarkable inhibitory action against CaSki, HeLa, and SK-OV-3, with $IC_{50}$ levels of 5.311, 5.474, and 32.61 µM, respectively, in comparison to the standard drug berberine. The electron-withdrawing group like cyano enhances their antitumor activity. These analogues can be very useful for developing other innovative antineoplastic drugs [142].

In the search for a more effective and efficient antitumor agent, the novel series of compounds containing mercapto functional groups along with aryl donor groups (like nitrogen or phosphorous) was designed by El-Asmy *et al.* The chemotherapeutic action was examined in different cancer cell lines such as ovarian (OVCAR-8) and breast (MDA-MB231). These derivatives were known to be of low cytotoxicity, *i.e.* > 100 µM. Further, the modification was done on this lead compound and incorporated platinum to make a complex that exhibited strong inhibition of the proliferation of tumour cells. Compound **67** displayed excellent cytotoxic potential towards human breast (MDA-MB-231) cell lines having an $IC_{50}$ of 2.87 μM and human ovarian cell lines (OVCAR-8) with an $IC_{50}$ of 2.39 μM cell lines, compared with cisplatin ($IC_{50}$ values of 1.97 and 1.86 μM, respectively [143]. Table **1** illustrates the structures of benzothiazole analogs and their action on cell lines with their IC50 values.

**Table 1. Recent advancement in the development of innovative compounds specific to target cells with their $IC_{50}$ value.**

| S. No. | Structures | Cellular Assay | Result | Reference |
|---|---|---|---|---|
| 1 | 51 | HeLa | $IC_{50}$ = 1.8 μM | [127] |
| 2 | 52 | MCF-7 | $IC_{50}$ = 9.26 μM | [128] |
| | | HeLa | $IC_{50}$ = 15.21 μM | |
| 3 | 53 | DLA | $IC_{50}$ = 22.6 μM | [129] |
| 4 | 54 | Hela | $IC_{50}$ = 2.41 μM/L | [130] |
| | | COS-7 | $IC_{50}$ = 4.31 μM/L | |
| 5 | 55 | MCF-7 | $IC_{50}$ = 5.15 μM | [131] |

(Table 1) cont.....

| 6 | 56 | HeLa | GI$_{50}$ = 0.1µM | [132] |
|---|---|---|---|---|
| 7 | 57 | Human U251 | IC$_{50}$= 3.5 µM | [133] |
| | | Rat C6 glioma | IC$_{50}$= 4 µM | |
| 8 | 58 | MCF-7 | IC$_{50}$ = 12.30 µM | [134] |
| | | A549 | IC$_{50}$ = 15.12 µM | |
| 9 | 59 | SW620 | IC$_{50}$= 7.05 µM | [135] |
| | | HepG2 | IC$_{50}$= 14.17 µM | |
| | | CFPAC- | IC$_{50}$= 5.04 µM | |
| | | HeLa | IC$_{50}$ = 1.16 µM | |
| | | WI-38 | IC$_{50}$= 4.24 µM | |
| 10 | 60 | Hepatoce llular carcinom a cells | IC$_{50}$ = 60.32 µM | [136] |
| 11 | 61 | MCF-7 | IC$_{50}$ = 20.2 µM | [137] |
| | | HepG2 | IC$_{50}$ = 4.0 µM | |

*(Table 1) cont.....*

| 12 | **62** | MCF-7 | IC$_{50}$= 6.72µM | [138] |
| | | HeLa | IC$_{50}$= 4.97µM | |
| | | HT-29 | IC$_{50}$= 3.90µM | |
| | | K-562 | IC$_{50}$= 40.5µM | |
| | | Neuro-2a | IC$_{50}$= 22.7µM | |
| 13 | **63** | A549 | IC$_{50}$ = 6.99 µM | [139] |
| | | | S.I = 5.27 µM | |
| | | MCF7 | IC$_{50}$ = 231.66 µM | |
| | | | S.I = 0.15 µM | |
| | | Hep3B | IC$_{50}$ = 81.49 uM | |
| | | | S.I = 0.45 µM | |
| 14 | **64** | U937 | IC$_{50}$ = 6.76µM | [140] |
| | | HL 60 | IC$_{50}$ = 7.21µM | |
| | | HeLa | IC$_{50}$= 8.67µM | |
| 15 | **65** | MCF-7 | IC$_{50}$= 20µM | [141] |
| 16 | **66** | CaSki | IC$_{50}$ = 81.49 µM | [142] |

(Table 1) cont.....

| 17 | | MDA-MB-231 | IC$_{50}$ = 2.87 μM | [143] |
|---|---|---|---|---|

## PATENT GRANTED ON BENZOTHIAZOLE SCAFFOLD

The benzothiazole scaffold has an imperative position over other bicyclic compounds like benzimidazole, quinazoline, *etc*. The BT core enhances the lipophilicity of the compound as well as its biological activity. A vast number of patents have been published, indicating the importance of the benzothiazole scaffold. Only a few researchers have applied to patent their invention.In the illustrated Table **2**, the recent patent granted on the benzothiazole scaffold was successfully discussed.

**Table 2. Recent patent granted on benzothiazole nucleus with their patent date and name of the inventor.**

| S.No. | Patent number | Patent date | Inventor | Reference |
|---|---|---|---|---|
| 1. | US7,087,761 | Aug 8, 2006 | Spur *et al.* | [144] |
| 2. | US7,091,227 | Aug 15, 2006 | Scott *et al.* | [145] |
| 3. | US8,143,258 | Dec 1, 2009 | Okaniwa *et al.* | [146] |
| 4. | US7,902,217 | Mar. 8, 2011 | Xie *et al.* | [147] |
| 5. | US7,943,773 | May 17, 2011 | Xie *et al.* | [148] |
| 6. | US7,994,337 | Aug.9, 2011 | Liu *et al.* | [149] |
| 7. | US8,063,204 | Nov.22, 2011 | Kamal *et al.* | [150] |
| 8. | US8,134,003 | Mar 13, 2012 | Xie *et al.* | [151] |
| 9. | US8,236,282 | Aug.7, 2012 | Klunk *et al.* | [152] |
| 10. | US8,252,811 | Aug.28, 2012 | Xie *et al.* | [153] |
| 11. | US8,263,610 | Sep.11, 2012 | Ali *et al.* | [154] |
| 12. | US8,410,272 | Apr. 2, 2013 | Zhang *et al.* | [155] |
| 13. | US8,486,937 | July 16, 2013 | Xie *et al.* | [156] |
| 14. | US8,501,938 | Aug.6, 2013 | Malefyt *et al.* | [157] |

*(Table 2) cont.....*

| S.No. | Patent number | Patent date | Inventor | Reference |
|-------|---------------|-------------|----------|-----------|
| 15. | US8,580,968 | Nov.12, 2013 | Black *et al.* | [158] |
| 16. | US8,691,185 B2 | Apr. 8, 2014 | Raje *et al.* | [159] |
| 17. | US8,754,233 | June17, 2014 | Zhang *et al.* | [160] |
| 18. | US8,993,580 | Mar 31, 2015 | Ren *et al.* | [161] |
| 19. | US9,592,224 | Mar 14, 2017 | Martinez Gil *et al.* | [162] |
| 20. | US 9,637,492 | May 2, 2017 | Ren *et al.* | [163] |

## ROLE OF BENZOTHIAZOLE-BEARING CLINICAL TRIAL DRUGS IN THE FUTURE

Cancer is one of the most dangerous diseases because if one cancerous cell remains after chemotherapy, it begins to proliferate again. According to the preceding research report, various benzothiazole and its analogues were tested, and it was determined that these compounds had a high potency against carcinoma cell lines. Furthermore, these compounds are in the clinical development stage and may yield potential chemotherapeutic compounds with high potency or promising properties. CJM126 was replaced with a benzothiazole analogue designed by Bradshaw *et al.*, and it demonstrated increased cytotoxicity against human breast cancer lines, particularly the MCF-7 cell line. Recently, the following compounds with high cytotoxicity against tumour cells have been shown to be in clinical trials: MKT077, YM-201627, 5F203, Phortress, and others are depicted in Table **3**.

In the future, the discovery of an innovative, more effective, and selective antineoplastic agent will be extremely beneficial. The optimization of a lead compound by changing a ring substitution resulted in varying levels of inhibition against various carcinoma cells Several breakthroughs around this benzothiazole nucleus tell us the relationship between SAR and their antitumor activity.

**Table 3. Drugs under clinical trial are depicted below along with the target site and their use.**

| S. No. | Compound/ Drug Name | Structure | Target site | Indication | Refs. |
|--------|---------------------|-----------|-------------|------------|-------|
| 1. | CJM126 | 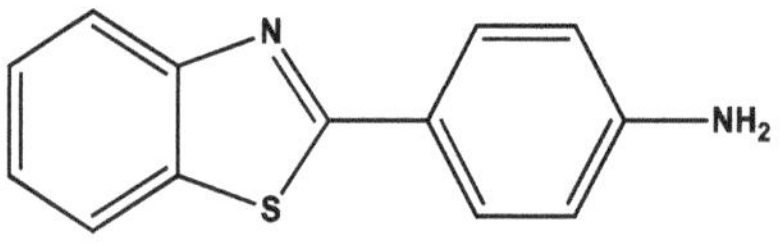 | DNA damage | Inhibitor of breast carcinoma | [164] |

(Table 3) cont.....

| S. No. | Compound/ Drug Name | Structure | Target site | Indication | Refs. |
|---|---|---|---|---|---|
| 2. | 5F203 | | AhR dependent activation of CYP1A1 enzyme | Breast and ovarian carcinoma therapy | [165] |
| 3. | Phortress (Prodrug) **Phase I** | | Induces CYP1A1 expression and by forming ROS. | Treatment of solid tumors. | [166] |
| 4. | YM-201627 | | Inhibiting endothelial surface receptor - VEGF-R, bFGF, FBS. | Treatment of solid tumors. | [167] |
| 5. | PMX-610 **Phase I** | | - | Inhibiting tumor cell lines of colon, lung, and breast cancer. | [168] |
| 6. | MKT077 (Rhodacyanine dyes) **Phase I** | | Allosteric Hsp 70 inhibitor | Treating solid tumor Especially in the colon carcinoma cell line. | [169] |
| 7. | Riluzole | | Induces apoptosis | For treating prostate and breast cancer. | [170] |

## CONCLUSION

This chapter describes the various segments that rely on the benzothiazole scaffold in detail. It depicts the SAR of benzothiazole analogues against various biological targets, as well as several synthetic routes and their anticancer activity. Mitotic inhibitors, topoisomerase I and II inhibitors, Bcr-abl kinase inhibitors, Braf inhibitors, HDAC inhibitors, EGFR kinase inhibitors, and PI3K/mTOR inhibitors are important targets for cancer therapy. Researchers recently used nanotechnology to easily and safely synthesize benzothiazole analogues using a nanocatalyst.

Cancer cells, where sustained abnormal cell growth occurs, are analogous to the sustained efforts of researchers or medicinal chemists in cancer treatment. The goal of developing novel compounds is to have better and more selective cytotoxicity against cancer cells than normal cells, as well as to overcome rapid resistance problems. Furthermore, it provides information relevant to the recently approved or granted patent to prevent tumorigenesis based on the benzothiazole nucleus. Aside from that, it shed some light on various benzothiazole molecules that are currently in various stages of clinical trials.

## CONSENT FOR PUBLICATION

All authors have given their consent for the publication of this manuscript.

## CONFLICT OF INTEREST

The authors declare no conflict of interest, financial or otherwise.

## ACKNOWLEDGEMENT

The author wishes to acknowledge the Management, Shivalik College of Pharmacy, Nangal for the constant encouragement and support for writing this chapter.

## REFERENCES

[1]   Smith, C.E.P.; Prasad, V. Targeted Cancer Therapies. *Am. Fam. Physician,* **2021,** *103*(3), 155-163. [PMID: 33507053]

[2]   Padma, V.V. An overview of targeted cancer therapy. *Biomedicine (Taipei),* **2015,** *5*(4), 19. [http://dx.doi.org/10.7603/s40681-015-0019-4] [PMID: 26613930]

[3]   Raval, S.H.; Singh, R.D.; Joshi, D.V.; Patel, H.B.; Mody, S.K. Recent developments in receptor tyrosine kinases targeted anticancer therapy. *Vet. World,* **2016,** *9*(1), 80-90. [http://dx.doi.org/10.14202/vetworld.2016.80-90] [PMID: 27051190]

[4]   Kumari, A.; Singh, R.K. Medicinal chemistry of indole derivatives: Current to future therapeutic prospectives. *Bioorg. Chem.,* **2019,** *89*103021 [http://dx.doi.org/10.1016/j.bioorg.2019.103021] [PMID: 31176854]

[5]     Kumari, A.; Singh, R.K. Morpholine as ubiquitous pharmacophore in medicinal chemistry: Deep insight into the structure-activity relationship (SAR). *Bioorg. Chem.,* **2020**, *96*103578
[http://dx.doi.org/10.1016/j.bioorg.2020.103578] [PMID: 31978684]

[6]     Sethi, N.S.; Prasad, D.N.; Singh, R.K. An Insight into the Synthesis and SAR of 2,4-Thiazolidinediones (2,4-TZD) as Multifunctional Scaffold: A Review. *Mini Rev. Med. Chem.,* **2020**, *20*(4), 308-330.
[http://dx.doi.org/10.2174/1389557519666191029102838] [PMID: 31660809]

[7]     Kumar, S.; Singh, R.K.; Patial, B.; Goyal, S.; Bhardwaj, T.R. Recent advances in novel heterocyclic scaffolds for the treatment of drug-resistant malaria. *J. Enzyme Inhib. Med. Chem.,* **2016**, *31*(2), 173-186.
[http://dx.doi.org/10.3109/14756366.2015.1016513] [PMID: 25775094]

[8]     Yadav, P.S.; Prakash, D.; Kumar, S.G.P. Benzothiazole: Different Methods of Synthesis and Diverse Biological activities. *Int. J. Pharm. Sci. Drug Res.,* **2011**, *3*(10), 1-7.

[9]     Ruhi, A.; Nadeem, S. Biological aspects of emerging benzothiazoles: a short review. *J. Chem. Article ID,* **2013**, *345198*, 1-12.

[10]    Stierle, A.A.; Cardellinall, J.H.; Singleton, F.L. Benzothiazoles from a putative bacterial symbiont of the marine sponge Tedania ignis. *Tetrahedron Lett.,* **1991**, *32*, 4847-4848.
[http://dx.doi.org/10.1016/S0040-4039(00)93476-2]

[11]    Irfan, A.; Batool, F.; Zahra Naqvi, S.A.; Islam, A.; Osman, S.M.; Nocentini, A.; Alissa, S.A.; Supuran, C.T. Benzothiazole derivatives as anticancer agents. *J. Enzyme Inhib. Med. Chem.,* **2020**, *35*(1), 265-279.
[http://dx.doi.org/10.1080/14756366.2019.1698036] [PMID: 31790602]

[12]    Pathak, N.; Rathi, E.; Kumar, N.; Kini, S.G.; Rao, C.M. A Review on Anticancer Potentials of Benzothiazole Derivatives. *Mini Rev. Med. Chem.,* **2020**, *20*(1), 12-23.
[http://dx.doi.org/10.2174/1389557519666190617153213] [PMID: 31288719]

[13]    Fan, X.; He, Y.; Wang, Y.; Zhang, X.; Wang, J. A novel and practical synthesis of 2-benzoylbenzothiazoles and 2-benzylbenzothiazoles. *Tetrahedron Lett.,* **2011**, *52*, 899-902.
[http://dx.doi.org/10.1016/j.tetlet.2010.12.057]

[14]    Ali, A.; Taylor, G.E.; Graham, D.W. *PCT Int*; , **2001**. WO2001028561.

[15]    Bose, D.S.; Idrees, M. Metal-free cascade intramolecular S-arylation: regioselective synthesis of substituted benzothiazoles. *J. Org. Chem.,* **2011**, *76*(18), 7630.
[http://dx.doi.org/10.1021/jo802826x] [PMID: 21902272]

[16]    Moghadhan, F.M.; Ismaili, H.; Bardajee, G.R. Zirconium (IV) oxide chloride and anhydrous copper (II) sulfate mediated synthesis of 2-substituted benzothiazoles. *Heteroatom Chem.,* **2006**, *17*, 136-141.
[http://dx.doi.org/10.1002/hc.20191]

[17]    Ryabukhin, S.V.; Plaskon, A.S.; Volochnyuk, D.M.; Tolmachev, A.A. Synthesis of fused imidazoles and benzothiazoles from (hetero) aromatic ortho-diamines or ortho-aminothiophenols and aldehydes promoted by chlorotrimethylsilane. *Synthesis,* **2006**, *21*, 3715-3726.

[18]    Praveen, C.; Hemanthkumar, K.; Muralidharan, D.; Perumal, P.T. Oxidative cyclization of thiophenolic and phenolic Schiff's bases promoted by PCC anew oxidant for 2-substituted benzothiazoles and benzoxazoles. *Tetrahedron,* **2008**, *64*, 2369-2374.
[http://dx.doi.org/10.1016/j.tet.2008.01.004]

[19]    Shelkar, R.; Sarode, S.; Nagarkar, J. Nano ceria catalyzed synthesis of substituted benzimidazole, benzothiazole, and benzoxazole in aqueous media. *Tetrahedron Lett.,* **2013**, *54*, 6986-6990.
[http://dx.doi.org/10.1016/j.tetlet.2013.09.092]

[20]    Cho, Y.H.; Lee, C.Y.; Cheon, C.H. Cyanide as a powerful catalyst for facile synthesis of benzofused heteroaromatic compounds *via* aerobic oxidation. *Tetrahedron,* **2013**, *69*, 6565-6573.

[http://dx.doi.org/10.1016/j.tet.2013.05.138]

[21]  Bommegowdaa, Y.K.; Lingarajua, G.S.; Thamasb, S.; Kumara, K.S.V.; Kumaraa, C.S.P.; Rangappaa, K.S.; Sadashiva, M.P. Weinreb amide as an efficient reagent in the one-pot synthesis of benzimidazoles and benzothiazoles. *Tetrahedron Lett.,* **2013**, *54*, 2693-2695.
[http://dx.doi.org/10.1016/j.tetlet.2013.03.075]

[22]  Das, S.; Samanta, S.; Maji, S.; Samanta, P.; Dutta, A.; Srivastava, D.N.; Biswas, B.A.P. Visible-ligh-
-driven synthesis of 2-substituted benzothiazoles using CdS nanosphere as heterogeneous recyclable catalyst. *Tetrahedron Lett.,* **2013**, *54*, 1090-1096.
[http://dx.doi.org/10.1016/j.tetlet.2012.12.044]

[23]  Inamdara, S.M.; Morea, V.K.; Mandal, S.K. CuO nanoparticles supported on silica, a new catalyst for facile synthesis of benzimidazoles, benzothiazoles, and benzoxazoles. *Tetrahedron Lett.,* **2013**, *54*, 579-583.
[http://dx.doi.org/10.1016/j.tetlet.2012.11.091]

[24]  Ranu, B.C.; Jana, R.; Dey, S.S. An efficient and green synthesis of *2*-arylbenzothiazoles in an ionic liquid [PmIm]Br under microwave irradiation. *Chem. Lett.,* **2004**, *33*, 286-287.
[http://dx.doi.org/10.1246/cl.2004.274]

[25]  Bahrami, K.; Khodaei, M.M.; Naali, F. Mild and highly efficient method for the synthesis of 2-arylbenzimidazoles and 2-arylbenzothiazoles. *J. Org. Chem.,* **2008**, *73*(17), 6835-6837.
[http://dx.doi.org/10.1021/jo8010232] [PMID: 18652508]

[26]  Bose, D.S.; Idrees, M. Dess-martin periodinane mediated intramolecular cyclization of phenolic azomethines: a solution-phase strategy toward benzoxazoles and benzothiazoles. *Synthesis,* **2010**, *3*, 398-402.
[http://dx.doi.org/10.1055/s-0029-1217136]

[27]  Bose, D.S.; Idrees, M.; Srikanth, B. Synthesis of 2-arylbenzothiazoles by DDQ-promoted cyclization of thioformanilides; a solution-phase strategy for library. *Synthesis,* **2007**, *6*, 819-823.
[http://dx.doi.org/10.1055/s-2007-965929]

[28]  Li, Y.; Wang, Y.L.; Wang, J.Y. A simple iodine promoted synthesis of 2- substituted benzothiazoles by condensation of aldehydes with 2-aminothiophenol. *Chem. Lett.,* **2006**, *35*, 460-461.
[http://dx.doi.org/10.1246/cl.2006.460]

[29]  Seijas, J.A.; Tato, M.P.V.; Reboredo, M.R.C.; Campo, J.C.; Lopez, L.R. Lawesson's reagent and microwaves: a new efficient access to benzoxazoles and benzothiazoles from carboxylic acids under solvent-free conditions. *Synlett,* **2007**, *2*, 313-316.
[http://dx.doi.org/10.1055/s-2007-967994]

[30]  Bose, D.S.; Idrees, M. Hypervalent iodine mediated intramolecular cyclization of thioformanilides: expeditious approach to 2-substituted benzothiazoles. *J. Org. Chem.,* **2006**, *71*(21), 8261-8263.
[http://dx.doi.org/10.1021/jo0609374] [PMID: 17025321]

[31]  Luo, K.; Yang, W-C.; Wei, K.; Liu, Y.; Wang, J-K.; Wu, L. Di-*tert*-butyl Peroxide-Mediated Radical $C(sp^2/sp^3)$-S Bond Cleavage and Group-Transfer Cyclization. *Org. Lett.,* **2019**, *21*(19), 7851-7856.
[http://dx.doi.org/10.1021/acs.orglett.9b02837] [PMID: 31524412]

[32]  Xing, Q.; Ma, Y.; Xie, H.; Xiao, F.; Zhang, F.; Deng, G.J. Iron-Promoted Three-Component 2-Substituted Benzothiazole Formation via Nitroarene ortho-C-H Sulfuration with Elemental Sulfur. *J. Org. Chem.,* **2019**, *84*(3), 1238-1246.
[http://dx.doi.org/10.1021/acs.joc.8b02619] [PMID: 30606012]

[33]  Dey, A.; Hajra, A. Metal-Free Synthesis of 2-Arylbenzothiazoles from Aldehydes, Amines, and Thiocyanate. *Org. Lett.,* **2019**, *21*(6), 1686-1689.
[http://dx.doi.org/10.1021/acs.orglett.9b00245] [PMID: 30811211]

[34]  Huang, Y.; Zhou, P.; Wu, W.; Jiang, H. Selective Construction of 2-Substituted Benzothiazoles from o-Iodoaniline Derivatives $S_8$ and N-Tosylhydrazones. *J. Org. Chem.,* **2018**, *83*(4), 2460-2466.

[http://dx.doi.org/10.1021/acs.joc.7b03118] [PMID: 29337553]

[35]  Bouchet, L.M.; Heredia, A.A.; Argüello, J.E.; Schmidt, L.C. Riboflavin as Photoredox Catalyst in the Cyclization of Thiobenzanilides: Synthesis of 2-Substituted Benzothiazoles. *Org. Lett.,* **2020**, *22*(2), 610-614.
[http://dx.doi.org/10.1021/acs.orglett.9b04384] [PMID: 31887062]

[36]  Wang, X.; Li, X.; Hu, R.; Yang, Z.; Gu, R.; Ding, S.; Li, P.; Han, S. Elemental sulfur-mediated decarboxylative redox cyclization reaction; Copper-catalyzed synthesis of 2-substituted benzothiazoles. *Synlett,* **2018**, *29*, 219-224.
[http://dx.doi.org/10.1055/s-0036-1589112]

[37]  Zhang, J.; Zhao, X.; Liu, P.; Sun, P. TBHP/KI-Promoted Annulation of Anilines, Ethers, and Elemental Sulfur: Access to 2-Aryl-, 2-Heteroaryl-, or 2-Alkyl-Substituted Benzothiazoles. *J. Org. Chem.,* **2019**, *84*(19), 12596-12605.
[http://dx.doi.org/10.1021/acs.joc.9b02145] [PMID: 31502839]

[38]  Chander Sharma, P.; Sharma, D.; Sharma, A.; Bansal, K.K.; Rajak, H.; Sharma, S.; Thakur, V.K. New Horizons in benzothiazole scaffold for cancer therapy: Advances in bioactivity, functionality, and chemistry. *Appl. Mater. Today,* **2020**, *20*, 1-39.
[http://dx.doi.org/10.1016/j.apmt.2020.100783]

[39]  Banerjee, S.; Payra, S.; Saha, A.; Sereda, G. ZnO nanoparticles: a green efficient catalyst for the room temperature synthesis of biologically active 2-aryl-1, 3-benzothiazole and 1, 3-benzoxazole derivatives. *Tetrahedron Lett.,* **2014**, *55*(40), 5515-5520.
[http://dx.doi.org/10.1016/j.tetlet.2014.07.123]

[40]  Satish, G.; Reddy, K.H.V.; Anil, B.S.P.; Ramesh, K.; Kumar, R.U.; Nageswar, Y.V.D. Direct C-H arylation of benzothiazoles by magnetically separable nano copper ferrite, a recyclable catalyst. *Tetrahedron Lett.,* **2015**, *56*(34), 4950-4953.
[http://dx.doi.org/10.1016/j.tetlet.2015.07.002]

[41]  Ghafuri, H.; Esmaili, E.; Talebi, M. FeO@SiO$_2$/collagen: an efficient magnetic nanocatalyst for the synthesis of benzimidazole and benzothiazole derivatives. *C. R. Chim.,* **2016**, *19*(8), 942-950.
[http://dx.doi.org/10.1016/j.crci.2016.05.003]

[42]  Karimian, A.; Beidokhti, H.K.; Kakhki, R.M. Magnetic Co-doped NiFeOnanocomposite, A heterogeneous and recyclable catalyst for the one-pot synthesis of benzimidazoles, benzoxazoles and benzothiazoles under solvent-free conditions. *J. Chin. Chem. SOC-TAIP,* **2017**, *64*(11), 1316-1325.

[43]  Kommula, D.; Madugula, S.R.M. Synthesis of benzimidazoles/benzothiazoles by using recyclable, magnetically separable nano-Fe$_2$O$_3$ in aqueous medium. *J. Iran.Chem.Soc.,* **2017**, *14*(8), 1665-1671.
[http://dx.doi.org/10.1007/s13738-017-1107-z]

[44]  Xie, M.; Ujjinamatada, R.K.; Sadowska, M.; Lapidus, R.G.; Edelman, M.J.; Hosmane, R.S. A novel, broad-spectrum anticancer compound containing the imidazo[4,5-e][1,3]diazepine ring system. *Bioorg. Med. Chem. Lett.,* **2010**, *20*(15), 4386-4389.
[http://dx.doi.org/10.1016/j.bmcl.2010.06.061] [PMID: 20594843]

[45]  Bhaskar, V.H.; Mohite, P.B. Synthesis characterization and evaluation of anticancer activity of some tetrazole derivatives. *J. Optoelectron. Biomed. Mater.,* **2010**, *2*, 249-259.

[46]  Zhang, N.; Ayral-Kaloustian, S.; Nguyen, T.; Afragola, J.; Hernandez, R.; Lucas, J.; Gibbons, J.; Beyer, C. Synthesis and SAR of [1,2,4]triazolo[1,5-*a*]pyrimidines, a class of anticancer agents with a unique mechanism of tubulin inhibition. *J. Med. Chem.,* **2007**, *50*(2), 319-327.
[http://dx.doi.org/10.1021/jm060717i] [PMID: 17228873]

[47]  Yue, Q.X.; Liu, X.; Guo, D.A. Microtubule-binding natural products for cancer therapy. *Planta Med.,* **2010**, *76*(11), 1037-1043.
[http://dx.doi.org/10.1055/s-0030-1250073] [PMID: 20577942]

[48]  Hour, M.J.; Huang, L.J.; Kuo, S.C.; Xia, Y.; Bastow, K.; Nakanishi, Y.; Hamel, E.; Lee, K.H. 6-

Alkylamino- and 2,3-dihydro-3′-methoxy-2-phenyl-4-quinazolinones and related compounds: their synthesis, cytotoxicity, and inhibition of tubulin polymerization. *J. Med. Chem.,* **2000**, *43*(23), 4479-4487.
[http://dx.doi.org/10.1021/jm000151c] [PMID: 11087572]

[49]   De Martino, G.; La Regina, G.; Coluccia, A.; Edler, M.C.; Barbera, M.C.; Brancale, A.; Wilcox, E.; Hamel, E.; Artico, M.; Silvestri, R. Arylthioindoles, potent inhibitors of tubulin polymerization. *J. Med. Chem.,* **2004**, *47*(25), 6120-6123.
[http://dx.doi.org/10.1021/jm049360d] [PMID: 15566282]

[50]   Kamal, A.; Mallareddy, A.; Janaki Ramaiah, M.; Pushpavalli, S.N.; Suresh, P.; Kishor, C.; Murty, J.N.; Rao, N.S.; Ghosh, S.; Addlagatta, A.; Pal-Bhadra, M. Synthesis and biological evaluation of combretastatin-amidobenzothiazole conjugates as potential anticancer agents. *Eur. J. Med. Chem.,* **2012**, *56*, 166-178.
[http://dx.doi.org/10.1016/j.ejmech.2012.08.021] [PMID: 22982122]

[51]   Subba Rao, A.V.; Swapna, K.; Shaik, S.P.; Lakshma Nayak, V.; Srinivasa Reddy, T.; Sunkari, S.; Shaik, T.B.; Bagul, C.; Kamal, A. Synthesis and biological evaluation of *cis*-restricted triazole/tetrazole mimics of combretastatin-benzothiazole hybrids as tubulin polymerization inhibitors and apoptosis inducers. *Bioorg. Med. Chem.,* **2017**, *25*(3), 977-999.
[http://dx.doi.org/10.1016/j.bmc.2016.12.010] [PMID: 28034647]

[52]   Ashraf, M.; Shaik, T.B.; Malik, M.S.; Syed, R.; Mallipeddi, P.L.; Vardhan, M.V.P.S.V.; Kamal, A. Design and synthesis of *cis*-restricted benzimidazole and benzothiazole mimics of combretastatin A-4 as antimitotic agents with apoptosis inducing ability. *Bioorg. Med. Chem. Lett.,* **2016**, *26*(18), 4527-4535.
[http://dx.doi.org/10.1016/j.bmcl.2016.06.044] [PMID: 27515320]

[53]   a)Haider, K.; Rahaman, S.; Yar, M.S.; Kamal, A. Tubulin inhibitors as novel anticancer agents: an overview on patents (2013-2018*). Expert Opin. Ther. Pat.,* **2019**, *29*(8), 623-641.
[http://dx.doi.org/10.1080/13543776.2019.1648433] [PMID: 31353978] b)Kremmidiotis, G.; Leske, A.F.; Lavranos, T.C.; Beaumont, D.; Gasic, J.; Hall, A.; O'Callaghan, M.; Matthews, C.A.; Flynn, B. BNC105: a novel tubulin polymerization inhibitor that selectively disrupts tumor vasculature and displays single-agent antitumor efficacy. *Mol. Cancer Ther.,* **2010**, *9*(6), 1562-1573.
[http://dx.doi.org/10.1158/1535-7163.MCT-09-0815] [PMID: 20515948]

[54]   Shaik, T.B.; Hussaini, S.M.A.; Nayak, V.L.; Sucharitha, M.L.; Malik, M.S.; Kamal, A. Rational design and synthesis of 2-anilinopyridinyl-benzothiazole Schiff bases as antimitotic agents. *Bioorg. Med. Chem. Lett.,* **2017**, *27*(11), 2549-2558.
[http://dx.doi.org/10.1016/j.bmcl.2017.03.089] [PMID: 28400235]

[55]   Bhat, M.; Belagali, S.L.; Kumar, N.K.H.; Jagannath, S. Anti-mitotic Activity of the Benzothiazole-pyrazole Hybrid Derivatives. *Antiinfect. Agents,* **2019**, *17*, 66-73.
[http://dx.doi.org/10.2174/2211352516666180914101758]

[56]   Song, J.; Gao, Q.L.; Wu, B.W.; Zhu, T.; Cui, X.X.; Jin, C.J.; Wang, S.Y.; Wang, S.H.; Fu, D.J.; Liu, H.M.; Zhang, S.Y.; Zhang, Y.B.; Li, Y.C. Discovery of tertiary amide derivatives incorporating benzothiazole moiety as anti-gastric cancer agents *in vitro via* inhibiting tubulin polymerization and activating the Hippo signaling pathway. *Eur. J. Med. Chem.,* **2020**, *203*112618
[http://dx.doi.org/10.1016/j.ejmech.2020.112618] [PMID: 32682200]

[57]   Broekman, F.; Giovannetti, E.; Peters, G.J. Tyrosine kinase inhibitors: Multi-targeted or single-targeted? *World J. Clin. Oncol.,* **2011**, *2*(2), 80-93.
[http://dx.doi.org/10.5306/wjco.v2.i2.80] [PMID: 21603317]

[58]   Cohen, P. Protein kinases--the major drug targets of the twenty-first century? *Nat. Rev. Drug Discov.,* **2002**, *1*(4), 309-315.
[http://dx.doi.org/10.1038/nrd773] [PMID: 12120282]

[59]   Hunter, T. Tyrosine phosphorylation: thirty years and counting. *Curr. Opin. Cell Biol.,* **2009**, *21*(2), 140-146.

[http://dx.doi.org/10.1016/j.ceb.2009.01.028] [PMID: 19269802]

[60]   Fabbro, D.; Parkinson, D.; Matter, A. Protein tyrosine kinase inhibitors: new treatment modalities? *Curr. Opin. Pharmacol.,* **2002**, *2*(4), 374-381.
[http://dx.doi.org/10.1016/S1471-4892(02)00179-0] [PMID: 12127869]

[61]   Kumar, M.; Nagpal, R.; Hemalatha, R.; Verma, V.; Kumar, A.; Singh, S.; Marotta, F.; Jain, S.; Yadav, H. Targeted cancer therapies: the future of cancer treatment. *Acta Biomed.,* **2012**, *83*(3), 220-233.
[PMID: 23762999]

[62]   Yamaoka, T.; Kusumoto, S.; Ando, K.; Ohba, M.; Ohmori, T. Receptor tyrosine kinase targeted cancer therapy. *Int. J. Mol. Sci.,* **2018**, *19*(11), 3491-3525.
[http://dx.doi.org/10.3390/ijms19113491] [PMID: 30404198]

[63]   Chen, D.; Jansson, A.; Sim, D.; Larsson, A.; Nordlund, P. Structural analyses of human thymidylate synthase reveal a site that may control conformational switching between active and inactive states. *J. Biol. Chem.,* **2017**, *292*(32), 13449-13458.
[http://dx.doi.org/10.1074/jbc.M117.787267] [PMID: 28634233]

[64]   Bhuva, H.A.; Kini, S.G. Synthesis, anticancer activity and docking of some substituted benzothiazoles as tyrosine kinase inhibitors. *J. Mol. Graph. Model.,* **2010**, *29*(1), 32-37.
[http://dx.doi.org/10.1016/j.jmgm.2010.04.003] [PMID: 20493747]

[65]   Noolvi, M.N.; Patel, H.M.; Kaur, M. Benzothiazoles: search for anticancer agents. *Eur. J. Med. Chem.,* **2012**, *54*, 447-462.
[http://dx.doi.org/10.1016/j.ejmech.2012.05.028] [PMID: 22703845]

[66]   Gabr, M.T.; El-Gohary, N.S.; El-Bendary, E.R.; El-Kerdawy, M.M. New series of benzothiazole and pyrimido [2,1-b] benzothiazole derivatives: Synthesis, Antitumor activity, EGFR tyrosine kinase inhibitory activity and molecular modeling studies. *Med. Chem. Res.,* **2014**, 1-19.

[67]   Labib, M.B.; Philoppes, J.N.; Lamie, P.F.; Ahmed, E.R. Azole-hydrazone derivatives: Design, synthesis, *in vitro* biological evaluation, dual EGFR/HER2 inhibitory activity, cell cycle analysis and molecular docking study as anticancer agents. *Bioorg. Chem.,* **2018**, *76*, 67-80.
[http://dx.doi.org/10.1016/j.bioorg.2017.10.016] [PMID: 29153588]

[68]   Abdellatif, K.R.A.; Belal, A.; El-Saadi, M.T.; Amin, N.H.; Said, E.G.; Hemeda, L.R. Design, synthesis, molecular docking and antiproliferative activity of some novel benzothiazole derivatives targeting EGFR/HER2 and TS. *Bioorg. Chem.,* **2020**, *101*103976
[http://dx.doi.org/10.1016/j.bioorg.2020.103976] [PMID: 32506018]

[69]   Mokhtar, A.M.; El-Messery, S.M.; Ghaly, M.A.; Hassan, G.S. Targeting EGFR tyrosine kinase: Synthesis, in vitro antitumor evaluation, and molecular modeling studies of benzothiazole-based derivatives. *Bioorg. Chem.,* **2020**, *104*104259
[http://dx.doi.org/10.1016/j.bioorg.2020.104259] [PMID: 32919134]

[70]   Hong, S.; Kim, J.; Yun, S.M.; Lee, H.; Park, Y.; Hong, S-S.; Hong, S. Discovery of new benzothiazole-based inhibitors of breakpoint cluster region-Abelson kinase including the T315I mutant. *J. Med. Chem.,* **2013**, *56*(9), 3531-3545.
[http://dx.doi.org/10.1021/jm301891t] [PMID: 23600806]

[71]   El-Damasy, A.K.; Jin, H.; Seo, S.H.; Bang, E.K.; Keum, G. Design, synthesis, and biological evaluations of novel 3-amino-4-ethynyl indazole derivatives as Bcr-Abl kinase inhibitors with potent cellular antileukemic activity. *Eur. J. Med. Chem.,* **2020**, *207*112710
[http://dx.doi.org/10.1016/j.ejmech.2020.112710] [PMID: 32961435]

[72]   Ivanova, E.S.; Tatarskiy, V.V.; Yastrebova, M.A.; Khamidullina, A.I.; Shunaev, A.V.; Kalinina, A.A.; Zeifman, A.A.; Novikov, F.N.; Dutikova, Y.V.; Chilov, G.G.; Shtil, A.A. PF□114, a novel selective inhibitor of BCR□ABL tyrosine kinase, is a potent inducer of apoptosis in chronic myelogenous leukemia cells. *Int. J. Oncol.,* **2019**, *55*(1), 289-297.
[http://dx.doi.org/10.3892/ijo.2019.4801] [PMID: 31115499]

[73]    Hofmann, W.K.; Jones, L.C.; Lemp, N.A.; de Vos, S.; Gschaidmeier, H.; Hoelzer, D.; Ottmann, O.G.; Koeffler, H.P. Ph(+) acute lymphoblastic leukemia resistant to the tyrosine kinase inhibitor STI571 has a unique BCR-ABL gene mutation. *Blood,* **2002**, *99*(5), 1860-1862.
        [http://dx.doi.org/10.1182/blood.V99.5.1860] [PMID: 11861307]

[74]    El-Damasy, A.K.; Cho, N.C.; Kang, S.B.; Pae, A.N.; Keum, G. ABL kinase inhibitory and antiproliferative activity of novel picolinamide based benzothiazoles. *Bioorg. Med. Chem. Lett.,* **2015**, *25*(10), 2162-2168.
        [http://dx.doi.org/10.1016/j.bmcl.2015.03.067] [PMID: 25881828]

[75]    Han, M.W.; Ryu, I.S.; Lee, J.C.; Kim, S.H.; Chang, H.W.; Lee, Y.S.; Lee, S.; Kim, S.W.; Kim, S.Y. Phosphorylation of PI3K regulatory subunit p85 contributes to resistance against PI3K inhibitors in radioresistant head and neck cancer. *Oral Oncol.,* **2018**, *78*, 56-63.
        [http://dx.doi.org/10.1016/j.oraloncology.2018.01.014] [PMID: 29496059]

[76]    Hanker, A.B.; Kaklamani, V.; Arteaga, C.L. Challenges for the Clinical Development of PI3K Inhibitors: Strategies to Improve Their Impact in Solid Tumors. *Cancer Discov.,* **2019**, *9*(4), 482-491.
        [http://dx.doi.org/10.1158/2159-8290.CD-18-1175] [PMID: 30867161]

[77]    Dienstmann, R.; Rodon, J.; Serra, V.; Tabernero, J. Picking the point of inhibition: a comparative review of PI3K/AKT/mTOR pathway inhibitors. *Mol. Cancer Ther.,* **2014**, *13*(5), 1021-1031.
        [http://dx.doi.org/10.1158/1535-7163.MCT-13-0639] [PMID: 24748656]

[78]    Paplomata, E.; O'Regan, R. The PI3K/AKT/mTOR pathway in breast cancer: targets, trials and biomarkers. *Ther. Adv. Med. Oncol.,* **2014**, *6*(4), 154-166.
        [http://dx.doi.org/10.1177/1758834014530023] [PMID: 25057302]

[79]    Bauer, T.M.; Patel, M.R.; Infante, J.R. Targeting PI3 kinase in cancer. *Pharmacol. Ther.,* **2015**, *146*, 53-60.
        [http://dx.doi.org/10.1016/j.pharmthera.2014.09.006] [PMID: 25240910]

[80]    Slomovitz, B.M.; Coleman, R.L. The PI3K/AKT/mTOR pathway as a therapeutic target in endometrial cancer. *Clin. Cancer Res.,* **2012**, *18*(21), 5856-5864.
        [http://dx.doi.org/10.1158/1078-0432.CCR-12-0662] [PMID: 23082003]

[81]    Li, H.; Wang, X.M.; Wang, J.; Shao, T.; Li, Y.P.; Mei, Q.B.; Lu, S.M.; Zhang, S.Q. Combination of 2-methoxy-3-phenylsulfonylaminobenzamide and 2-aminobenzothiazole to discover novel anticancer agents. *Bioorg. Med. Chem.,* **2014**, *22*(14), 3739-3748.
        [http://dx.doi.org/10.1016/j.bmc.2014.04.064] [PMID: 24878359]

[82]    Xie, X.X.; Li, H.; Wang, J.; Mao, S.; Xin, M.H.; Lu, S.M.; Mei, Q.B.; Zhang, S.Q. Synthesis and anticancer  effects  evaluation  of  1-alkyl-3-(6-(2-methoxy-3-sulfonylaminopyridin-5 -yl)benzo[*d*]thiazol-2-yl)urea as anticancer agents with low toxicity. *Bioorg. Med. Chem.,* **2015**, *23*(19), 6477-6485.
        [http://dx.doi.org/10.1016/j.bmc.2015.08.013] [PMID: 26321603]

[83]    Collier, P.N.; Martinez-Botella, G.; Cornebise, M.; Cottrell, K.M.; Doran, J.D.; Griffith, J.P.; Mahajan, S.; Maltais, F.; Moody, C.S.; Huck, E.P.; Wang, T.; Aronov, A.M. Structural basis for isoform selectivity in a class of benzothiazole inhibitors of phosphoinositide 3-kinase γ. *J. Med. Chem.,* **2015**, *58*(1), 517-521.
        [http://dx.doi.org/10.1021/jm500362j] [PMID: 24754609]

[84]    Wan, P.T.C.; Garnett, M.J.; Roe, S.M.; Lee, S.; Niculescu-Duvaz, D.; Good, V.M.; Jones, C.M.; Marshall, C.J.; Springer, C.J.; Barford, D.; Marais, R. Mechanism of activation of the RAF-ERK signaling pathway by oncogenic mutations of B-RAF. *Cell,* **2004**, *116*(6), 855-867.
        [http://dx.doi.org/10.1016/S0092-8674(04)00215-6] [PMID: 15035987]

[85]    Thiel, A.; Ristimäki, A. Toward a molecular classification of colorectal cancer: the role of BRAF. *Front. Oncol.,* **2013**, *3*, 281.
        [http://dx.doi.org/10.3389/fonc.2013.00281] [PMID: 24298448]

[86] Madhunapantula, S.V.; Robertson, G.P. Is B-Raf a good therapeutic target for melanoma and other malignancies? *Cancer Res.,* **2008**, *68*(1), 5-8.
[http://dx.doi.org/10.1158/0008-5472.CAN-07-2038] [PMID: 18172288]

[87] Kamal, A.; Faazil, S.; Ramaiah, M.J.; Ashraf, M.; Balakrishna, M.; Pushpavalli, S.N.; Patel, N.; Pal-Bhadra, M. Synthesis and study of benzothiazole conjugates in the control of cell proliferation by modulating Ras/MEK/ERK-dependent pathway in MCF-7 cells. *Bioorg. Med. Chem. Lett.,* **2013**, *23*(20), 5733-5739.
[http://dx.doi.org/10.1016/j.bmcl.2013.07.068] [PMID: 23999041]

[88] Song, E.Y.; Kaur, N.; Park, M.Y.; Jin, Y.; Lee, K.; Kim, G.; Lee, K.Y.; Yang, J.S.; Shin, J.H.; Nam, K.Y.; No, K.T.; Han, G. Synthesis of amide and urea derivatives of benzothiazole as Raf-1 inhibitor. *Eur. J. Med. Chem.,* **2008**, *43*(7), 1519-1524.
[http://dx.doi.org/10.1016/j.ejmech.2007.10.008] [PMID: 18023932]

[89] El-Damasy, A.K.; Lee, J.H.; Seo, S.H.; Cho, N.C.; Pae, A.N.; Keum, G. Design and synthesis of new potent anticancer benzothiazole amides and ureas featuring pyridylamide moiety and possessing dual B-Raf(V600E) and C-Raf kinase inhibitory activities. *Eur. J. Med. Chem.,* **2016**, *115*, 201-216.
[http://dx.doi.org/10.1016/j.ejmech.2016.02.039] [PMID: 27017549]

[90] Okaniwa, M.; Hirose, M.; Arita, T.; Yabuki, M.; Nakamura, A.; Takagi, T.; Kawamoto, T.; Uchiyama, N.; Sumita, A.; Tsutsumi, S.; Tottori, T.; Inui, Y.; Sang, B-C.; Yano, J.; Aertgeerts, K.; Yoshida, S.; Ishikawa, T. Discovery of a selective kinase inhibitor (TAK-632) targeting pan-RAF inhibition: design, synthesis, and biological evaluation of C-7-substituted 1,3-benzothiazole derivatives. *J. Med. Chem.,* **2013**, *56*(16), 6478-6494.
[http://dx.doi.org/10.1021/jm400778d] [PMID: 23906342]

[91] Monneret, C. Histone deacetylase inhibitors. *Eur. J. Med. Chem.,* **2005**, *40*(1), 1-13.
[http://dx.doi.org/10.1016/j.ejmech.2004.10.001] [PMID: 15642405]

[92] Kumboonma, P.; Senawong, T.; Saenglee, S.; Senawong, G.; Somsakeesit, L. Yenjai, C.; Phaosiri, C. New histone deacetylase inhibitors and anticancer agents from Curcuma longa. *Med. Chem. Res.,* **2019**, *28*, 1773-1782.

[93] Zagni, C.; Citarella, A.; Oussama, M.; Rescifina, A.; Maugeri, A.; Navarra, M.; Scala, A.; Piperno, A.; Micale, N. Hydroxamic Acid-Based Histone Deacetylase (HDAC) Inhibitors Bearing a Pyrazole Scaffold and a Cinnamoyl Linker. *Int. J. Mol. Sci.,* **2019**, *20*(4), 945.
[http://dx.doi.org/10.3390/ijms20040945] [PMID: 30795625]

[94] Oanh, D.T.; Hai, H.V.; Park, S.H.; Kim, H.J.; Han, B.W.; Kim, H.S.; Hong, J.T.; Han, S.B.; Hue, V.T.; Nam, N.H. Benzothiazole-containing hydroxamic acids as histone deacetylase inhibitors and antitumor agents. *Bioorg. Med. Chem. Lett.,* **2011**, *21*(24), 7509-7512.
[http://dx.doi.org/10.1016/j.bmcl.2011.07.124] [PMID: 22036991]

[95] Rajak, H.; Singh, A.; Raghuwanshi, K.; Kumar, R.; Dewangan, P.K.; Veerasamy, R.; Sharma, P.C.; Dixit, A.; Mishra, P. A structural insight into hydroxamic acid based histone deacetylase inhibitors for the presence of anticancer activity. *Curr. Med. Chem.,* **2014**, *21*(23), 2642-2664.
[http://dx.doi.org/10.2174/09298673113209990191] [PMID: 23895688]

[96] Munster, P.N.; Troso-Sandoval, T.; Rosen, N.; Rifkind, R.; Marks, P.A.; Richon, V.M. The histone deacetylase inhibitor suberoylanilide hydroxamic acid induces differentiation of human breast cancer cells. *Cancer Res.,* **2001**, *61*(23), 8492-8497.
[PMID: 11731433]

[97] Rajak, H.; Singh, A.; Dewangan, P.K.; Patel, V.; Jain, D.K.; Tiwari, S.K.; Veerasamy, R.; Sharma, P.C. Peptide based macrocycles: selective histone deacetylase inhibitors with antiproliferative activity. *Curr. Med. Chem.,* **2013**, *20*(14), 1887-1903.
[http://dx.doi.org/10.2174/0929867311320140006] [PMID: 23409715]

[98] West, A.C.; Johnstone, R.W. New and emerging HDAC inhibitors for cancer treatment. *J. Clin. Invest.,* **2014**, *124*(1), 30-39.

[http://dx.doi.org/10.1172/JCI69738] [PMID: 24382387]

[99]    Yang, F.; Zhao, N.; Hu, Y.; Jiang, C-S.; Zhang, H. The development process: from SAHA to hydroxamate HDAC inhibitors with branched CAP region and linear linker. *Chem. Biodivers.,* **2020**, *17*(1), e1900427.
[PMID: 31793143]

[100]   Staker, B.L.; Feese, M.D.; Cushman, M.; Pommier, Y.; Zembower, D.; Stewart, L.; Burgin, A.B. Structures of three classes of anticancer agents bound to the human topoisomerase I-DNA covalent complex. *J. Med. Chem.,* **2005**, *48*(7), 2336-2345.
[http://dx.doi.org/10.1021/jm049146p] [PMID: 15801827]

[101]   Pommier, Y. DNA topoisomerase I inhibitors: chemistry, biology, and interfacial inhibition. *Chem. Rev.,* **2009**, *109*(7), 2894-2902.
[http://dx.doi.org/10.1021/cr900097c] [PMID: 19476377]

[102]   Kaur, P.; Kaur, V.; Kaur, S. DNA Topoisomerase II: promising target for anticancer drugs. In: *In Multi-Targeted Approach to Treatment of Cancer*; , **2015**; pp. 323-338.

[103]   Weller, M.; Winter, S.; Schmidt, C.; Esser, P.; Fontana, A.; Dichgans, J.; Groscurth, P. Topoisomerase-I inhibitors for human malignant glioma: differential modulation of p53, p21, bax and bcl-2 expression and of CD95-mediated apoptosis by camptothecin and beta-lapachone. *Int. J. Cancer,* **1997**, *73*(5), 707-714.
[http://dx.doi.org/10.1002/(SICI)1097-0215(19971127)73:5<707::AID-IJC16>3.0.CO;2-2] [PMID: 9398050]

[104]   Kamal, A.; Kumar, B.A.; Suresh, P.; Shankaraiah, N.; Kumar, M.S. An efficient one-pot synthesis of benzothiazolo-4β-anilino-podophyllotoxin congeners: DNA topoisomerase-II inhibition and anticancer activity. *Bioorg. Med. Chem. Lett.,* **2011**, *21*(1), 350-353.
[http://dx.doi.org/10.1016/j.bmcl.2010.11.002] [PMID: 21144748]

[105]   Nagaraju, B.; Kovvuri, J.; Kumar, C.G.; Routhu, S.R.; Shareef, M.A.; Kadagathur, M.; Adiyala, P.R.; Alavala, S.; Nagesh, N.; Kamal, A. Synthesis and biological evaluation of pyrazole linked benzothiazole-β-naphthol derivatives as topoisomerase I inhibitors with DNA binding ability. *Bioorg. Med. Chem.,* **2019**, *27*(5), 708-720.
[http://dx.doi.org/10.1016/j.bmc.2019.01.011] [PMID: 30679134]

[106]   Sankara, Rao N; Nagesh, N; Lakshma Nayak, V; Sunkari, S; Tokala, R; Kiranmai, G; Regur, P; Shankaraiah N, N; Kamal, A Design and synthesis of DNA-intercalative naphthalimide-benzothiazole/cinnamide derivatives: cytotoxicity evaluation and topoisomerase-IIα inhibition. In: *Medchemcomm*; , **2018**; 10, pp. (1)72-79.

[107]   Tokala, R.; Mahajan, S.; Kiranmai, G.; Sigalapalli, D.K.; Sana, S.; John, S.E.; Nagesh, N.; Shankaraiah, N. Development of β-carboline-benzothiazole hybrids *via* carboxamide formation as cytotoxic agents: DNA intercalative topoisomerase IIα inhibition and apoptosis induction. *Bioorg. Chem.,* **2020**.

[108]   Hay, A.E.; Murugesan, A.; DiPasquale, A.M.; Kouroukis, T.; Sandhu, I.; Kukreti, V.; Bahlis, N.J.; Lategan, J.; Reece, D.E.; Lyons, J.F.; Sederias, J.; Xu, H.; Powers, J.; Seymour, L.K.; Reiman, T. A Phase II Study of AT9283, an Aurora Kinase Inhibitor, in Patients with Relapsed or Refractory Multiple Myeloma: NCIC Clinical Trials Group IND.191. *Leuk. Lymphoma,* **2015**, 1-10.
[PMID: 26376958]

[109]   Bavetsias, V.; Linardopoulos, S. Aurora Kinase Inhibitors: Current Status and Outlook. *Front. Oncol.,* **2015**, *5*, 278.
[http://dx.doi.org/10.3389/fonc.2015.00278] [PMID: 26734566]

[110]   Dar, A.A.; Goff, L.W.; Majid, S.; Berlin, J.; El-Rifai, W. Aurora kinase inhibitors--rising stars in cancer therapeutics? *Mol. Cancer Ther.,* **2010**, *9*(2), 268-278.
[http://dx.doi.org/10.1158/1535-7163.MCT-09-0765] [PMID: 20124450]

[111]   Lee, E.; An, Y.; Kwon, J.; Kim, K.I.; Jeon, R. Optimization and biological evaluation of 2-

aminobenzothiazole derivatives as Aurora B kinase inhibitors. *Bioorg. Med. Chem.,* **2017**, *25*(14), 3614-3622.
[http://dx.doi.org/10.1016/j.bmc.2017.04.004] [PMID: 28529042]

[112]   Tasler, S.; Müller, O.; Wieber, T.; Herz, T.; Pegoraro, S.; Saeb, W.; Lang, M.; Krauss, R.; Totzke, F.; Zirrgiebel, U.; Ehlert, J.E.; Kubbutat, M.H.; Schächtele, C. Substituted 2-arylbenzothiazoles as kinase inhibitors: hit-to-lead optimization. *Bioorg. Med. Chem.,* **2009**, *17*(18), 6728-6737.
[http://dx.doi.org/10.1016/j.bmc.2009.07.047] [PMID: 19692247]

[113]   Borisa, A.C.; Bhatt, H.G. A comprehensive review on Aurora kinase: Small molecule inhibitors and clinical trial studies. *Eur. J. Med. Chem.,* **2017**, *140*, 1-19.
[http://dx.doi.org/10.1016/j.ejmech.2017.08.045] [PMID: 28918096]

[114]   Gaikwad, D.D.; Pawar, C.D.; Pansare, D.N.; Chavan, S.L.; Pawar, U.D.; Shelke, R.N.; Chavan, S.L.; Pawar, R.P.; Zine, A.M. Synthesis of novel substituted-benzothiazole-2,4-dicarboxamides having kinase inhibition and anti-proliferative activity. *Eur. Chem. Bull.,* **2019**, *8*(4), 78-84.
[http://dx.doi.org/10.17628/ecb.2019.8.78-84]

[115]   Fowler, C.J. Monoacylglycerol lipase - a target for drug development? *Br. J. Pharmacol.,* **2012**, *166*(5), 1568-1585.
[http://dx.doi.org/10.1111/j.1476-5381.2012.01950.x] [PMID: 22428756]

[116]   Granchi, C.; Caligiuri, I.; Minutolo, F.; Rizzolio, F. andTuccinardi, T. A patent review of Monoacylglycerol Lipase (MAGL) inhibitors (2013-2017). *Expert Opin. Ther. Pat.,* **2012**, 1-12.

[117]   Vila, A.; Rosengarth, A.; Piomelli, D.; Cravatt, B.; Marnett, L.J. Hydrolysis of prostaglandin glycerol esters by the endocannabinoid-hydrolyzing enzymes, monoacylglycerol lipase and fatty acid amide hydrolase. *Biochemistry,* **2007**, *46*(33), 9578-9585.
[http://dx.doi.org/10.1021/bi7005898] [PMID: 17649977]

[118]   Afzal, O.; Akhtar, M.S.; Kumar, S.; Ali, M.R.; Jaggi, M.; Bawa, S. Hit to lead optimization of a series of N-[4-(1,3-benzothiazol-2-yl)phenyl]acetamides as monoacylglycerol lipase inhibitors with potential anticancer activity. *Eur. J. Med. Chem.,* **2016**, *121*, 318-330.
[http://dx.doi.org/10.1016/j.ejmech.2016.05.038] [PMID: 27267002]

[119]   Enchev, R.I.; Schulman, B.A.; Peter, M. Protein neddylation: beyond cullin-RING ligases. *Nat. Rev. Mol. Cell Biol.,* **2015**, *16*(1), 30-44.
[http://dx.doi.org/10.1038/nrm3919] [PMID: 25531226]

[120]   Song, J.; Cui, X-X.; Wu, B-W.; Li, D.; Wang, S-H.; Shi, L.; Zhu, T.; Zhang, Y-B.; Zhang, S-Y. Discovery of 1, 2, 4-triazine-based derivatives as novel neddylation inhibitors and anticancer activity studies against gastric cancer MGC-803 cells. *Bioorg. Med. Chem. Lett.,* **2019**, 1-20.
[PMID: 31740251]

[121]   Kee, Y.; Huang, M.; Chang, S.; Moreau, L.A.; Park, E.; Smith, P.G.; D'Andrea, A.D. Inhibition of the Nedd8 system sensitizes cells to DNA interstrand cross-linking agents. *Mol. Cancer Res.,* **2012**, *10*(3), 369-377.
[http://dx.doi.org/10.1158/1541-7786.MCR-11-0497] [PMID: 22219386]

[122]   Zhou, L.; Jiang, Y.; Luo, Q.; Li, L.; Jia, L. Neddylation: a novel modulator of the tumor microenvironment. *Mol. Cancer,* **2019**, *18*(1), 77.
[http://dx.doi.org/10.1186/s12943-019-0979-1] [PMID: 30943988]

[123]   Ma, H.; Zhuang, C.; Xu, X.; Li, J.; Wang, J.; Min, X.; Zhang, W.; Zhang, H.; Miao, Z. Discovery of benzothiazole derivatives as novel non-sulfamide NEDD8 activating enzyme inhibitors by target-based virtual screening. *Eur. J. Med. Chem.,* **2017**, *133*, 174-183.
[http://dx.doi.org/10.1016/j.ejmech.2017.03.076] [PMID: 28388520]

[124]   Dutta Gupta, S.; Bommaka, M.K.; Banerjee, A. Inhibiting protein-protein interactions of Hsp90 as a novel approach for targeting cancer. *Eur. J. Med. Chem.,* **2019**, *178*, 48-63.
[http://dx.doi.org/10.1016/j.ejmech.2019.05.073] [PMID: 31176095]

[125] Tutar, L.; Tunoglu, E.N.Y.; Kiyak, B.Y.; Tutar, Y. *Heat Shock Protein and Cancer Based Therapies*; Springer, **2020**, pp. 1-25.
[http://dx.doi.org/10.1007/7515_2020_14]

[126] Pugh, K.W.; Zhang, Z.; Wang, J.; Xu, X.; Munthali, V.; Zuo, A.; Blagg, B.S.J. From Bacteria to Cancer: A Benzothiazole-Based DNA Gyrase B Inhibitor Redesigned for Hsp90 C-Terminal Inhibition. *ACS Med. Chem. Lett.,* **2020**, *11*(8), 1535-1538.
[http://dx.doi.org/10.1021/acsmedchemlett.0c00100] [PMID: 32832020]

[127] Venkatesh, P.; Tiwari, V.S. Design and synthesis of quinazolinone, benzothiazole derivatives bearing guanidinopropanoic acid moiety and their Schiff bases as cytotoxic and antimicrobial agents. *A. J. Chemistry,* **2016**, *9*(1), S914-S925.
[http://dx.doi.org/10.1016/j.arabjc.2011.09.004]

[128] Chhabra, M.; Sinha, S.; Banerjee, S.; Paira, P. An efficient green synthesis of 2-arylbenzothiazole analogues as potent antibacterial and anticancer agents. *Bioorg. Med. Chem. Lett.,* **2016**, *26*(1), 213-217.
[http://dx.doi.org/10.1016/j.bmcl.2015.10.087] [PMID: 26590102]

[129] Al-Ghorbani, M.; Pavankumar, G.S.; Naveen, P.; Thirusangu, P.; Prabhakar, B.T.; Khanum, S.A. Synthesis and an angiolytic role of novel piperazine-benzothiazole analogues on neovascularization, a chief tumoral parameter in neoplastic development. *Bioorg. Chem.,* **2016**, *65*, 110-117.
[http://dx.doi.org/10.1016/j.bioorg.2016.02.006] [PMID: 26918263]

[130] Gabr, M.T.; El-Gohary, N.S.; El-Bendary, E.R.; El-Kerdawy, M.M.; Ni, N. Synthesis, *in vitro* antitumor activity and molecular modeling studies of a new series of benzothiazole Schiff bases. *Chin. Chem. Lett.,* **2016**, *27*, 380-386.
[http://dx.doi.org/10.1016/j.cclet.2015.12.033]

[131] Mohamed, L.W.; Taher, A.T.; Rady, G.S.; Ali, M.M.; Mahmoud, A.E. Synthesis and cytotoxic activity of certain benzothiazole derivatives against human MCF-7 cancer cell line. *Chem. Biol. Drug Des.,* **2017**, *89*(4), 566-576.
[http://dx.doi.org/10.1111/cbdd.12879] [PMID: 27700014]

[132] Lad, N.P.; Manohar, Y.; Mascarenhas, M.; Pandit, Y.B.; Kulkarni, M.R.; Sharma, R.; Salkar, K.; Suthar, A.; Pandit, S.S. Methylsulfonyl benzothiazoles (MSBT) derivatives: Search for new potential antimicrobial and anticancer agents. *Bioorg. Med. Chem. Lett.,* **2017**, *27*(5), 1319-1324.
[http://dx.doi.org/10.1016/j.bmcl.2016.08.032] [PMID: 28188067]

[133] Lei, D.Q.; Deng, X.L.; Zhao, H.Y.; Zhang, F.C.; Liu, R.E. Inhibition of tumor growth and angiogenesis by 2-(4-aminophenyl)benzothiazole in orthotopic glioma C6 rat model. *Saudi. J. Bio. Sci,* **2017**, 1-10.

[134] Abdelgawad, M.A.; Bakr, R.B.; Omar, H.A. Design, synthesis and biological evaluation of some novel benzothiazole/benzoxazole and/or benzimidazole derivatives incorporating a pyrazole scaffold as antiproliferative agents. *Bioorg. Chem.,* **2017**, *74*, 82-90.
[http://dx.doi.org/10.1016/j.bioorg.2017.07.007] [PMID: 28772160]

[135] Cindrić, M.; Jambon, S.; Harej, A.; Depauw, S.; David-Cordonnier, M.H.; Kraljević Pavelić, S.; Karminski-Zamola, G.; Hranjec, M. Novel amidino substituted benzimidazole and benzothiazole benzo[b]thieno-2-carboxamides exert strong antiproliferative and DNA binding properties. *Eur. J. Med. Chem.,* **2017**, *136*, 468-479.
[http://dx.doi.org/10.1016/j.ejmech.2017.05.014] [PMID: 28525845]

[136] Chacko, S.; Samanta, S. A novel approach towards design, synthesis and evaluation of some Schiff base analogues of 2-aminopyridine and 2-aminobezothiazole against hepatocellular carcinoma. *Biomed. Pharmacother.,* **2017**, *89*, 162-176.
[http://dx.doi.org/10.1016/j.biopha.2017.01.108] [PMID: 28222397]

[137] Rubino, S.; Busà, R.; Attanzio, A.; Alduina, R.; Di Stefano, V.; Girasolo, M.A.; Orecchio, S.; Tesoriere, L. Synthesis, properties, antitumor and antibacterial activity of new Pt(II) and Pd(II)

complexes with 2,2′-dithiobis(benzothiazole) ligand. *Bioorg. Med. Chem.*, **2017**, *25*(8), 2378-2386.
[http://dx.doi.org/10.1016/j.bmc.2017.02.067] [PMID: 28336408]

[138]  Eshkil, F.; Eshghi, H.Sh.; Saljooghi, A.; Bakavoli, M.; Rahimizadeh, M. Benzothiazole thiourea derivatives as anticancer agents: design, synthesis, and biological screening. *Russian J. Bio.Chemi.*, **2017**, *43*(5), 576-582.
[http://dx.doi.org/10.1134/S1068162017050065]

[139]  Belal, A. Abdelgawad, M.A. New benzothiazole/benzoxazole-pyrazole hybrids with potential as COX inhibitors: design, synthesis and anticancer activity evaluation. *Res. Chem. Intermed.*, **2017**, *43*(7), 3859-3872.
[http://dx.doi.org/10.1007/s11164-016-2851-x]

[140]  Yang, L. M.; Zhang, H.; Wang, W.W.; Wang, X.J. Design, synthesis, and evaluation of bis-benzothiazole derivatives as DNA minor groove binding agents. In: *J. Heterocyclic Chem*; , **2017**; pp. 1-15.

[141]  Mavroidi, B.; Sagnou, M.; Stamatakis, K.; Paravatou-Petsotas, M.; Pelecanou, M.; Methenitis, C. Palladium-(II) and platinum-(II) complexes of derivatives of 2-(4′-aminophenyl)benzothiazole as potential anticancer agents. *Inorg. Chim. Acta*, **2016**, *444*, 63-75.
[http://dx.doi.org/10.1016/j.ica.2016.01.012]

[142]  Mistry, B.M.; Patel, R.V.; Keum, Y.; Kim, D.H. Evaluation of the biological potencies of newly synthesized berberine derivatives bearing benzothiazole moieties with substituted functionalities. *J. Saudi Chem. Soc.*, **2017**, *21*, 210-219.
[http://dx.doi.org/10.1016/j.jscs.2015.11.002]

[143]  El-Asmy, H.A.; Butler, I.S.; Mouhri, Z.S.; Jean-Claude, B.J.; Emmamc, M.; Mostafa, S.I. Synthesis, characterization and DNA interaction studies of new complexes containing 2-mercaptobenzothiazole and different dinitrogen or phosphorous aromatic donors. *Inorg. Chim. Acta*, **2016**, *441*, 20-33.
[http://dx.doi.org/10.1016/j.ica.2015.10.041]

[144]  Spurr, Paul; Riehen, C. Cyclization process for substituted benzothiazole derivatives. **2006**,

[145]  Scott, B.; Arnold, L.D.; Ericsson, A.M.; Cusack, K.P. Benzothiazole derivatives. **2006**,

[146]  Okaniwa, M.; Takag, T.; Hirose, M. Benzothiazole compounds useful for Raf inhibition. US8143258B2 **2009**.

[147]  Xie, W.; Herbert, B.; Schumacher, R.A.; Nguyen, T.M.; Ma, J.; Gauss, C.M.; Tehim, A. Indazoles, benzothiazoles, benzoisothiazoles, benzoisoxazoles, and preparation and use thereof. US 7,902,217 B2 **2011**.

[148]  Xie, W.; Herbert, B.; Nguyen, C.; Gauss, C.; Tehim, A. Indazoles, benzothiazoles and benzoisothiazoles, and preparation and uses thereof, US 7,943,773 B2. **2011**.

[149]  Liu, C.; Leftheris, K.; Lin, J. Benzothiazole and azobenzothiazole compounds useful as kinase inhibitors. US 7,994,337 B2 **2011**.

[150]  Kamal, A.; Reddy, K.S.; Khan, A.; Naseer, M.; Shetti, R.V. Benzothiazole and benzoxazole linked pyrrolo-[2, 1-c] [1, 4] benzodiazepine hybrids as novel antitumor agents and process for the preparation thereof. US 8,063,204 **2011**.

[151]  Xie, W.; Herbert, B.; Nguyen, C.; Gauss, C.; Tehim, A. Indazoles, benzothiazoles, and benzoisothiazoles, and preparation and uses thereof. US 8,134,003 B2. **2012**.

[152]  Klunk, W.E.; Mathis, C.A.; Wang, Y. Benzothiazole derivative compounds, compositions and uses. US 8,236,282 B2 **2012**.

[153]  Xie, W.; Herbert, B.; Schumacher, R.A.; Nguyen, T.M.; Ma, J.; Gauss, C.M.; Tehim, A. Indazoles, benzothiazoles, benzoisothiazoles, benzoisoxazoles, and preparation and use thereof. US 8,252,811 B. **2012**.

[154]  Xie, W.; Herbert, B.; Schumacher, R.A.; Nguyen, T.M.; Ma, J.; Gauss, C.M.; Tehim, A. Indazoles,

benzothiazoles, benzoisothiazoles, benzoisoxazoles, and preparation and use thereof. US 8,263,619 B2. **2012**.

[155] Zhang, Z.; Daynard, T.S.; Wang, S.; Du, X.; Chopiuk, G.B.; Yan, J.; Chen, J.; Sviridov, S.V. Pyrazolyl-benzothiazole derivatives and their use as therapeutic agents. US 8,410,272 B2 **2013**.

[156] Xie, W.; Herbert, B.; Schumacher, R.A.; Nguyen, T.M.; Ma, J.; Gauss, C.M.; Tehim, A. Indazoles, benzothiazoles, benzoisothiazoles, benzoisoxazoles, and preparation and use thereof. US 8,486,937 B2. **2013**.

[157] Thomas, M.R.; Leslie, P. Benzothiazole derivatives. US 8,501,938 **2013**.

[158] Black, L.A.; Cowart, M.D.; Gfesser, G.A.; Wakefield, B.D.; Alterbach, R.J.; Zhao, C.; Heieh, G.C. Benzothiazole and benzooxazole derivative and methods of use. US 8,580,968 B2 **2013**.

[159] Klunk, W.E.; Jr, C.A.M.; Wang, Y. Benzothiazole derivative compounds, compositions and uses. US 8,691,185 B2 **2014**.

[160] Zhang, Z.; Daynard, T.S.; Wang, S.; Du, X.; Chopiuk, G.B.; Yan, J.; Chen, J.; Sviridov, S.V. Pyrazolyl-benzothiazole derivatives and their use as therapeutic agents. US 8,754,233 B2 **2014**.

[161] Ren, P.; Liu, Y.; Wilson, T.E.; Li, L.; Chan, K. Benzothiazole kinase inhibitors and methods of use. **2015**.

[162] Gil, A.M.; Fernández, D.I.P.; Gil, C.; Gontán, A.; Salado, I.G.; Sancho, M.R.; Martínez, C.P. Substituted benzothiazoles and therapeutic uses thereof for the treatment of human diseases. **2017**.

[163] Ren, P.; Liu, Y.; Wilson, T.E.; Li, L.; Chan, K. Benzothiazole kinase inhibitors and methods of use. **2017**.

[164] Bradshaw, T.D.; Chua, M.S.; Orr, S.; Matthews, C.S.; Stevens, M.F.G. Mechanisms of acquired resistance to 2-(4-aminophenyl)benzothiazole (CJM 126, NSC 34445). *Br. J. Cancer,* **2000**, *83*(2), 270-277.
[http://dx.doi.org/10.1054/bjoc.2000.1231] [PMID: 10901382]

[165] Callero, M.A.; Luzzani, G.A.; De Dios, D.O.; Bradshaw, T.D.; Perez, A.I.L. Biomarkers of sensitivity to potent and selective antitumor 2-(4-amino-3-methylphenyl)-5-fluorobenzothiazole (5F203) in ovarian cancer. *J. Cell. Biochem.,* **2013**, *114*(10), 2392-2404.
[http://dx.doi.org/10.1002/jcb.24589] [PMID: 23696052]

[166] Chua, M.S.; Kashiyama, E.; Bradshaw, T.D.; Stinson, S.F.; Brantley, E.; Sausville, E.A.; Stevens, M.F. Role of Cyp1A1 in modulation of antitumor properties of the novel agent 2-(4-amin-3-methylphenyl)benzothiazole (DF 203, NSC 674495) in human breast cancer cells. *Cancer Res.,* **2000**, *60*(18), 5196-5203.
[PMID: 11016648]

[167] Amino, N.; Ideyama, Y.; Yamano, M.; Kuromitsu, S.; Tajinda, K.; Samizu, K.; Matsuhisa, A.; Kudoh, M.; Shibasaki, M. YM-201627: an orally active antitumor agent with selective inhibition of vascular endothelial cell proliferation. *Cancer Lett.,* **2006**, *238*(1), 119-127.
[http://dx.doi.org/10.1016/j.canlet.2005.06.037] [PMID: 16095812]

[168] Mondal, J.; Sreejith, S.; Borah, P.; Zhao, Y. One-Pot Synthesis of Antitumor Agent PMX 610 by a Copper (II)-Incorporated Mesoporous Catalyst. *ACS Sustain. Chem.& Eng.,* **2014**, *3*(4), 934.
[http://dx.doi.org/10.1021/sc400530a]

[169] Kawakami, M.; Koya, K.; Ukai, T.; Tatsuta, N.; Ikegawa, A.; Ogawa, K.; Shishido, T.; Chen, L.B. Structure-activity of novel rhodacyanine dyes as antitumor agents. *J. Med. Chem.,* **1998**, *41*(1), 130-142.
[http://dx.doi.org/10.1021/jm970590k] [PMID: 9438030]

[170] https://ClinicalTrials.gov/show/NCT01303341

# CHAPTER 4

# Structure-Activity-Relationship (SAR) Studies of Novel Hybrid Quinoline and Quinolone Derivatives as Anticancer Agents

**Pravati Panda[1], Subhendu Chakroborty[2],\* and M.V. B. Unnamatla[3]**

[1] *Department of Chemistry, Ravenshaw University, Cuttack, Odisha753 003, India*

[2] *Department of Basic Sciences, IITM, IES University, Bhopal, India*

[3] *Universidad autonoma del estado de Mexico, Toluca de Lerdo, Mexico*

**Abstract:** Cancer, caused by uncontrolled cell growth in any part of the body, is a significant life-threatening burden for the growing civilization. Though cancer research has reached a high level, considering the high cost of the available therapies to treat various cancers, the morbidity and mortality rates are still high. Organ toxicity, lack of cell specificity, drug resistance, and short half-life with adverse side effects are the major hurdles associated with currently used therapeutics. Therefore, there is a high need to search for new anticancer agents with minimal side effects and toxicity. In this connection, nature always acts as a treasury for scientists by offering its natural sources to fight the war against various life-harvesting diseases. Nowadays, hybrid molecule drug designs attract much attention among organic and medicinal chemists. What is more interesting about the hybrid molecule is that, depending upon the target disease-creating protein, scientists are designing and optimising the target molecule by considering their structure-activity relationship studies (SARs). Among the different natural sources, quinoline, quinolone, and their hybrid derivatives are the most privileged ones. They are found as the central core of many bioactive natural products as well as drug molecules (camptothecin, bosutinib, cabozantinib, pelitinib, lenvatinib, levofloxacin, voreloxin, ciprofloxacin, garenofloxacin, *etc.*) acting as anticancer agents. Literature is enriched with the excellent achievements of hybrid quinoline and quinolone derivatives which function as anticancer agents through various mechanisms such as Bcl-2 inhibition, ALDH inhibition, kinase inhibition, topo-II, and EGFR-TK inhibition, *etc.* Given the excellent performance of quinoline and quinolone hybrid derivatives, it will be worthwhile to continue researching them.

**Keywords:** Anticancer, Hybrid, Quinoline, Quinolone, SARs.

\* **Corresponding author Subhendu Chakroborty:** IES University, Bhopal, Madhya Pradesh, 462044, India; E-mail: subhendu.cy@gmail.com

**Rajesh Kumar Singh (Ed.)**

## INTRODUCTION

Nowadays, cancer is the second leading cause of death, affecting millions of people worldwide. It is caused by the cell's uncontrolled growth in any part of the body [1]. This deadly poisonous disease is found to affect all ages of people. If we look at the statistics of cancer around the globe, then it can be seen that, as compared to men, cancer is more common in women [2]. Breast cancer, cervical cancer, prostate cancer, *etc.*, are the most frequently diagnosed types of cancer in women of all ages. Chemotherapy, surgery, radiation therapy, and hormonal therapies are the primary treatments available for cancer [3]. Though cancer research has reached the pillars, the medicines used for the treatment are associated with some limitations, *i.e.*, drug resistance, organ toxicity, short half-life, lack of cell specificity, adverse side effects, *etc.* Due to the high cost and drug resistance, the mortality and morbidity rates are still high due to cancer [4 - 8]. Therefore, the design and development of drug molecules (*in silico* modeling) by understanding protein-ligand binding through SAR analysis is imperative for the day to sustain cancer.

Natural history and its sources always give enthusiasm to medicinal chemists for discovering new innovative drug entities. Nitrogen-containing heterocycles are highly precious [9 - 12]. This constitutes the fundamental units of nucleic acids such as DNA and RNA, as well as most of the life-saving drug molecules. Considering the significance of nitrogen-containing heterocycles, quinoline/quinolone and its derivatives are the most important. The quinoline/quinolone scaffold is the fusion of benzene and pyridine (Fig. **1**) [13 - 15].

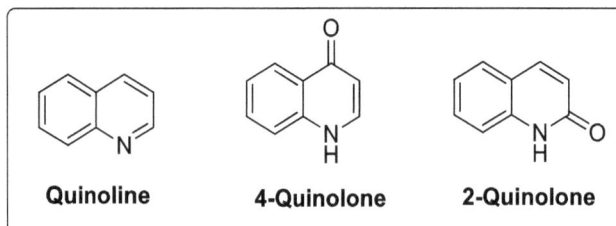

Fig. **(1).** Structure of quinoline/quinolone.

Quinoline and quinolone belong to the benzo-pyridine family. It is one of the most ubiquitous and privileged scaffolds found in many pharmaceutically active compounds associated with versatile biological activities, *i.e.*, antibacterial, antimalarial, anticancer, anti-tubercular, anti-inflammatory, and many more [16 - 21]. The analogues of quinoline and quinolone have been reported to have multiple anticancer potencies involving various mechanisms, including anti-proliferation by the arrest of the cell cycle, apoptosis, angiogenesis inhibition, *etc*

[22, 23]. Camptothecin, topotecan, mappicine, flindersine, haplamine, graveoline, *etc.*, are the most highlighted examples of familiar anticancer drugs bearing quinoline or quinolone as the central moiety [24 - 28]. Due to the development of multidrug resistance over time, there is a need to design and develop novel anticancer agents with high efficacy (Fig. **2**).

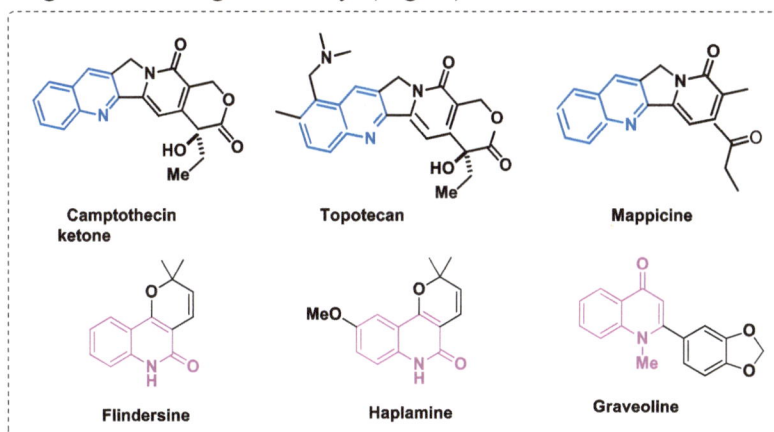

**Fig. (2).** Quinoline/quinolone nuclei present in different natural products and anticancer drugs.

To synthesise multifunctional pharmacophores and avoid the limitations associated with single bioactive entities, nowadays, most researchers are emphasizing the technique of hybridization. It is the phenomenon of intermixing two bioactive pharmacophores into a single molecule called a hybrid molecule, with more potential biological properties than its parent analogue [29]. Voreloxin, quarfloxin, cefatrizine, and AT-3639 are some common examples of anticancer drugs [30, 31]. To avoid drug resistance and toxicity while increasing drug specificity, scientists are using in silico drug design (depending on SAR studies) to create novel anticancer drug molecules by combining quinoline or quinolone with other biologically active cores, which could eventually lead to next-generation anticancer drugs.

This book chapter discussed the design, synthesis, and potential anticancer abilities of various hybrid quinoline/quinolone derivatives against cancer cell lines. The SAR of the active molecules was also explained, providing a charming pathway to explore new dimensions for quinoline/quinolone-based hybrid drug discovery.

## QUINOLINE-COUMARIN/CHROME HYBRIDS

Both quinoline and chromene derivatives have been found to possess a wide range of biological properties such as anticancer, antitumor, antibacterial, anti-inflammatory, *etc.* [32]. The literature contains many reports regarding the versatile efficiency offered by the hybrid analogues derived from quinoline and coumarin [33]. Therefore, Taheri *et al.* synthesised quinoline-coumarin hybrids (**1a-n**) *via* the Ugi reaction and studied their *in vitro* cytotoxicity.

Among the series of compounds tested, quinoline-coumarin hybrid **1k** showed the highest anticancer activity with an $IC_{50}$ of 25 µg/mL towards A2780 cells with a P-value of ≤0.5, causing apoptosis by the downregulation of Bcl2 and survivin through the formation of enzyme-substrate complex and activation of caspase 3 and 9. Both Bcl2 and survivin are the proteins responsible for causing apoptosis. Overexpression of these proteins in the cell causes multidrug resistance and prevents apoptosis by the deactivation of caspase 3 and 9 [34]. In general, the quinoline ring with di-substitution remarkably enhances the hybrid molecules' anticancer potential, as predicted by SAR studies (Fig. **3**) [35].

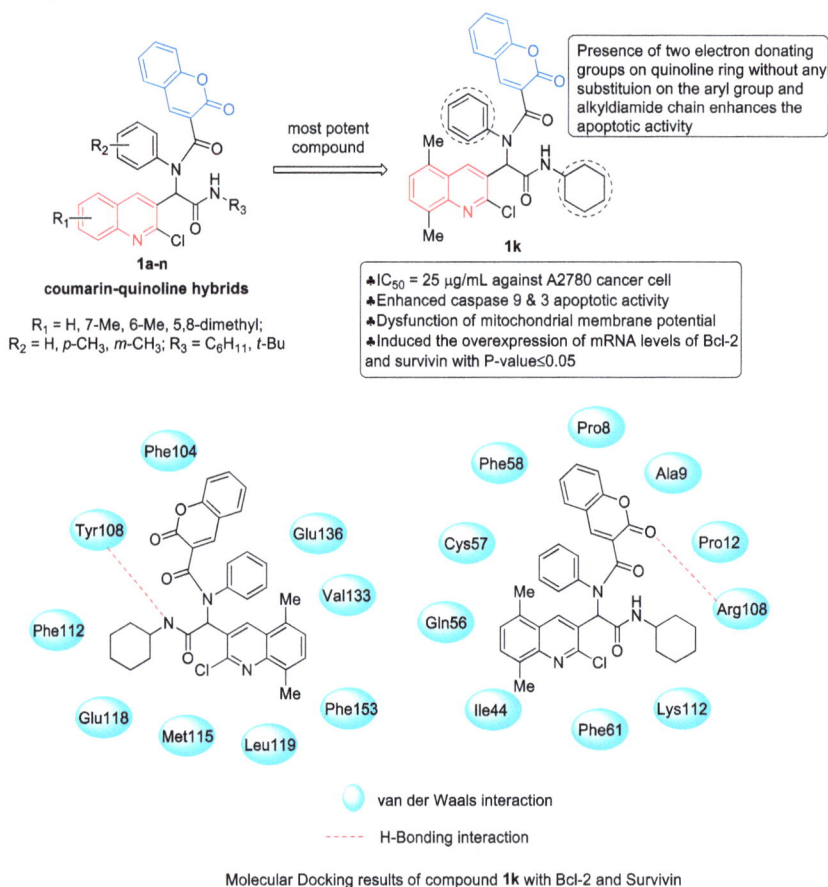

**Fig. (3).** Quinoline-coumarin hybrids as anticancer agents.

Chromene or benzopyran derivatives were discovered to have significant biological properties, most notably anticancer [36, 37]. Inspired by chromene's versatility, Sultana *et al*. planned to fuse it with quinoline to find a new anticancer drug with high efficacy. With this intention, the authors synthesised quinoline-chromene hybrids **4(a-r)** and studied their *in vitro* anticancer efficiency towards MCF7, B16F10, and A549 cells. The hybrids were found to be more effective against the MCF7 cell line. In particular, compounds **4i** and **4m** of the series were seen as the most active molecules in the series and caused apoptosis with $IC_{50}$ = 6.10±1.23 µM and $IC_{50}$ = 8.21±2.31 µM against MCF7 cells (Fig. **4**) [38].

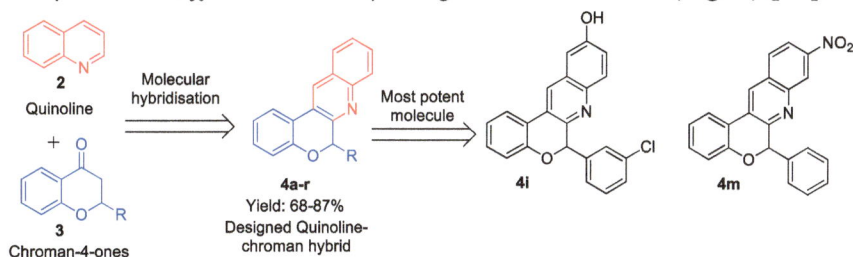

**Fig. (4).** Quinoline-chromene hybrids as anticancer agents.

## QUINOLINE-AZOLE HYBRIDS

### Quinoline-pyrazole Hybrids

Pyrazoles have gained much attention due to their interesting pharmacological properties, making them unique candidates and inspiring chemists to think more about them [39, 40]. Therefore, Nagarapu *et al*. reported the synthesis of quinoline-pyrazole hybrids **5(a-o)** and explored their anticancer potential towards MCF7, HeLa, HepG2, SKNSH, and A549 cells. Compound **5g** was found as the most active molecule (highest antiproliferative activity) of the series with an $IC_{50}$ of 6.01 µM towards the MCF7 cell line (Fig. **5**) [41].

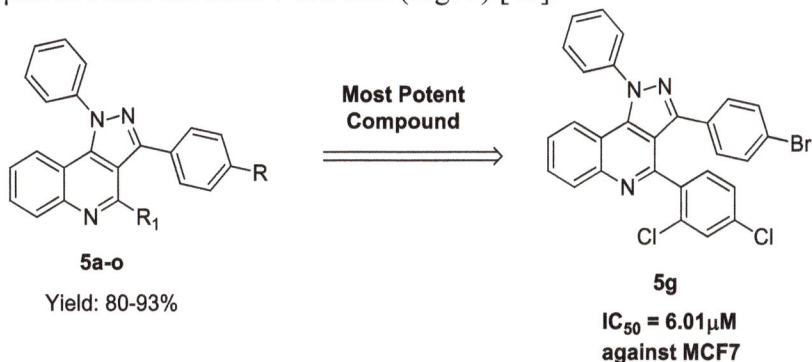

**Fig. (5).** Pyrazole-quinoline hybrids as an anticancer agent.

George *et al.* synthesised quinolinyl-pyrazolyl thiazole hybrids **6a-d**, **7a-c,** and **8a-d** and studied their *in vitro* antiproliferative and EGFR inhibitory activities against HeLa, DLD1, and MCF7 cancer cell lines. The majority of the compounds in the series were discovered to be effective against DLD1 cancer cells. Hybrid **6b** and **7c** were discovered to be active EGFR pannel inhibitors with $IC_{50}$ = 31.8 nM and $IC_{50}$ = 42.5 nM (Fig. **6**) [42].

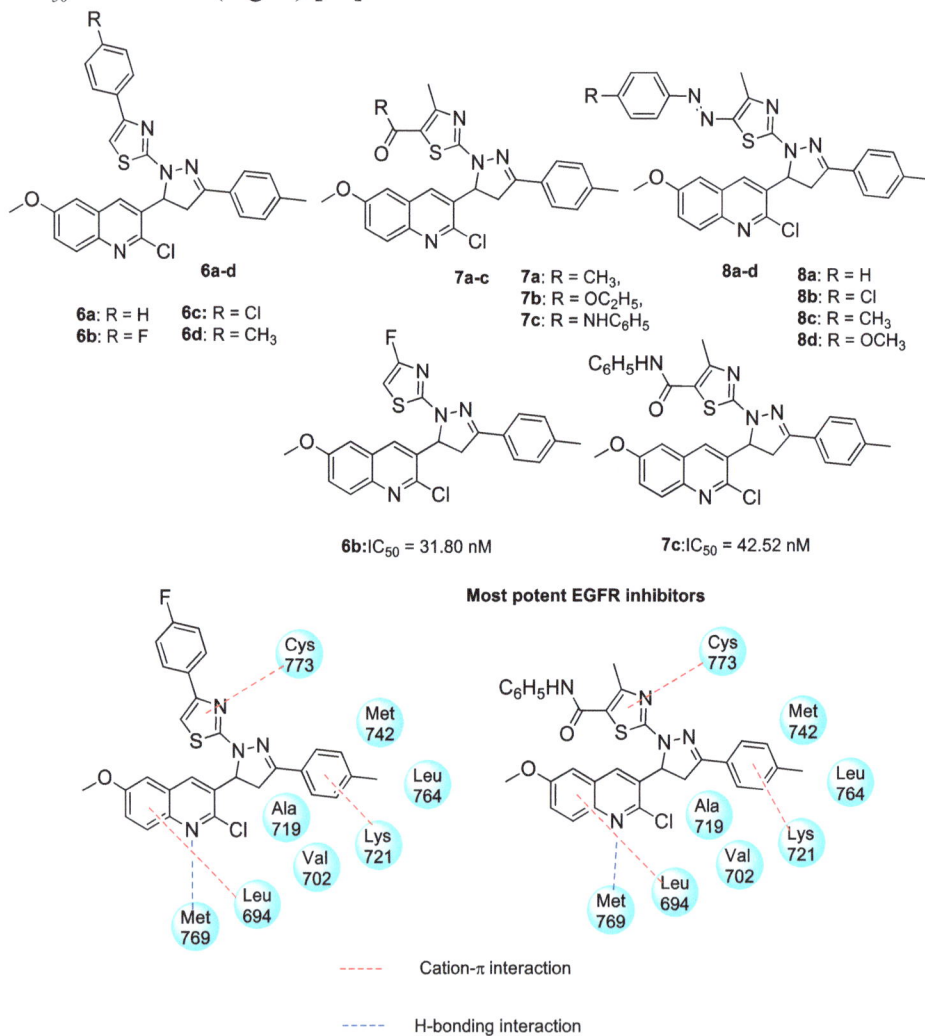

**6a-d**

**6a**: R = H    **6c**: R = Cl
**6b**: R = F    **6d**: R = CH_3

**7a-c**

**7a**: R = CH_3,
**7b**: R = OC_2H_5,
**7c**: R = NHC_6H_5

**8a-d**

**8a**: R = H
**8b**: R = Cl
**8c**: R = CH_3
**8d**: R = OCH_3

**6b**:$IC_{50}$ = 31.80 nM      **7c**:$IC_{50}$ = 42.52 nM

**Most potent EGFR inhibitors**

----- Cation-π interaction

----- H-bonding interaction

Molecular docking results of **6b** and **7c** at the active site of EGFR

**Fig. (6).** Quinoline-pyrazolylthiazole hybrids as inhibitors of EGFR.

## Quinoline-oxazole Hybrids

Oxazole is a five-membered heterocyclic moiety containing both oxygen and nitrogen. Its derivatives were discovered to have a wide range of biological properties, including anticancer properties [43, 44].Therefore, Katariya *et al.* synthesised quinoline-fused oxazole hybrids **9a-l** and demonstrated their anticancer and Topo-I inhibitory properties. Compound **9d** of the series was found to have the highest Topo-I inhibitor activity, with a $GI_{50}$ of 0.26 µM. The phenyl ring-bearing oxadiazole core substituted with electron-donating groups (R = $CH_3/OCH_3$) was found to actively enhance the anticancer activity, as confirmed by SAR (Fig. **7**) [45].

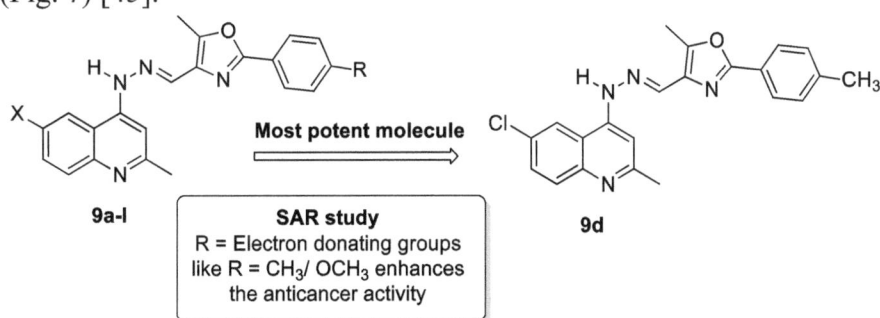

**Fig. (7).** Quinoline-oxazole hybrids as anticancer agents.

The oxyazoline core is found to be present in a number of bioactive molecules exhibiting a range of versatile pharmacological properties [46]. Taking advantage of oxazoline, Bernal *et al.* synthesised tetrahydroquinoline fused oxazoline hybrids **10a-p** *via* a 1,3-dipolar cycloaddition reaction and explained their antiproliferative activities towards a group of cancer cell lines. Hybrid **10a** and **10i** were found active against the B16F10 cell line with $CC_{50}$ = 11.37 µM and $CC_{50}$ = 25.59 µM. Also, hybrid **10h** showed the highest anticancer activity ($CC_{50}$ = 10.21 µM) towards the HeLa cell line (Fig. **8**) [47].

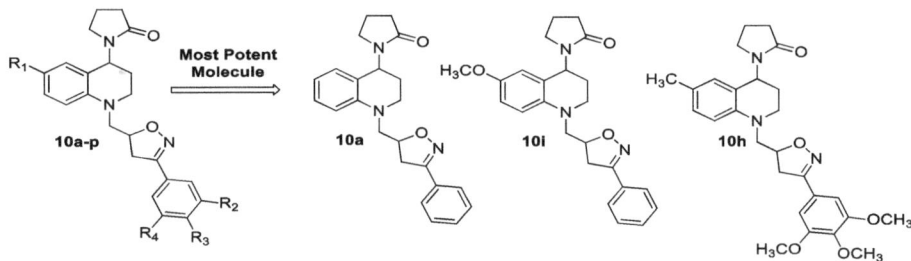

**Fig. (8).** Tetrahydroquinoline-isoxazoline hybrids as anticancer agents.

## Quinoline-oxadiazole Hybrids

Oxadiazole is a privileged heterocyclic scaffold associated with a countless number of bioactivities. Zibotentan is an oxadiazole-based anticancer drug that is under clinical trial [48]. Inspired by the efficacy of oxadiazole derivatives, Westwell *et al.* synthesised quinoline-fused oxazole hybrids **11a–k** and studied their antiproliferative activities against HeLa, MDA-MB-231, Jurkat, and KG1a cancer cell lines. A number of compounds from the series were found to have good inhibitory activity towards HeLa and MDA-MB-231 cell lines, moderate potency towards KG1a, and almost null potency towards the Jurkat cancer cell line. Hybrid **11i** was found as the most active Bcl2 inhibitor of the series, with an $IC_{50}$ of 0.15 μM (Fig. **9**) [49].

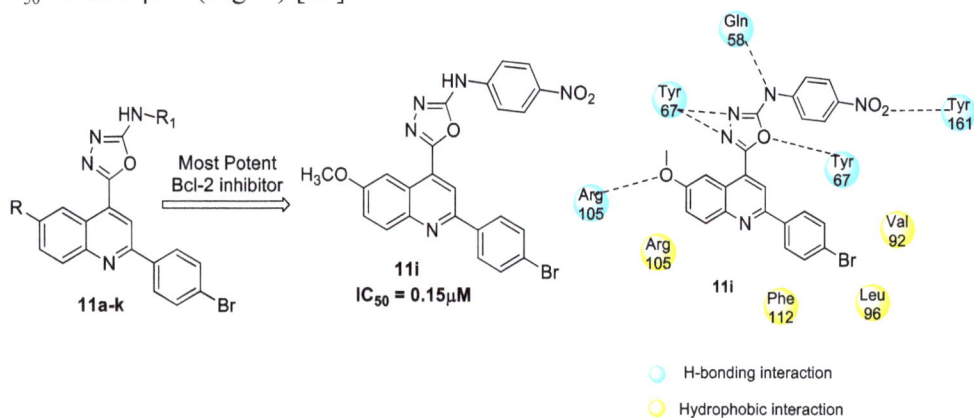

**Fig. (9).** Quinoline-oxadiazoles as inhibitors of Bcl-2.

Abid *et al.* synthesised quinoline-oxadiazole-triazole hybrids and analysed their antiproliferative properties towards HeLa, A-549, HepG2, and SiHa cancer cell lines. Unfortunately, not many compounds were detected to have impressive anticancer abilities. Only one compound from the series, *i.e.*, **12,** was effective in the A549 cell line, with an $IC_{50}$ of 5.6 μM (Fig. **10**) [50].

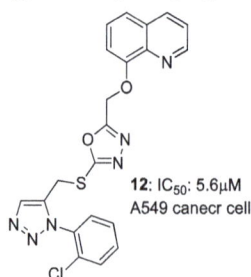

**Fig. (10).** Quinoline-oxadiazole-triazole hybrids as an anticancer agent.

# QUINOLINE-TRIAZOLE HYBRIDS

## Quinoline-1,2,3-triazole Hybrids

Triazoles are well known due to their easy synthesis strategies and numerous bioactivities [51]. Maračić *et al.* synthesized quinoline triazole fused ferrocene hybrids **13a-d** following azide-alkyne coupling reaction involving [3+2] cycloaddition reaction. Hybrid analog **13c** with $IC_{50}$ = 7.9µM was found as the active molecule of the panel towards Raji and K562 cell line with negligible toxicity towards MDCK1 (normal cells) (Fig. **11**) [52].

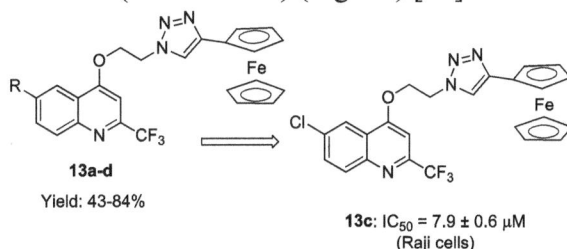

**Fig. (11).** Quinoline-ferrocene hybrids as anticancer agents.

Jadhav and Naidu synthesised quinoline-triazine hybrids **14a-g** and **15a-f** and studied their anticancer activities against HEK, MDA-MB-231, and B16F10 cell lines. The hybrids **14c, 14e, 14f, 14g, 15a, 15c,** and **15d** exhibited significant activity against B16F10 and MDA-MB-231, with $IC_{50}$ values ranging from 13.4 µM to 38.2 µM (Fig. **12**) [53].

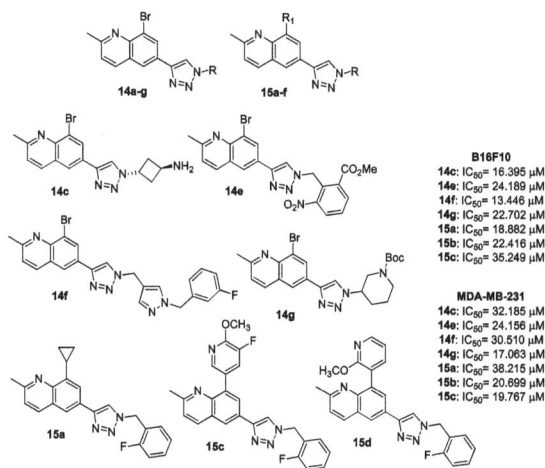

**Fig. (12).** Quinoline-triazole hybrids as an anticancer agent.

Liu and Huang synthesised quinoline/steroidal/coumarin fused triazole nucleobase hybrids and estimated the anticancer potential against SGC-7901 and MGC-803 cells and towards normal epithelial cells (GES-1). Compound **19** was detected as the active anticancer agent of the group of molecules with an $IC_{50}$ of 2.28 µM (SGC-7901) and an $IC_{50}$ of 1.48 µM (MGC-803) towards both the cell lines by the inhibition of over-expression of TGF1 and no toxicity against the normal cell. Fragment A with –F and –Cl substituents was found to enhance the anticancer activity, and fragment B with quinoline/coumarin/steroids also enhanced the anti-gastric potency of the hybrids suggested by SAR (Fig. **13**) [54].

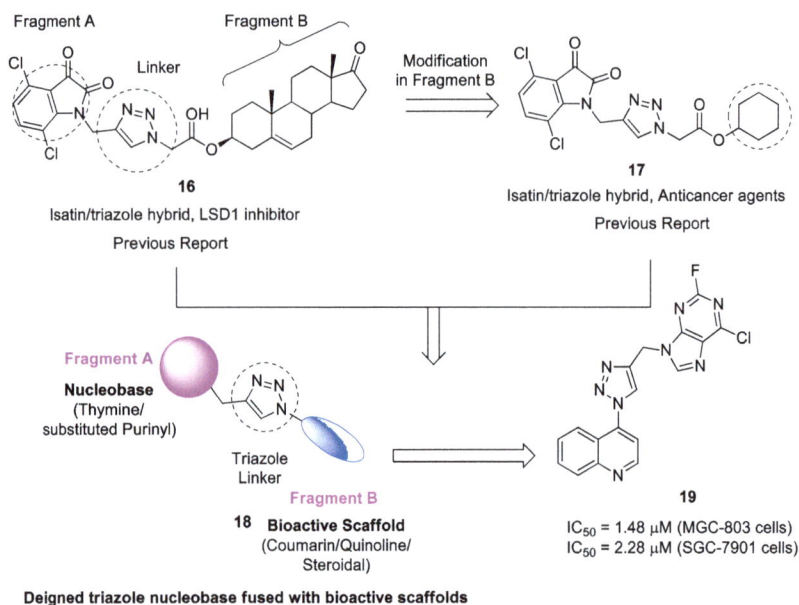

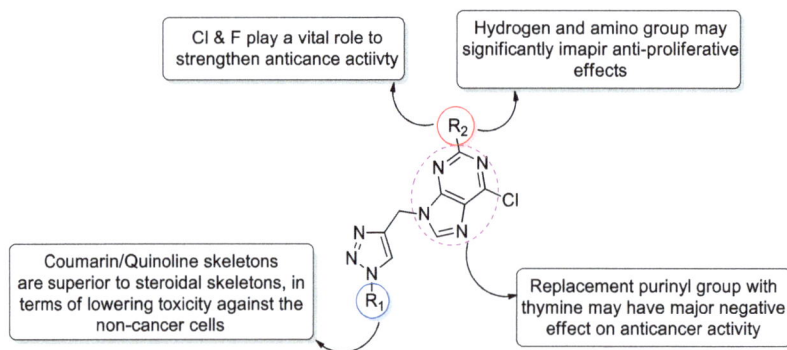

**Fig. (13).** Quinoline-triazole fused nucleobase derivatives as anticancer agents.

## Quinoline-1,2,4-triazole Hybrids

Kamble *et al.* synthesised quinoline-1,2,4-triazole hybrids **23a-f** by molecular hybridising compounds **20** and **21** and evaluated their anticancer potency. Hybrids **23a** and **23b** with $GI_{50}$ = 9.67 µM (**23a**) and $GI_{50}$ = 9.50 µM (**23b**) were found to have the highest anticancer potency in the HeLa cell line. The benzene ring of the quinoline moiety-bearing halogens at the $6^{th}$ position and triazole having R = Ph were acting as the active enhancers for anticancer potential as predicted by SAR (Fig. **14**) [55].

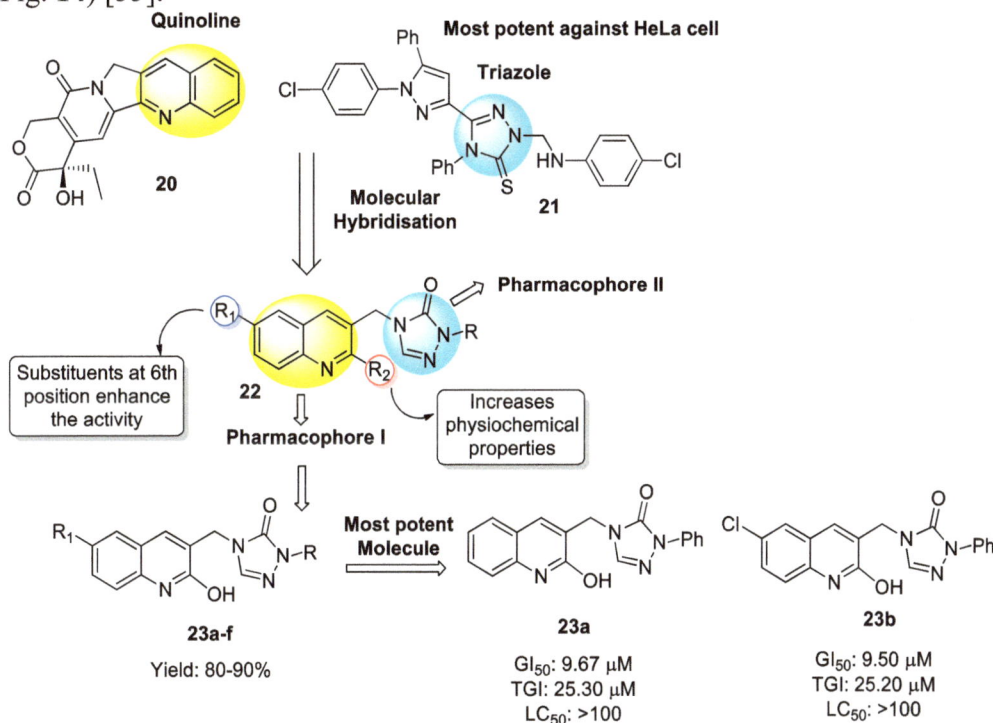

**Fig. (14).** Quinoline-triazole hybrids as potent anticancer agents.

Satyanarayan *et al.* synthesised quinoline-1,2,4-triazole hybrids **24a-o** and evaluated their anticancer activity. A number of compounds from the series (**24a, 24b, 24c**, and **24k**) were found to possess good anticancer potencies with $IC_{50}$ = 6.2-11.3 µg/mL and $IC_{50}$ = 2.9–7.8 µg/mL towards MDA-MB-231 and A375 cells. The presence of halogens at the *p*-position of aldehyde significantly enhances the anticancer activity, which was confirmed by SAR (Fig. **15**) [56].

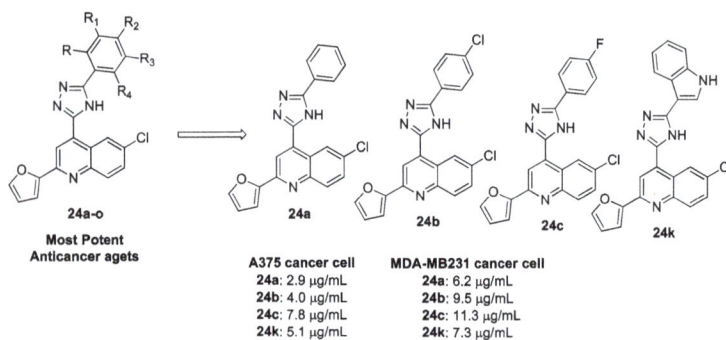

**Fig. (15).** Quinoline-triazole hybrids as cytotoxic agents.

## Quinoline-tetrazole Hybrids

According to the literature, both tetrazole quinoline nuclei and napthopyran nuclei had significant anticancer activities with $IC_{50}$ values of 100 µM and 43.6 µM, respectively.Therefore, Nasr *et al*. planned to fuse both the pharmacophores with the hope of getting a new, higher efficacy anticancer drug as compared to the parent nuclei. Therefore, the authors synthesised a series of quinoline-tetrazol--chromene hybrids and tested their cytotoxicity against HL-60, SR, and MDA-MB-435 cells. HL-60 ($GI_{50}$ = 0.26 µM, SR: $GI_{50}$ = 0.23 µM, and MDA-MB-435: $GI_{50}$ = 0.30 µM) was found to have pronounced anticancer activity. Also, it inhibited Topo I by forming an enzyme-substrate complex with an $IC_{50}$ of 0.27 µM (Fig. **16**) [57].

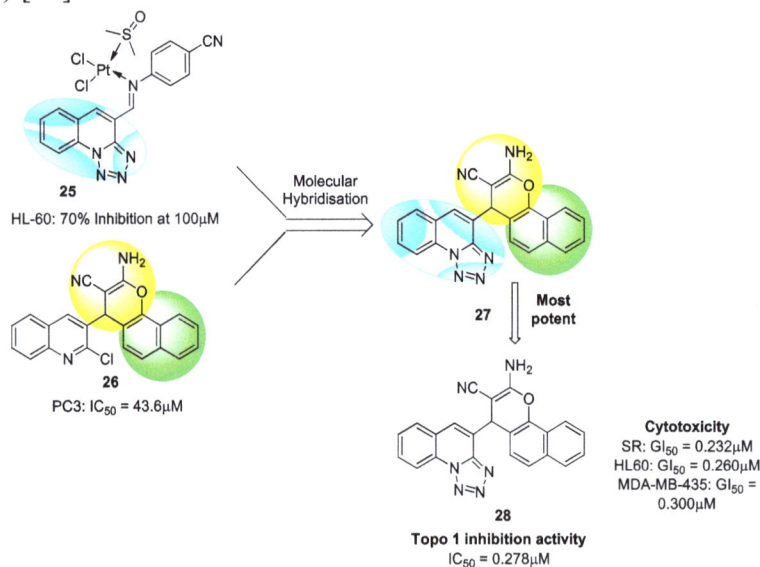

**Fig. (16).** Quinoline-tetrazole-chromene hybrids as inhibitors of Topo I.

## QUINOLINE-PIPERAZINE HYBRIDS

Solomon *et al.* synthesised quinoline-sulfonyl hybrids **33** and **34** containing diamine linkage by molecular hybridising compounds **29, 30, 31,** and 32. The synthesised molecules' cytotoxicity was evaluated against MDA-MB-231, MDA-MB-468, and MCF7 and against normal epithelial cells (184B5 and MCF710A). Hybrid **33g** was found to possess pronounced anticancer properties with an $IC_{50}$ of 0.7 μM towards MDA-MB-468 by causing apoptosis through the inactivation of kinase Cdk1 and non-toxicity towards non-cancer cells (MCF10A: $IC_{50}$ = 12.3 μM). In comparison to flexible aliphatic amine, fixed cyclic piperazine linkage and the presence of electron-withdrawing substituents in the aryl-sulfonyl moiety significantly enhance the anticancer potency predicted by SAR (Fig. **17**) [58].

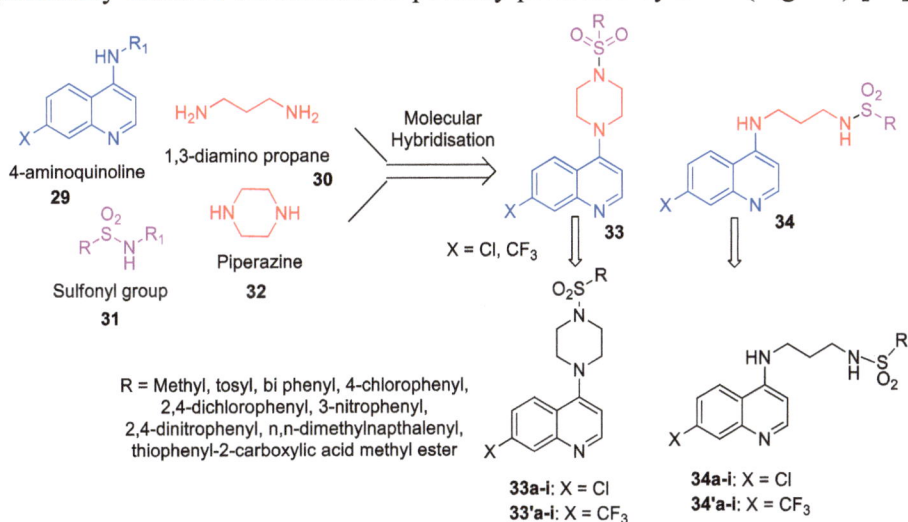

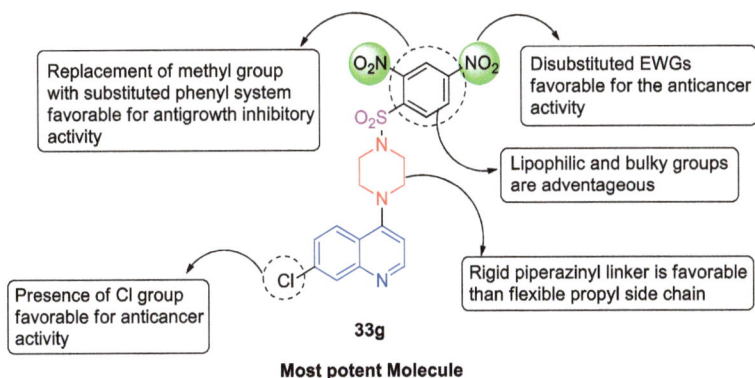

**Fig. (17).** Quinoline-piperazine-sulfonyl hybrids as anticancer agents.

Yang and Maloney synthesised quinoline-sulfonyl-piperazine/piperidine hybrids by the molecular fusion of compounds **35** and **36** and further studied their ALDH inhibitory potential. Compound **37,** with an $IC_{50}$ of 7 nM, was found as the active inhibitor of ALDH (Fig. **18**) [59].

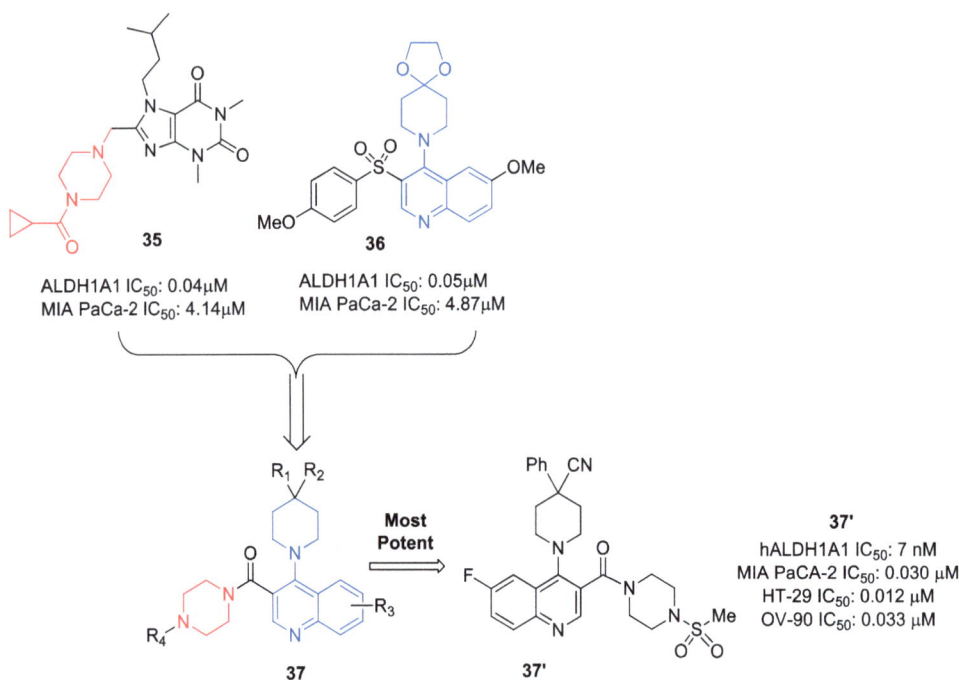

**Fig. (18).** Quinoline-sulfonyl-piperazine/piperidine hybrids as (ALDH1A1) inhibitors.

Solomon and Pundir synthesised quinoline-piperazine-urea/thiourea hybrids **40** and **41** by the hybridization of **38**, **39,** and **39,** and then studied their antiproliferative properties for cancerous (MDA-MB-231, MDA-MB-468, and MCF7) and non-cancerous (MCF10A and 184B5) cells. The number of molecules in the series **40a**, **40e**, **41a**, **41b**, **41e**, **41g**, and **41f** were found to possess considerable antiproliferative activities in all the tested cell lines. The derivative **41g** of the series was mainly found to have effective anticancer activities with an $IC_{50}$ of 3.0 μM towards the MDA-MB-231 cell line and non-toxic towards the normal cell line. Urea/thiourea derivatives bearing bulky substituents and quinoline having X = Cl act as the enhancer of anticancer potential over X = $CF_3$ as predicted by SAR (Fig. **19**) [60].

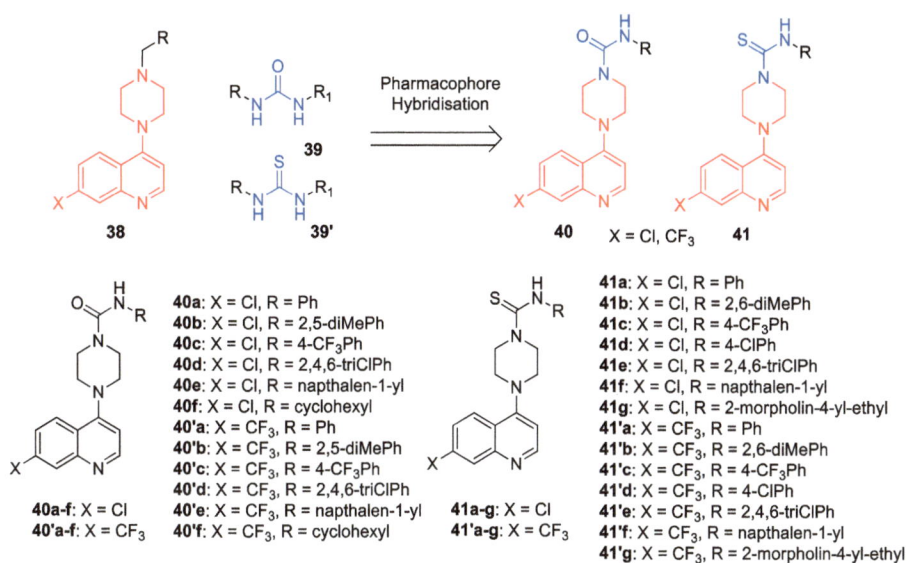

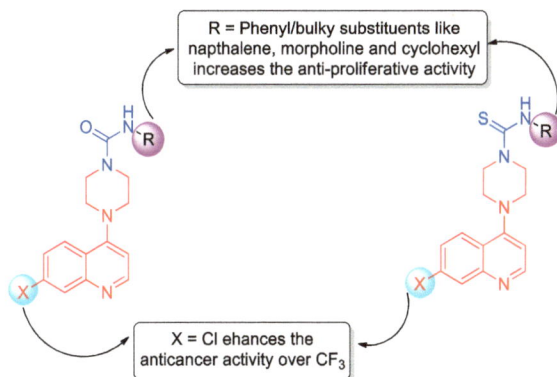

**Fig. (19).** Quinoline-4-piperazinyl-urea/thiourea hybrids as an anticancer agent.

## QUINOLINE-CHALCONE HYBRIDS

Chalcone is a well-known scaffold in the literature known for its anticancer ability through the apoptosis pathway [61]. Using the chalcone advancement, El-Hafeez and Hassan synthesised and investigated the anticancer activity of quinoline-chalcone hybrids **42a**. The panel's A549 (IC50 = 3.91 μM) and **42j** (K562: $IC_{50}$ = 2.67 μM, A549: $IC_{50}$ = 5.29 μM) compounds were found to be the most effective against both K-562 and A549 when compared to the reference drug cisplatin (K562: $IC_{50}$ = 2.71 μM, A549: $IC_{50}$ = 15.3 μM). These compounds cause apoptosis and act as PI3Kγ inhibitors (Fig. **20**) [62].

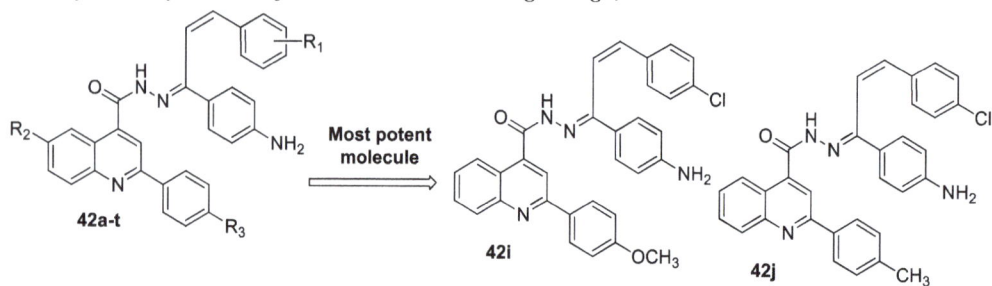

**Fig. (20).** Quinoline-chalcone hybrids as inhibitors of PI3K.

Ghodsi *et al.* synthesised quinoline-chalcone hybrids **45a-j** by the hybridization of **43** and **44** and further studied their *in vitro* anticancer potency against a cell line group. Hybrid **45j** with an $IC_{50}$ of 2.32 µM exhibited the highest cytotoxicity towards MCF-7MX and A2780 cell lines. Docking studies revealed the anti-tubulin and antimitotic activities of compound **45j** through non-covalent interaction and cell cycle arrest at the G2/M phase. SAR (Fig. **21**) depicted a quinoline ring substituted with a benzoyl group at C-6 and C-8 positions, and R1' = R2' = R3' = OMe acted as an enhancer of anticancer potential [63].

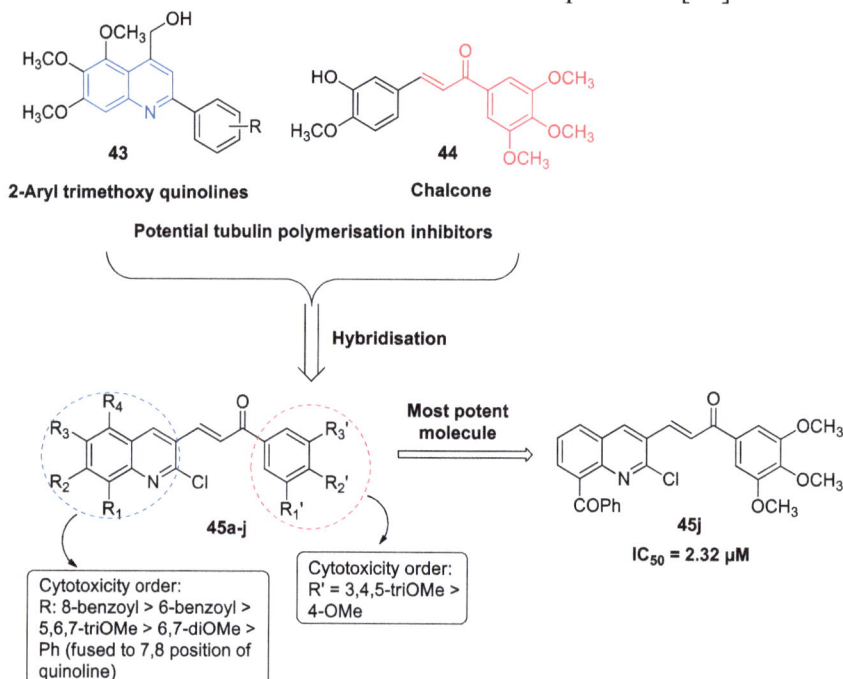

**Fig. (21).** Quinoline-chalcone hybrids as tubulin polymerization inhibitors.

## QUINOLINE-THIOPHENE HYBRIDS

Othman *et al*. synthesised quinoline-thiophene hybrids **49** and **50a-f** by the hybridization of **46** and **47** and then studied their anticancer activity. Quinoline-thiophene hybrids containing OH **49** (IC$_{50}$ = 17.5 μM) and benzyloxyl functionalization with C-4 position substituted with halogens **50d** (IC$_{50}$ = 38.4 μM) and 50e (IC$_{50}$ = 28.3 μM) were found to have the highest anticancer potential over other analogs. This was explained by SAR. These hybrids also act as potential inhibitors of EGFR-TK and Topo IIenzymes (a type of protein that helps in DNA replication) (Fig. **22**) [64].

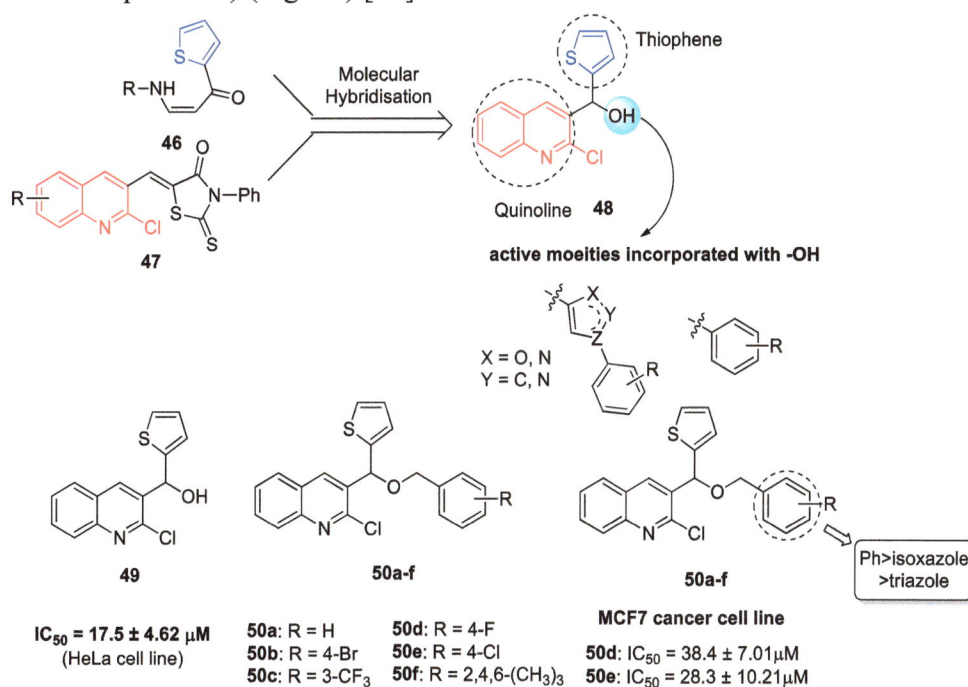

**Fig. (22).** Quinoline-thiophene hybrids as inhibitors of EGFR-TK and Topo II.

## QUINOLINE-GALACTOSE HYBRIDS

Nilsson *et al*. synthesised quinoline-galactose hybrids and studied the in vitro anticancer activity. Quinoline-galactose hybrid **51** was the most active inhibitor of galectin-8N through hydrogen bonding interaction between N-atom and –COOH group (Fig. **23**) [65].

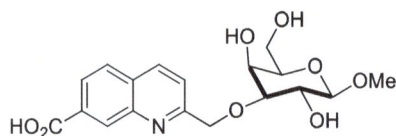

**51**

**Fig. (23).** Quinoline-galactose hybrids as an inhibitor of galectin-8N.

## MISCELLANEOUS QUINOLINE HYBRIDS

Bhat *et al.* synthesised quinoline-triazine hybrids **52a-j** and evaluated their EGFR-TK inhibitory activity. Hybrid **52c** was found to exhibit highest EGFR-TK inhibition (96.3%) at $IC_{50} = 10$ μM (Fig. 24) [66].

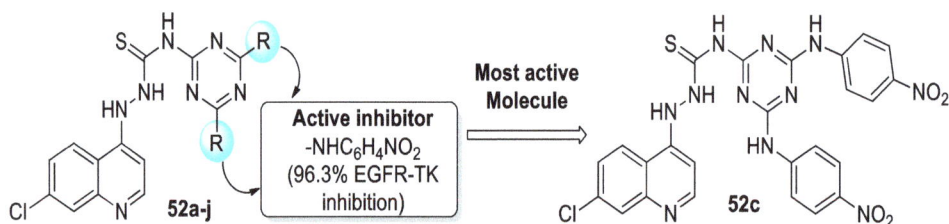

**Fig. (24).** Quinoline-triazine hybrids as inhibitors of EGFR-TK.

Fiorot and Greco synthesised quinoline-triazine/morpholine/1,4-naphthoquinone scaffolds **53** and **54** and evaluated their *in vitro* cytotoxicity (Fig. **25**). These compounds were found to exhibit pronounced anticancer activity towards the SKMEL-103 cell line with an $IC_{50}$ of 25 μM. As was evident from SAR data, the presence of morpholine and triazine plays a key role in enhancing anticancer activity, as was depicted by SAR data. These compounds form an enzyme-substrate complex present in the core site of AMPK and PI3K *via* different non-covalent bonding interactions (Fig. **26**) [67].

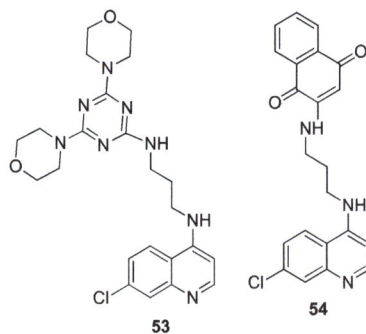

**53**

**54**

**Fig. (25).** Quinoline-triazine/morpholine/naphthoquinone scaffold **53** and **54** as potent inhibitors of PI3K and AMPK.

Molecular docking of hybrid **53** and **54** at the active site of PI3Kγ

Molecular docking of hybrid **53** and **54** at the active site of AMPK

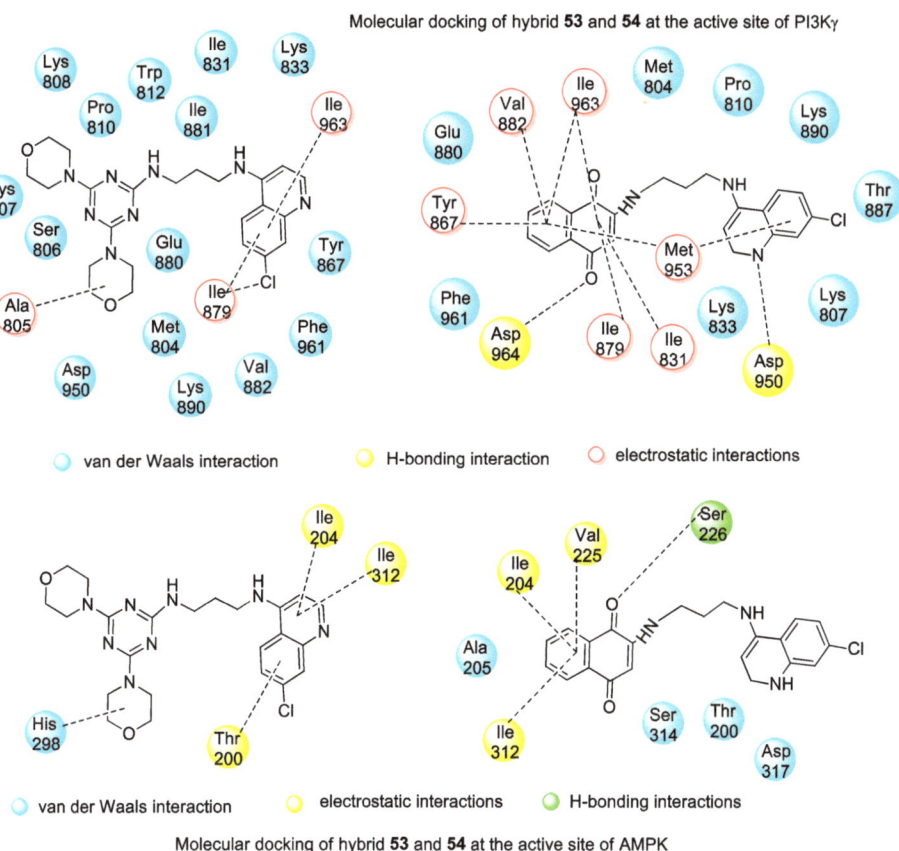

**Fig. (26).** Quinoline-triazine/morpholine/naphthoquinone hybrids as inhibitors of PI3K and AMPK.

Jing-Ping Liou *et al.* synthesised quinoline-resorcinol hybrids by the hybridization of **55** and **56** and evaluated their HSP90 inhibitory activity. Hybrid **57**'exhibited maximum anti-proliferative potential with an $IC_{50}$ of 0.14-0.33 nM and HSP90 inhibition with an $IC_{50}$ of 149nM. It acts as an antimitotic agent by arresting the cell cycle at the G2/M phase. As predicted by SAR (Fig. **27**), ethylation at C-3 and C-6 positions and NH ethylation of amide played a considerable function in enhancing the anticancer ability predicted by SAR (Fig. **27**) [68].

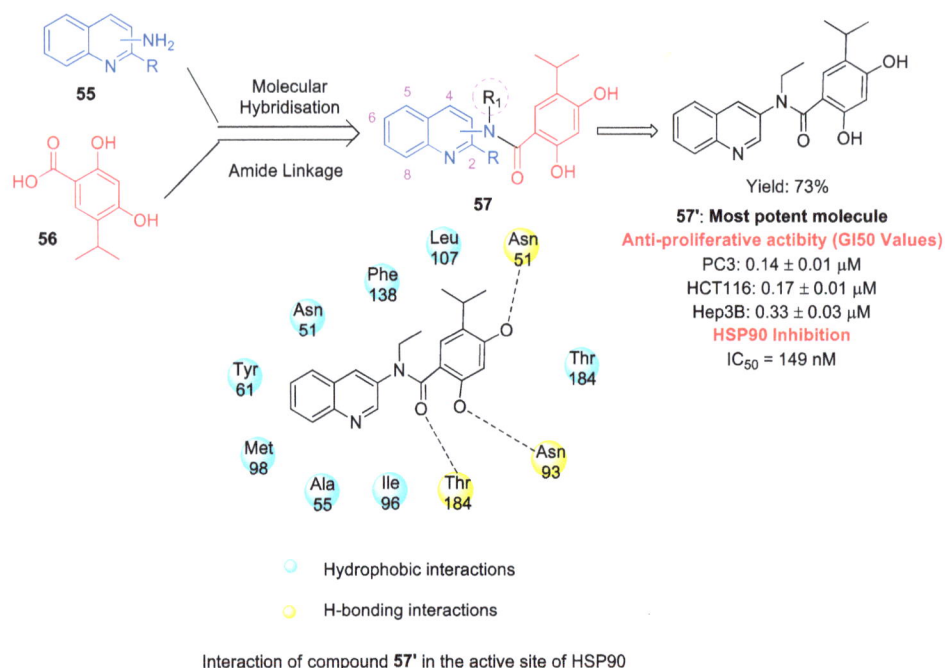

**Fig. (27).** quinoline-resorcinol hybrids as an inhibitor of HSP90.

Saczewski *et al.* synthesised quinoline-hydrazone hybrids **58a-e** and studied their *in vitro* cytotoxicity against LCLC-103H, SISO, and DAN-G cancer cell lines. Compound **58e** showed the highest anti-proliferative activity with an $IC_{50}$ of 1.23 µM (LCLC-103H), 1.35 µM (DAN-G) and 1.49 µM (SISO). As predicted by SAR (Fig. **28**), the C-2 position substituted with benzotriazole works as an enhancer of anticancer potential compared to triazole substitution [69].

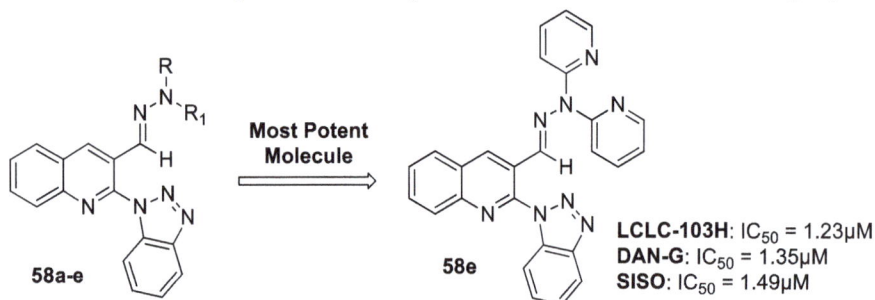

**Fig. (28).** Quinoline-benzotriazoles as anticancer agents.

Ravi *et al.* synthesized quinoline-hydrazide hybrids 61a-l and studied their cytotoxicity towards the K562 cancer cell line. Derivative **61e** exhibited maximum anticancer potential with an $IC_{50}$ of 26.93 µg/mL. The presence of electron-donating groups at the p-position of aldehyde moiety significantly enhances the anticancer potential over electron-withdrawing groups was predicted by SAR (Fig. **29**) [70].

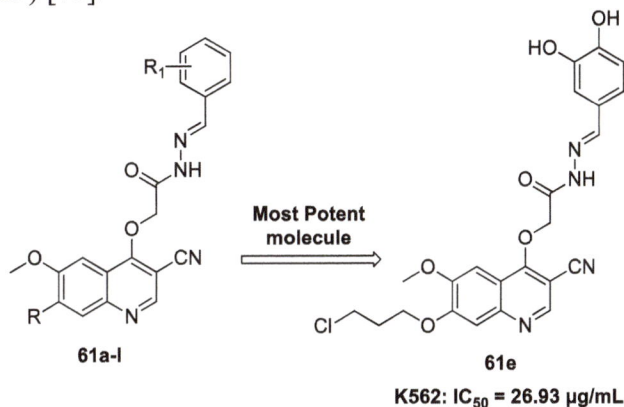

**Fig. (29).** Quinoline-hydrazides as an inhibitor of tyrosine kinase.

Katariya *et al.* prepared quinoline hydrazone hybrids **64a-p** by the hybridization of **62** and **63** and evaluated their antiproliferative ability. **64b, 64d, 64e, 64f, 64g, 64h, 64i, 64j, 64l** exhibited fine anti-proliferative potential at $IC_{50}$ =10 µM, $GI_{50}$= 0.33 to 4.87 µM and $LC_{50}$= 4.67 µM to>100 µM.. Furthermore, derivative **64j** causes apoptosis and shows topoI inhibitory activity with $GI_{50}$ = 0.50 µM (Fig. **30**) [71].

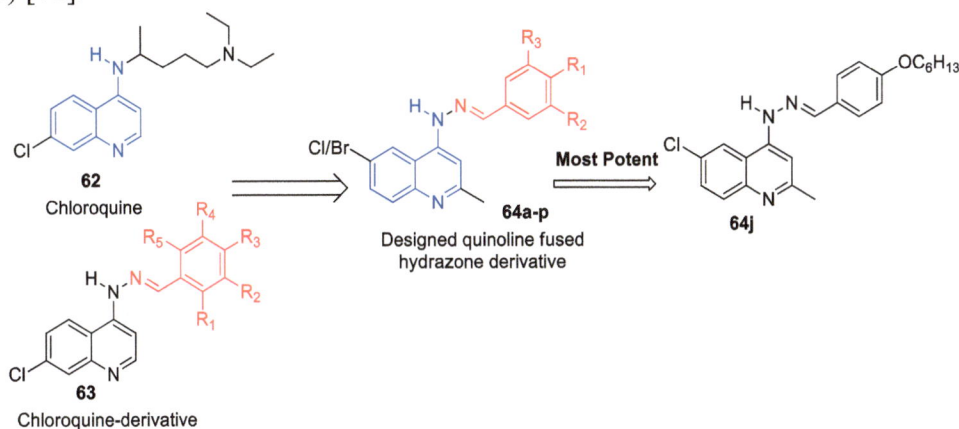

**Fig. (30).** Quinoline-hydrazone hybrids as an inhibitor of topo I.

# QUINOLONE DERIVATIVES AS ANTICANCER AGENTS

## Pyrano[3,2-c]quinolone Analogs as Anticancer Agents

The Pyran core merged with quinolone is consistently exciting for pharmaceutical people because of its outstanding biological properties, particularly against cancer [72]. Upadhyay *et al.* (2018) were inspired by the beautiful architecture of pyranoquinolones and studied in vitro anticancer abilities against different cancer cell lines using gemcitabine and flavopiridol as reference drugs for cytotoxicity measurement.Screening results suggested that compounds **65a**, **65b**, **65c,** and **65d** were the active agents of the series, showing suitable anticancer activities against all the tested cell lines. SAR predicted a critical role in enhancing anticancer ability at the C4 position of pyranoquinolone (Fig. **31**) [73].

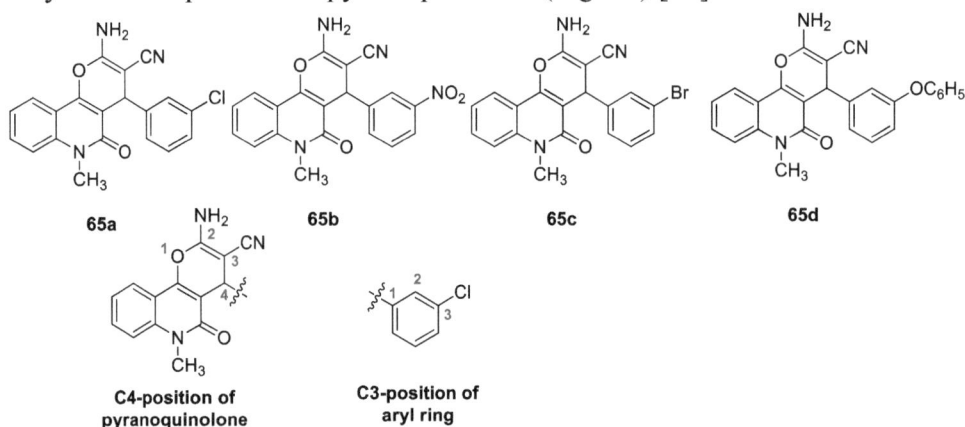

**65a**          **65b**          **65c**          **65d**

**C4-position of pyranoquinolone**          **C3-position of aryl ring**

**Fig. (31).** Pyranoquinolone hybrids as anticancer agents.

## Ciprofloxacin Hybrids as Anticancer Agents

Ciprofloxacin, a quinolone derivative, is the most commonly known antibiotic. Besides its antibacterial properties, it also possesses a broad spectrum of antiproliferative activities. Through SAR studies, it was suggested that the F-atom and the quinolone-3-carboxylic acid part of the ciprofloxacin derivative play a significant role in enhancing the anticancer activity of the molecule through their H-bonding ability with different components of DNA [74]. To further improve its lipophilicity and enhance its drug-likeness, Kassab *et al.* (2018) designed the synthesis of a novel series of ciprofloxacin derivatives by functionalizing the C4 N-atom of the piperazine core of ciprofloxacin with different aryl/heteroaryl hydrazones. After successful synthesis, the authors explored their anticancer ability against fifty-nine other cancer cell lines. Five compounds from the series (**66e**, **66f**, **66h**, **66o,** and **66p**) were found to possess significant anticancer potencies in all the tested cell lines with an $IC_{50}$ of 0.72–4.92 µM, which suggests that the synthesised hybrids are 9 to 1.5 folds more efficient than the referral drug doxorubicin.

Further studies revealed that particular compounds **66f** and **66o** were found to have better antiproliferative ability than others and showed significant Topo II inhibitory ability with $IC_{50}$ = 0.58 and 0.86 µM. It is worthwhile to note that compound **66f** was 1.5 times more effective than etoposide, 5 times more effective than amsacrine, and 6 folds more effective than doxorubicin. Furthermore, derivative 66o was three times more effective than amsacrine, four times more effective against Topo II than doxorubicin, and nearly as effective as etoposide.The compound causes apoptosis by the arrest of the cell cycle at the G2/M phase (Fig. **32**) [75].

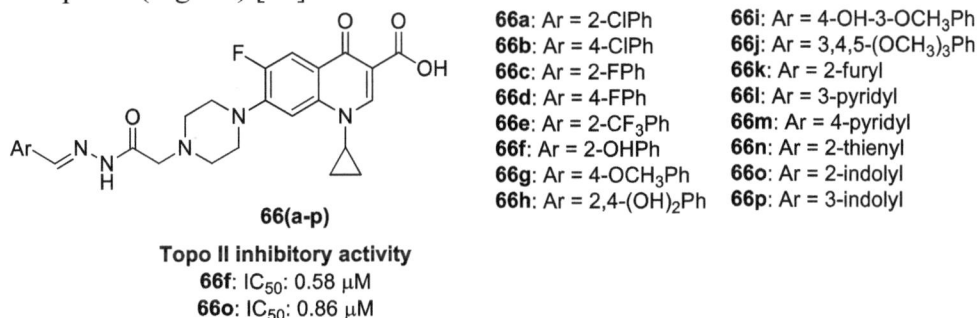

66a: Ar = 2-ClPh
66b: Ar = 4-ClPh
66c: Ar = 2-FPh
66d: Ar = 4-FPh
66e: Ar = 2-CF₃Ph
66f: Ar = 2-OHPh
66g: Ar = 4-OCH₃Ph
66h: Ar = 2,4-(OH)₂Ph

66i: Ar = 4-OH-3-OCH₃Ph
66j: Ar = 3,4,5-(OCH₃)₃Ph
66k: Ar = 2-furyl
66l: Ar = 3-pyridyl
66m: Ar = 4-pyridyl
66n: Ar = 2-thienyl
66o: Ar = 2-indolyl
66p: Ar = 3-indolyl

**66(a-p)**

**Topo II inhibitory activity**
**66f**: $IC_{50}$: 0.58 µM
**66o**: $IC_{50}$: 0.86 µM

**Fig. (32).** Ciprofloxacin hybrids as anticancer agents.

## Quinolone-Benzimidazole Hybrids as Anticancer Agents

The universal nature of imidazole derivatives, from amino acids to life-saving drug molecules, makes them unique and desirable candidates and inspires chemists and biologists to optimise them more. Chen, Liang, and Zhang (2018) synthesised quinolone-benzimidazole hybrids and evaluated their antitumor ability. A few compounds showed moderate to high inhibition towards SK-OV-3, HepG2, BEL-7404, and NCI-H460, whereas most of them showed negligible toxicity towards normal cells (HL-7702) compared to cisplatin and 5-FU. *In vivo* studies predicted that compounds 67c and 67u were mainly found as potential anticancer drug candidates in the NCI-H460 and BEL-7402 xenograft mouse models. Antitumor activity of the compound was demonstrated by intracellular $Ca^{2+}$ release, up-regulation of Bax, down-regulation of Bcl-2, activation of caspase-3 and caspase-9, ROS generation, inhibition of CDK by p53 protein activation, and subsequent cleavage of PARP (Fig. **33**) [76].

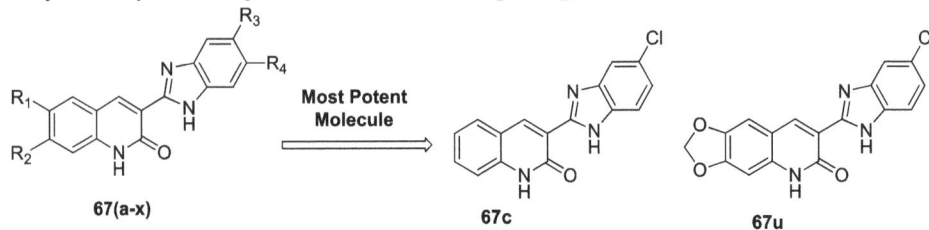

**Fig. (33).** Quinolone-benzimidazole hybrid as anticancer agent.

## Ferrocene-quinolone Hybrids as Anticancer Agents

Ferrocene's discovery and massive success as an analogue of tamoxifen, acting as a female oestrogen modulator, the chemistry of ferrocene derivatives has triggered a great deal of interest among researchers recently, as it serves as a highly demanding research topic [77]. With the hope of synthesising a ferrocene-mediated highly active drug entity with minimal side effects, AnkaPejovi and Marcin Cieslak *et al.* in 2018 synthesised allyl ferrocene-quinolone hybrids. They evaluated the *in vitro* anticancer potential of HeLa, K562, and HUVEC cell lines. Among the series of compounds studied, the quinolone derivative **68c** exhibited the highest cytotoxicity with an $IC_{50}$ of 28 µM towards HeLa cells, and **68f** showed the highest toxicity with an $IC_{50}$ of 19 µM toward the K562 cell line (Fig. **34**) [78].

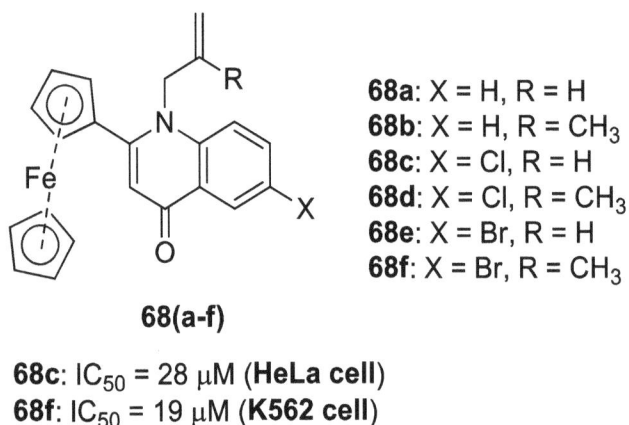

**68a**: X = H, R = H
**68b**: X = H, R = CH$_3$
**68c**: X = Cl, R = H
**68d**: X = Cl, R = CH$_3$
**68e**: X = Br, R = H
**68f**: X = Br, R = CH$_3$

**68(a-f)**

**68c**: $IC_{50}$ = 28 µM (**HeLa cell**)
**68f**: $IC_{50}$ = 19 µM (**K562 cell**)

**Fig. (34).** Ferrocene-quinolone hybrids as anticancer agents.

## Carbohydrate Fused Pyrano[3,2-c]quinolone Hybrids as Anticancer Agents

Taking into consideration the presence of a pyranoquinolone core in a number of natural products associated with relevant pharmacological properties [79], Ashish Gupta and Ram Sagar *et al.* in 2018 synthesised carbohydrate-fused pyranoquinolone hybrids in order to enhance the lipophilicity, selectivity and to reduce the toxicity most commonly encountered in other anticancer drugs. The antiproliferative activities of the synthesised compounds were studied. Delightfully, the compounds show anticancer abilities with an $IC_{50}$ of 3.53–9.68 µM (Fig. **35**) [80].

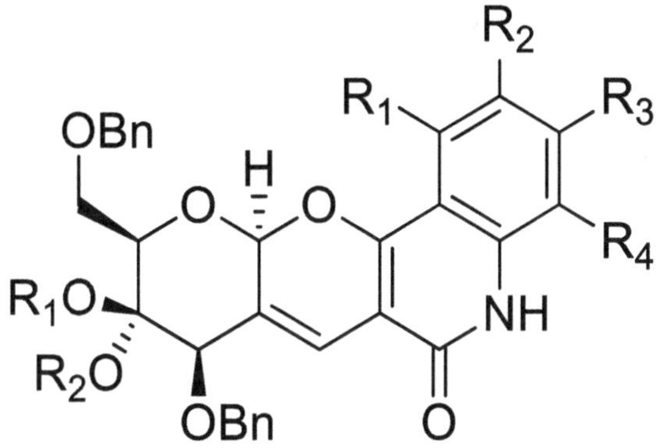

**69**
**Anticancer activity:**
$IC_{50}$ = 3.53-9.68 µM

**Fig. (35).** Pyrano[3,2-c]quinolone fused carbohydrate hybrids as anticancer agents.

## Oxindole-quinolone Hybrids as Anticancer Agents

Spiro oxindole fused pyrrolidine skeletons are most desirous because of their occurrence in many bioactive value-added molecules as well as for their pronounced anticancer potencies [81]. Taking this into consideration, Palathurai Subramaniam Mohan *et al.* in 2019 synthesised dispiro fused oxindole pyrrolidine-8-nitro-quinolone hybrids and evaluated them for their *in vitro* anticancer potential against the HeLa cell line by taking doxorubicin as the referral drug. The number of compounds in the series (**70a, 70b, 70d, 70e,** and **70h**) showed potent inhibitory action towards HeLa and less toxicity to normal cells. Notably, compound **70d** with $IC_{50}$ = 16 µM showed the highest anticancer potential compared to the reference drug doxorubicin ($IC_{50}$ = 14 µM) by increasing the generation of ROS-induced apoptosis by the activation of caspase-3. SAR results revealed that substituents on the aromatic ring play a key role in enhancing the activity. Similarly, oxindole moiety bearing –Cl substitution increased the anticancer potency over other halogen substituents. The order of cytotoxicity of the compounds as per the SAR analysis was **70d > 70a > 70h > 70b > 70e** (Fig. **36**) [82].

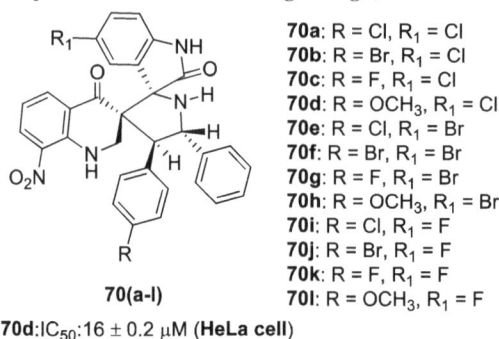

**70a**: R = Cl, R$_1$ = Cl
**70b**: R = Br, R$_1$ = Cl
**70c**: R = F, R$_1$ = Cl
**70d**: R = OCH$_3$, R$_1$ = Cl
**70e**: R = Cl, R$_1$ = Br
**70f**: R = Br, R$_1$ = Br
**70g**: R = F, R$_1$ = Br
**70h**: R = OCH$_3$, R$_1$ = Br
**70i**: R = Cl, R$_1$ = F
**70j**: R = Br, R$_1$ = F
**70k**: R = F, R$_1$ = F
**70l**: R = OCH$_3$, R$_1$ = F

**70(a-l)**

**70d**:IC$_{50}$:16 ± 0.2 μM (**HeLa cell**)

**Fig. (36).** Oxindole-quinolone hybrids as an anticancer agent.

## Fluoroquinolone-Boron Complexes as Anticancer Agents

The advancement associated with the metal complexes helps improve the physicochemical properties of the desired molecules by increasing their bioavailabilities, solubilities, and pharmacokinetic properties with fewer side effects [83]. Therefore, metal complexes merged into hybrid drug discovery are highly desirable. In this regard, Hiram Hernandez-Lopez *et al.* in 2019 reported the synthesis of a series of fluoroquinolone-boron complexes through the selective activation of the C7 position of fluoroquinolone by the different electron-withdrawing groups and evaluated their in *vitro* cancer inhibitory efficiency against SiHa and CasKi cancer cells. All four compounds in the panel (**71a**, **71b**, **71d,** and **71e**) were found to have potential anticancer activity against SiHa cells, whereas only one compound (**71a**) was active towards CasKi cells. The authors also synthesised fluoroquinolone-uracil complexes. But, dissatisfactory, it did not show significant inhibitory activity (Fig. **37**) [84].

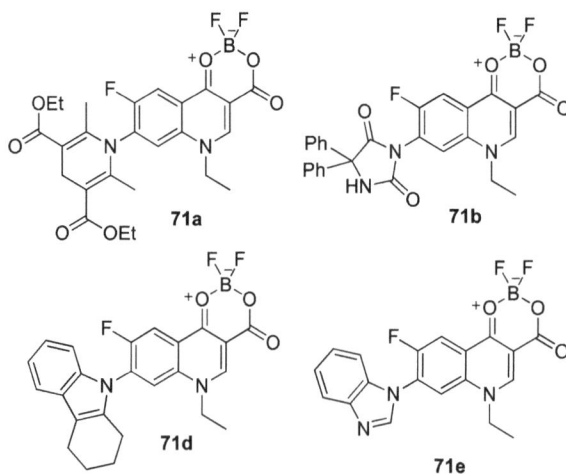

**71a**

**71b**

**71d**

**71e**

**Fig. (37).** Fluoroquinolone-boron complexes as anticervical cancer agents.

## Quinolone-pyrimidine Hybrids

Pyrimidine constitutes the central core structure of many bioactive natural products and pharmaceuticals and attracts a great deal of attention by offering its beneficial biological properties, particularly anticancer [85]. With the aspiration to synthesise a potentially active anticancer agent, Thanh *et al.* in 2020 synthesised 2-amino-4-(4'-hydroxy-*N*-methylquinolin-2'-on-3'-yl) pyrimidines **72a-i** and evaluated their *in vitro* cancer inhibition potential against HepG2 and KB cell lines with reference to Ellipticine (standard drug). Among the series of compounds studied, compounds **72b** and **72e** showed the highest anticancer potential, with an $IC_{50}$ of 1.33 μM towards KB cells. *In silico* studies showed that compounds **72b**, **72e,** and **72f** possessed drug-like behaviour through hydrogen bonding and *pi-pi*-stacking interactions with the proteins present at the active site of the human topoisomerase II present in DNA. In general, topoisomerases are the enzymes that play a crucial role in DNA replication and transcription and hence help in cell division. Therefore, most anticancer drugs are designed to target DNA topoisomerase to stop mitosis in cancerous cells. Substituents with the +I effect possessed higher cytotoxicity against the tested cell lines than electron-withdrawing substituents (Fig. **38**) [86].

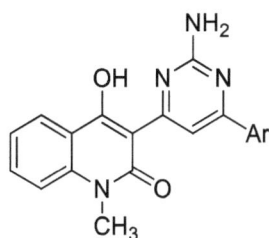

| | |
|---|---|
| **72a**: Ar = Ph | **72f**: Ar = 4-OHPh |
| **72b**: Ar = 4-ClPh | **72g**: Ar = 4-MePh |
| **72c**: Ar = 3-ClPh | **72h**: Ar = 3-MePh |
| **72d**: Ar = 4-BrPh | **72i**: Ar = 2-thienyl |
| **72e**: Ar = 4-OMePh | |

**72a-i**

**KB cell**: $IC_{50}$: 1.32 - 23.46 μM
HepG2 cell: $IC_{50}$: 1.38 - 12.60 μM

*(Fig. 38) contd.....*

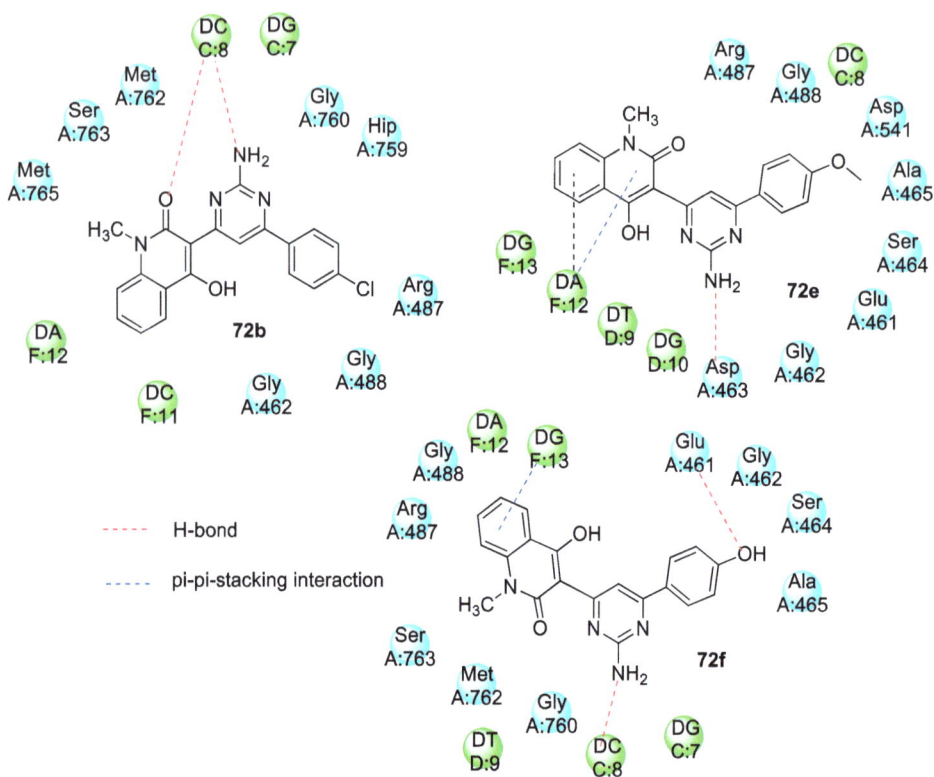

**Interaction of compound 72b, 72e and 72f with human topoisomerase IIa in complex with DNA (5GWK)**

**Fig. (38).** Quinolone-pyrimidine hybrids as anticancer agents.

## Benzo[d]thiazolyl Substituted-2-quinolone Hybrids as Anticancer Agents

Pages of literature are enriched with the magical anticancer potencies offered by benzothiazolyl and its derivatives [87]. Bolakatti et al. in 2020 synthesised 3-(-(4-(substituted benzo[d]thiazol-2-yl)phenylamino)acetyl)-4-hydroxy-1-methyl/ phenyl quinolone derivatives **73(a-f)** and **74(a-f)** and tested their cytotoxicity against MCF-7 and WRL68 cell lines. **74f** displayed the most promising anticancer activity among the tested compounds and acted as an EGFR tyrosine kinase inhibitor. SAR revealed that electronegative groups on the benzo[d]thiazole nucleus boost anticancer efficacy (Fig. **39**) [88].

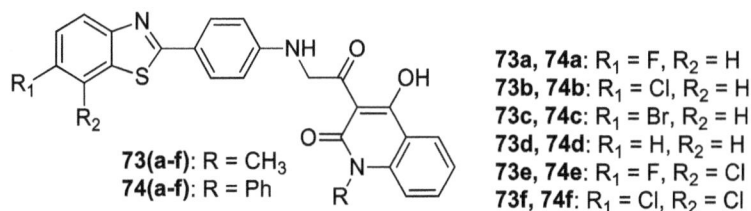

73a, 74a: $R_1$ = F, $R_2$ = H
73b, 74b: $R_1$ = Cl, $R_2$ = H
73c, 74c: $R_1$ = Br, $R_2$ = H
73d, 74d: $R_1$ = H, $R_2$ = H
73e, 74e: $R_1$ = F, $R_2$ = Cl
73f, 74f: $R_1$ = Cl, $R_2$ = Cl

73(a-f): R = CH₃
74(a-f): R = Ph

**Fig. (39).** Quinolone benzo[*d*]thiazolyl hybrids as EGFR inhibitors.

## Indeno-quinoxaline Pyrrolidine Quinolone Hybrids as Anticancer Agents

Nitrogen-containing heterocycles constitute the core structure of many natural products, such as alkaloids and pharmaceuticals. The widespread nature of versatile bioactivity makes them highly demanded candidates for synthesising more active therapeutics. Among the different nitrogen-containing heterocycles, quinoxaline derivatives are famous for their potential anticancer potencies through multiple mechanisms. Also, the biological prospects of spirocyclic molecules are quite more interesting due to their rigid three-dimensional structures. Promoted by the bulletins of literature, Mohan *et al.* in 2020 synthesised phenyl and thiophene substituted dispiroindeno quinoxaline pyrrolidine quinolone hybrids and evaluated their cytotoxicity towards HeLa and MCF-7 cells using doxorubicin as the referral following an MTT assay. Compound **75e** was found to exhibit potential anticancer abilities towards both the cancer cell lines with an $IC_{50}$ of 17 µM (MCF-7) and 19 µM (HeLa) by causing apoptosis arrest of the cell cycle at G1/S and G2/M phases by binding with estrogen. The SAR study revealed that the electron-donating group, *i.e.*, the $CH_3$ group in the phenyl ring, enhances the anticancer properties. The decreasing trend for the anticancer abilities of the substituents follows the order of $CH_3$ > $OCH_3$ > H > F > Cl > Br (Fig. **40**) [89].

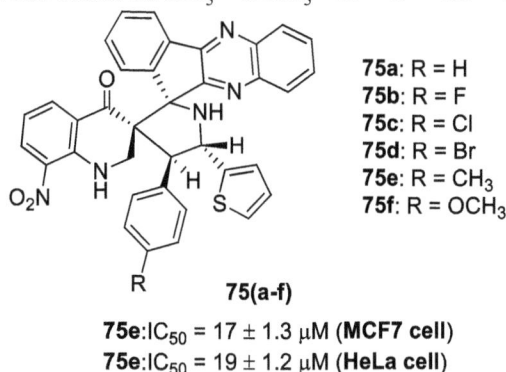

75a: R = H
75b: R = F
75c: R = Cl
75d: R = Br
75e: R = CH₃
75f: R = OCH₃

75(a-f)

75e: $IC_{50}$ = 17 ± 1.3 µM (**MCF7 cell**)
75e: $IC_{50}$ = 19 ± 1.2 µM (**HeLa cell**)

**Fig. (40).** Indeno-quinoxaline pyrrolidine quinolone hybrids as anticancer agents.

## Quinolone-1,5-benzothiazepines Hybrids as Anticancer Agents

Benzothiapines and their derivatives have been linked to remarkable pharmacological properties, which have always prompted researchers to investigate these compounds [90]. Toan and Thanhin 2020 created quinolone-benzothiazepine derivatives **76(a-g)** inspired by the versatility of benzothiazepines. They studied the *in vitro* anticancer efficacy against HepG2 and KB cell lines with reference to Ellipticine. Among the series of compounds evaluated, compounds **76c** and **76g** showed the best activity in both the cell lines, with an $IC_{50}$ of 0.25-0.27 μM (KB cell) and $IC_{50}$ of 0.26-0.28 μM (HepG2 cell) by the inhibition of topoisomerase (Fig. **41**) [91].

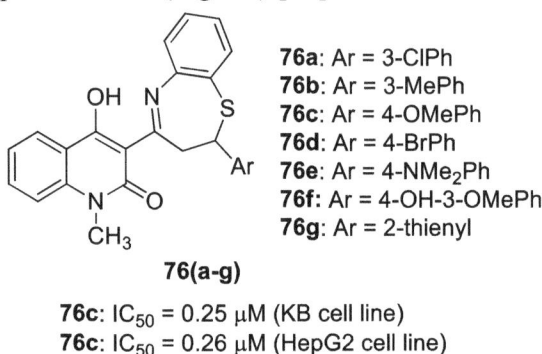

**76a**: Ar = 3-ClPh
**76b**: Ar = 3-MePh
**76c**: Ar = 4-OMePh
**76d**: Ar = 4-BrPh
**76e**: Ar = 4-NMe$_2$Ph
**76f**: Ar = 4-OH-3-OMePh
**76g**: Ar = 2-thienyl

**76(a-g)**

**76c**: $IC_{50}$ = 0.25 μM (KB cell line)
**76c**: $IC_{50}$ = 0.26 μM (HepG2 cell line)

**Fig. (41).** Quinolone-benzothiazepines hybrids as potential anticancer agents

## CONCLUSION

The growing population is under the influence of various deadly poisonous diseases. Among the different life-harvesting diseases, cancer is the second leading cause of death, affecting all ages of people worldwide. Multidrug resistance, organ toxicity, and lack of specificity are the major limitations of the currently available therapeutics. Thus, the morbidity and mortality rates are greatly increasing due to cancer because of the high cost of existing treatments. To fight cancer, researchers are focusing on designing drug molecules that are of natural origin. In this connection, the literature survey reveals that nitrogen-containing heterocycles, particularly quinoline and quinolone, are highly fascinating due to their advantageous biological properties. Anticancer properties are well known, along with other glorious jobs offered by quinoline/quinolone and its derivatives. To avoid the drawbacks of a single pharmacophore and with the concept of "one bullet, two targets" in mind, scientific communities are focusing on the design and synthesis of hybrid molecules, which can be synthesised by shuffling two or more bioactive pharmacophores. Based upon the literature precedent, it has been found that quinoline pyrazolylthiazole hybrid **6b** and **7c**, quinoline oxadiazole hybrid **11i**, quinoline tetrazole chromene **28**, quinoline-sulfonyl-piperazine hybrid **33g**, quinoline-sulfonyl-piperazi-e-piperidine hybrid **37'**, quinoline-resorcinol conjugate **57'**, ciprofloxacin hybrid **66f** and **66o**, quinoline-benzothiazepine hybrid **76c** showed more prominent anticancer properties through Bcl-2 inhibition, ALDH inhibition, kinase inhibition, topo-II and EGFR-TK inhibition in nanomolar and micromolar IC50 values. As a result, the authors believe that this book chapter will aid future researchers in gathering knowledge on designing new and valuable novel quinoline/quinolone hybrids based on structure-activity-relationship studies, resulting in future potent anticancer drug discoveries.

## CONSENT FOR PUBLICATION

All authors have given their consent for the publication of this manuscript.

## CONFLICT OF INTEREST

The authors declare no conflict of interest, financial or otherwise.

## ACKNOWLEDGEMENTS

PP is thankful to the Department of Chemistry, Ravenshaw University, Cuttack, Odisha, India. SC is grateful to the Department of Basic Sciences, IES University, Bhopal, Madhya Pradesh, India.

## REFERENCES

[1]     Brown, S.B.; Brown, E.A.; Walker, I. The present and future role of photodynamic therapy in cancer treatment. *Lancet Oncol.,* **2004**, *5*(8), 497-508.
[http://dx.doi.org/10.1016/S1470-2045(04)01529-3] [PMID: 15288239]

[2]     Maajani, K.; Jalali, A.; Alipour, S.; Khodadost, M.; Tohidinik, H.R.; Yazdani, K. The global and regional survival rate of women with breast cancer: A systematic review and meta-analysis. *Clin. Breast Cancer,* **2019**, *19*(3), 165-177.
[http://dx.doi.org/10.1016/j.clbc.2019.01.006] [PMID: 30952546]

[3]     Singh, R.K.; Kumar, S.; Prasad, D.N.; Bhardwaj, T.R. Therapeutic journery of nitrogen mustard as alkylating anticancer agents: Historic to future perspectives. *Eur. J. Med. Chem.,* **2018**, *151*, 401-433.
[http://dx.doi.org/10.1016/j.ejmech.2018.04.001] [PMID: 29649739]

[4]     Sahoo, C.R.; Paidesetty, S.K.; Padhy, R.N. Norharmane as a potential chemical entity for development of anticancer drugs. *Eur. J. Med. Chem.,* **2019**, *162*, 752-764.
[http://dx.doi.org/10.1016/j.ejmech.2018.11.024] [PMID: 30496990]

[5]     Sahoo, C.R.; Paidesetty, S.K.; Padhy, R.N. Nornostocine congeners as potential anticancer drugs: An overview. *Drug Dev. Res.,* **2019**, *80*(7), 878-892.
[http://dx.doi.org/10.1002/ddr.21577]

[6]     Panda, P.; Nayak, S.; Sahoo, S.K.; Mohapatra, S.; Nayak, D.; Pradhan, R.; Kundu, C.N. Diastereoselective synthesis of novel spiro indanone fused pyrano[3,2-c]chromene derivatives following hetero-Diels–Alder reaction and *in vitro* anticancer studies. *RSC Advances,* **2018**, *8*(30), 16802-16814.

[http://dx.doi.org/10.1039/C8RA02729C]

[7]     Panda, P.; Nayak, S.; Bhakta, S.; Mohapatra, S.; Murthy, T.R. Design and synthesis of (*Z/E*)-2-phenyl/*H*-3-styryl-2*H*-chromene derivatives as antimicrotubule agents. *J. Chem. Sci.,* **2018,** *130*(9), 127-142.
        [http://dx.doi.org/10.1007/s12039-018-1520-6]

[8]     Blagosklonny, M.V. Analysis of FDA approved anticancer drugs reveals the future of cancer therapy. *Cell Cycle,* **2004,** *3*(8), 1035-1042.
        [http://dx.doi.org/10.4161/cc.3.8.1023] [PMID: 15254418]

[9]     Kumari, A.; Singh, R.K. Medicinal chemistry of indole derivatives: Current to future therapeutic prospectives. *Bioorg. Chem.,* **2019,** *89*, 103021.
        [http://dx.doi.org/10.1016/j.bioorg.2019.103021] [PMID: 31176854]

[10]    Kumari, A.; Singh, R.K. Morpholine as ubiquitous pharmacophore in medicinal chemistry: Deep insight into the structure-activity relationship (SAR). *Bioorg. Chem.,* **2020,** *96*, 103578.
        [http://dx.doi.org/10.1016/j.bioorg.2020.103578] [PMID: 31978684]

[11]    Sethi, N.S.; Prasad, D.N.; Singh, R.K. An Insight into the Synthesis and SAR of 2,4-Thiazolidinediones (2,4-TZD) as Multifunctional Scaffold: A Review. *Mini Rev. Med. Chem.,* **2020,** *20*(4), 308-330.
        [http://dx.doi.org/10.2174/1389557519666191029102838] [PMID: 31660809]

[12]    Kumar, S.; Singh, R.K.; Patial, B.; Goyal, S.; Bhardwaj, T.R. Recent advances in novel heterocyclic scaffolds for the treatment of drug-resistant malaria. *J. Enzyme Inhib. Med. Chem.,* **2016,** *31*(2), 173-186.
        [http://dx.doi.org/10.3109/14756366.2015.1016513] [PMID: 25775094]

[13]    Marella, A.; Tanwar, O.P.; Saha, R.; Ali, M.R.; Srivastava, S.; Akhter, M.; Shaquiquzzaman, M.; Alam, M.M. Quinoline: A versatile heterocyclic. *Saudi Pharm. J.,* **2013,** *21*(1), 1-12.
        [http://dx.doi.org/10.1016/j.jsps.2012.03.002] [PMID: 23960814]

[14]    Chakroborty, S.; Panda, P. A Comprehensive Overview of the Synthesis of Tetrahydrocarbazoles and its Biological Properties. *Mini-Reviews in Org. Chem,* **2020.**
        [http://dx.doi.org/10.2174/1570193X17999200820163532]

[15]    Chakroborty, S.; Panda, P.; Basavanag Unnamatla, M.V. *Bicyclic 6-6 Systems With One Bridgehead (Ring Junction) Nitrogen Atom: Two Extra Heteroatoms 2:0. Reference Module in Chemistry, Molecular Sciences and Chemical Engineering*; Elsevier, **2020.**
        [http://dx.doi.org/10.1016/B978-0-12-409547-2.14957-1]

[16]    Kaur, K.; Jain, M.; Reddy, R.P.; Jain, R. Quinolines and structurally related heterocycles as antimalarials. *Eur. J. Med. Chem.,* **2010,** *45*(8), 3245-3264.
        [http://dx.doi.org/10.1016/j.ejmech.2010.04.011] [PMID: 20466465]

[17]    Panda, P.; Chakroborty, S. Navigating the Synthesis of Quinoline Hybrid Molecules as Promising Anticancer Agents. *ChemistrySelect,* **2020,** *5*(33), 10187-10199.
        [http://dx.doi.org/10.1002/slct.202002790]

[18]    Mandewale, M.C.; Patil, U.C.; Shedge, S.V.; Dappadwad, U.R.; Yamgar, R.S. A review on quinoline hydrazone derivatives as a new class of potent antitubercular and anticancer agents. *Beni. Suef Univ. J. Basic Appl. Sci.,* **2017,** *6*(4), 354-361.
        [http://dx.doi.org/10.1016/j.bjbas.2017.07.005]

[19]    Keri, R.S.; Patil, S.A. Quinoline: a promising antitubercular target. *Biomed. Pharmacother.,* **2014,** *68*(8), 1161-1175.
        [http://dx.doi.org/10.1016/j.biopha.2014.10.007] [PMID: 25458785]

[20]    Mukherjee, S.; Pal, M. Quinolines: a new hope against inflammation. *Drug Discov. Today,* **2013,** *18*(7-8), 389-398.
        [http://dx.doi.org/10.1016/j.drudis.2012.11.003] [PMID: 23159484]

[21]   Wainwright, M.; Kristiansen, J.E. Quinoline and cyanine dyes--putative anti-MRSA drugs. *Int. J. Antimicrob. Agents,* **2003**, *22*(5), 479-486.
[http://dx.doi.org/10.1016/S0924-8579(03)00264-4] [PMID: 14602365]

[22]   Jain, S.; Chandra, V.; Kumar Jain, P.; Pathak, K.; Pathak, D.; Vaidya, A. Comprehensive review on current developments of quinoline-based anticancer agents. *Arab. J. Chem.,* **2019**, *12*(8), 4920-4946.
[http://dx.doi.org/10.1016/j.arabjc.2016.10.009]

[23]   Gao, F.; Zhang, X.; Wang, T.; Xiao, J. Quinolone hybrids and their anti-cancer activities: An overview. *Eur. J. Med. Chem.,* **2019**, *165*, 59-79.
[http://dx.doi.org/10.1016/j.ejmech.2019.01.017] [PMID: 30660827]

[24]   Venditto, V.J.; Simanek, E.E. Cancer therapies utilizing the camptothecins: a review of the in vivo literature. *Mol. Pharm.,* **2010**, *7*(2), 307-349.
[http://dx.doi.org/10.1021/mp900243b] [PMID: 20108971]

[25]   Boschelli, F.; Arndt, K.; Gambacorti-Passerini, C. Bosutinib: a review of preclinical studies in chronic myelogenous leukaemia. *Eur. J. Cancer,* **2010**, *46*(10), 1781-1789.
[http://dx.doi.org/10.1016/j.ejca.2010.02.032] [PMID: 20399641]

[26]   Reddy, V.P. *Fluorinated compounds in enzyme-catalyzed reactions*; Organofluorine Compounds in Bio. and Med, **2015**.
[http://dx.doi.org/10.1016/B978-0-444-53748-5.00002-2]

[27]   Hegedüs, C.; Truta-Feles, K.; Antalffy, G.; Várady, G.; Német, K.; Özvegy-Laczka, C.; Kéri, G.; Orfi, L.; Szakács, G.; Settleman, J.; Váradi, A.; Sarkadi, B. Interaction of the EGFR inhibitors gefitinib, vandetanib, pelitinib and neratinib with the ABCG2 multidrug transporter: implications for the emergence and reversal of cancer drug resistance. *Biochem. Pharmacol.,* **2012**, *84*(3), 260-267.
[http://dx.doi.org/10.1016/j.bcp.2012.04.010] [PMID: 22548830]

[28]   Frampton, J.E. Lenvatinib: a review in refractory thyroid cancer. *Target. Oncol.,* **2016**, *11*(1), 115-122.
[http://dx.doi.org/10.1007/s11523-015-0416-3] [PMID: 26867945]

[29]   Zhang, S.; Zhang, J.; Gao, P.; Sun, L.; Song, Y.; Kang, D.; Liu, X.; Zhan, P. Efficient drug discovery by rational lead hybridization based on crystallographic overlay. *Drug Discov. Today,* **2019**, *24*(3), 805-813.
[http://dx.doi.org/10.1016/j.drudis.2018.11.021] [PMID: 30529326]

[30]   Gao, F.; Sun, Z.; Kong, F.; Xiao, J. Artemisinin-derived hybrids and their anticancer activity. *Eur. J. Med. Chem.,* **2020**, *188*, 112044.
[http://dx.doi.org/10.1016/j.ejmech.2020.112044] [PMID: 31945642]

[31]   Abbot, V.; Sharma, P.; Dhiman, S.; Noolvi, M.N.; Patel, H.M.; Bhardwaj, V. Small hybrid heteroaromatics: resourceful biological tools in cancer research. *RSC Advances,* **2017**, *7*(45), 28313-28349.
[http://dx.doi.org/10.1039/C6RA24662A]

[32]   Duarte, Y.; Fonseca, A.; Gutiérrez, M.; Adasme-Carreño, F.; Muñoz-Gutierrez, C.; Alzate-Morales, J.; Santana, L.; Uriarte, E.; Álvarez, R.; Matos, M.J. Novel coumarin-quinoline hybrids: design of multitarget compounds for Alzheimer's disease. *ChemistrySelect,* **2019**, *4*(2), 551-558.
[http://dx.doi.org/10.1002/slct.201803222]

[33]   Sangani, C.B.; Makawana, J.A.; Zhang, X.; Teraiya, S.B.; Lin, L.; Zhu, H-L. Design, synthesis and molecular modeling of pyrazole-quinoline-pyridine hybrids as a new class of antimicrobial and anticancer agents. *Eur. J. Med. Chem.,* **2014**, *76*, 549-557.
[http://dx.doi.org/10.1016/j.ejmech.2014.01.018] [PMID: 24607998]

[34]   Ding, Y.; Nguyen, T.A. PQ1, a quinoline derivative, induces apoptosis in T47D breast cancer cells through activation of caspase-8 and caspase-9. *Apoptosis,* **2013**, *18*(9), 1071-1082.
[http://dx.doi.org/10.1007/s10495-013-0855-1] [PMID: 23677255]

[35]   Taheri, S.; Nazifi, M.; Mansourian, M.; Hosseinzadeh, L.; Shokoohinia, Y. Ugi efficient synthesis,

biological evaluation and molecular docking of coumarin-quinoline hybrids as apoptotic agents through mitochondria-related pathways. *Bioorg. Chem.,* **2019**, *91*, 103147.
[http://dx.doi.org/10.1016/j.bioorg.2019.103147] [PMID: 31377390]

[36]   Menezes, J.C.; Diederich, M. Translational role of natural coumarins and their derivatives as anticancer agents. *Future Med. Chem.,* **2019**, *11*(9), 1057-1082.
[http://dx.doi.org/10.4155/fmc-2018-0375] [PMID: 31140865]

[37]   Zhang, L.; Xu, Z. Coumarin-containing hybrids and their anticancer activities. *Eur. J. Med. Chem.,* **2019**, *181*, 111587.
[http://dx.doi.org/10.1016/j.ejmech.2019.111587] [PMID: 31404864]

[38]   Sultana, R.; Tippanna, R.R. A novel and different approach for the synthesis of quinoline derivatives starting directly from nitroarenes and their evaluation as anticancer agents. *Int. J. Chem.,* **2020**, *12*(1), 99.
[http://dx.doi.org/10.5539/ijc.v12n1p99]

[39]   Khan, M.F.; Alam, M.M.; Verma, G.; Akhtar, W.; Akhter, M.; Shaquiquzzaman, M. The therapeutic voyage of pyrazole and its analogs: A review. *Eur. J. Med. Chem.,* **2016**, *120*, 170-201.
[http://dx.doi.org/10.1016/j.ejmech.2016.04.077] [PMID: 27191614]

[40]   Yang, X.; Zhang, P.; Zhou, Y.; Wang, J.; Liu, H. Synthesis and Antioxidant Activities of Novel 4,4′□Arylmethylene□bis(1H□pyrazole□5□ol)s from Lignin. *Chin. J. Chem.,* **2012**, *30*(3), 670-674.
[http://dx.doi.org/10.1002/cjoc.201280009]

[41]   Kasaboina, S.; Ramineni, V.; Banu, S.; Bandi, Y.; Nagarapu, L.; Dumala, N.; Grover, P. Iodine mediated pyrazolo-quinoline derivatives as potent anti-proliferative agents. *Bioorg. Med. Chem. Lett.,* **2018**, *28*(4), 664-667.
[http://dx.doi.org/10.1016/j.bmcl.2018.01.023] [PMID: 29409753]

[42]   George, R.F.; Samir, E.M.; Abdelhamed, M.N.; Abdel-Aziz, H.A.; Abbas, S.E.S. Synthesis and anti-proliferative activity of some new quinoline based 4,5-dihydropyrazoles and their thiazole hybrids as EGFR inhibitors. *Bioorg. Chem.,* **2019**, *83*, 186-197.
[http://dx.doi.org/10.1016/j.bioorg.2018.10.038] [PMID: 30380447]

[43]   Zhang, H.Z.; Zhao, Z.L.; Zhou, C.H. Recent advance in oxazole-based medicinal chemistry. *Eur. J. Med. Chem.,* **2018**, *144*, 444-492.
[http://dx.doi.org/10.1016/j.ejmech.2017.12.044] [PMID: 29288945]

[44]   Yamamuro, D.; Uchida, R.; Ohtawa, M.; Arima, S.; Futamura, Y.; Katane, M.; Homma, H.; Nagamitsu, T.; Osada, H.; Tomoda, H. Synthesis and biological activity of 5-(4-methoxypheny-)-oxazole derivatives. *Bioorg. Med. Chem. Lett.,* **2015**, *25*(2), 313-316.
[http://dx.doi.org/10.1016/j.bmcl.2014.11.042] [PMID: 25488842]

[45]   Shah, S.R.; Katariya, K.D.; Reddy, D. Quinoline-1,3;oxazole hybrids: syntheses, anticancer activity and molecular docking studies. *ChemistrySelect,* **2020**, *5*(3), 1097-1102.
[http://dx.doi.org/10.1002/slct.201903763]

[46]   Zhang, P.; Wei, C.; Wang, E.; Wang, W.; Liu, M.; Yin, Q.; Chen, H.; Wang, K.; Li, X.; Zhang, J. Synthesis and biological activities of novel isoxazoline-linked pseudodisaccharide derivatives. *Carbohydr. Res.,* **2012**, *351*, 7-16.
[http://dx.doi.org/10.1016/j.carres.2011.11.025] [PMID: 22305409]

[47]   Bernal, C.C.; Vesga, L.C.; Mendez-Sánchez, S.C.; Romero Bohórquez, A.R. Synthesis and anticancer activity of new tetrahydroquinoline hybrid derivatives tethered to isoxazoline moiety. *Med. Chem. Res.,* **2020**, *29*(4), 675-689.
[http://dx.doi.org/10.1007/s00044-020-02513-8]

[48]   Morris, C.D.; Rose, A.; Curwen, J.; Hughes, A.M.; Wilson, D.J.; Webb, D.J. Specific inhibition of the endothelin A receptor with ZD4054: clinical and pre-clinical evidence. *Br. J. Cancer,* **2005**, *92*(12), 2148-2152.
[http://dx.doi.org/10.1038/sj.bjc.6602676] [PMID: 15956965]

[49]    Hamdy, R.; Elseginy, S.A.; Ziedan, N.I.; Jones, A.T.; Westwell, A.D. New quinoline-based heterocycles as anticancer agents targeting Bcl-2. *Molecules,* **2019**, *24*(7), 13.
        [http://dx.doi.org/10.3390/molecules24071274] [PMID: 30986908]

[50]    Shamsi, F.; Aneja, B.; Hasan, P.; Zeya, B.; Zafaryab, M.; Mehdi, S.H.; Rizvi, M.M.A.; Patel, R.; Rana, S.; Abid, M. Synthesis, anticancer evaluation and DNA-binding spectroscopic insights of quinoline-based 1,3,4-oxadiazole-1,2,3-triazole conjugates. *ChemistrySelect,* **2019**, *4*(41), 12176-12182.
        [http://dx.doi.org/10.1002/slct.201902797]

[51]    Malani, A.H.; Makwana, A.H.; Makwana, H. A brief review article: Various synthesis and therapeutic importance of 1, 2, 4-triazole and its derivatives. *Mor. J. Chem,* **2017**, *5*, 41-58.

[52]    Maračić, S.; Lapić, J.; Djaković, S.; Opačak-Bernardi, T.; Glavaš-Obrovac, L.; Vrček, V.; Raić-Malić, S. Quinoline and ferrocene conjugates: synthesis, computational study and biological evaluations. *Appl. Organomet. Chem.,* **2019**, *33*(1), 1-17.
        [http://dx.doi.org/10.1002/aoc.4628]

[53]    Venkata, S.R.G.; Narkhede, U.C.; Jadhav, V.D.; Naidu, C.G.; Addada, R.R.; Pulya, S.; Ghosh, B. Quinoline consists of 1*H*1,2,3-triazole hybrids: design, synthesis and anticancer evaluation. *ChemistrySelect,* **2019**, *4*, 14184-14190.
        [http://dx.doi.org/10.1002/slct.201903938]

[54]    Zhao, J.W.; Wu, Z.H.; Guo, J.W.; Huang, M.J.; You, Y.Z.; Liu, H.M.; Huang, L.H. Synthesis and anti-gastric cancer activity evaluation of novel triazole nucleobase analogues containing steroidal/coumarin/quinoline moieties. *Eur. J. Med. Chem.,* **2019**, *181*, 111520.
        [http://dx.doi.org/10.1016/j.ejmech.2019.07.023] [PMID: 31404863]

[55]    Somagond, S.M.; Kamble, R.R.; Kattimani, P.P.; Shaikh, S.K.J.; Dixit, S.R.; Joshi, S.D.; Devarajegowda, H.C. Design, Docking and synthesis of quinoline-2*H*-1,2,4-triazol-3(4*H*)-ones as potent anticancer and antitubercular agents. *ChemistrySelect,* **2018**, *3*(7), 2004-2016.
        [http://dx.doi.org/10.1002/slct.201702279]

[56]    Anantacharya, R.; Satyanarayan, N.D.; Sukhlal Kalal, B.; Pai, V.R. Cytotoxic, DNA cleavage and pharmacokinetic parameter study of substituted novel furan C-2 quinoline coupled 1, 2, 4-triazole and its analogs. *Open Med. Chem. J.,* **2018**, *12*(1), 60-72.
        [http://dx.doi.org/10.2174/1874104501812010060] [PMID: 30008962]

[57]    Nasr, E.E.; Mostafa, A.S.; El-Sayed, M.A.A.; Massoud, M.A.M. Design, synthesis, and docking study of new quinoline derivatives as antitumor agents. *Arch. Pharm. (Weinheim),* **2019**, *352*(7), e1800355.
        [http://dx.doi.org/10.1002/ardp.201800355] [PMID: 31081954]

[58]    Solomon, V.R.; Pundir, S.; Lee, H. Examination of novel 4-aminoquinoline derivatives designed and synthesized by a hybrid pharmacophore approach to enhance their anticancer activities. *Sci. Rep.,* **2019**, *9*(1), 6315.
        [http://dx.doi.org/10.1038/s41598-019-42816-4] [PMID: 31004122]

[59]    Yang, S.M.; Martinez, N.J.; Yasgar, A.; Danchik, C.; Johansson, C.; Wang, Y.; Baljinnyam, B.; Wang, A.Q.; Xu, X.; Shah, P.; Cheff, D.; Wang, X.S.; Roth, J.; Lal-Nag, M.; Dunford, J.E.; Oppermann, U.; Vasiliou, V.; Simeonov, A.; Jadhav, A.; Maloney, D.J. Discovery of orally bioavailable, quinoline-based aldehyde dehydrogenase 1A1 (ALDH1A1) inhibitors with potent cellular activity. *J. Med. Chem.,* **2018**, *61*(11), 4883-4903.
        [http://dx.doi.org/10.1021/acs.jmedchem.8b00270] [PMID: 29767973]

[60]    Viswas, R.S.; Pundir, S.; Lee, H. Design and synthesis of 4-piperazinyl quinoline derived urea/thioureas for anti-breast cancer activity by a hybrid pharmacophore approach. *J. Enzyme Inhib. Med. Chem.,* **2019**, *34*(1), 620-630.
        [http://dx.doi.org/10.1080/14756366.2019.1571055] [PMID: 30727782]

[61]    Karthikeyan, C.; Moorthy, N.S.; Ramasamy, S.; Vanam, U.; Manivannan, E.; Karunagaran, D.; Trivedi, P. Advances in chalcones with anticancer activities. *Recent Patents Anticancer Drug Discov.,* **2015**, *10*(1), 97-115.

[http://dx.doi.org/10.2174/1574892809666140819153902] [PMID: 25138130]

[62]   Abbas, S.H.; Abd El-Hafeez, A.A.; Shoman, M.E.; Montano, M.M.; Hassan, H.A. New quinoline/chalcone hybrids as anti-cancer agents: Design, synthesis, and evaluations of cytotoxicity and PI3K inhibitory activity. *Bioorg. Chem.,* **2019**, *82*, 360-377.
[http://dx.doi.org/10.1016/j.bioorg.2018.10.064] [PMID: 30428415]

[63]   Mirzaei, S.; Hadizadeh, F.; Eisvand, F.; Mosaffa, F.; Ghodsi, R. Synthesis, structure-activity relationship and molecular docking studies of novel quinoline-chalcone hybrids as potential anticancer agents and tubulin inhibitors. *J. Mol. Struct.,* **2020**, *1202*, 127310.
[http://dx.doi.org/10.1016/j.molstruc.2019.127310]

[64]   Othman, D.I.A.; Selim, K.B.; El-Sayed, M.A.A.; Tantawy, A.S.; Amen, Y.; Shimizu, K.; Okauchi, T.; Kitamura, M. Design, Synthesis and anticancer evaluation of new substituted thiophene-quinoline derivatives. *Bioorg. Med. Chem.,* **2019**, *27*(19), 115026.
[http://dx.doi.org/10.1016/j.bmc.2019.07.042] [PMID: 31416740]

[65]   Pal, K.B.; Mahanti, M.; Huang, X.; Persson, S.; Sundin, A.P.; Zetterberg, F.R.; Oredsson, S.; Leffler, H.; Nilsson, U.J. Quinoline-galactose hybrids bind selectively with high affinity to a galectin-8 N-terminal domain. *Org. Biomol. Chem.,* **2018**, *16*(34), 6295-6305.
[http://dx.doi.org/10.1039/C8OB01354C] [PMID: 30117507]

[66]   Bhat, H.R.; Masih, A.; Shakya, A.; Ghosh, S.K.; Singh, U.P. Design, synthesis, anticancer, antibacterial, and antifungal evaluation of 4-aminoquinoline-1, 3, 5-triazine derivatives. *J. Heterocycl. Chem.,* **2020**, *57*(1), 390-399.
[http://dx.doi.org/10.1002/jhet.3791]

[67]   Fiorot, R.G.; Westphal, R.; Lemos, B.C.; Romagna, R.A.; Gonçalves, P.R.; Fernandes, M.R.N.; Ferreira, C.V.; Tarantoe, A.G.; Greco, S.J. Synthesis, molecular modelling and anticancer activities of new molecular hybrids containing 1,4-naphthoquinone, 7-chloroquinoline, 1,3,5-triazine and morpholine cores as PI3K and AMPK inhibitors in the metastatic melanoma cells. *J. Braz. Chem. Soc.,* **2019**, *30*, 1860-1873.
[http://dx.doi.org/10.21577/0103-5053.20190096]

[68]   Nepali, K.; Lin, M.H.; Chao, M.W.; Peng, S.J.; Hsu, K.C.; Eight Lin, T.; Chen, M.C.; Lai, M.J.; Pan, S.L.; Liou, J.P. Amide-tethered quinoline-resorcinol conjugates as a new class of HSP90 inhibitors suppressing the growth of prostate cancer cells. *Bioorg. Chem.,* **2019**, *91*, 103119.
[http://dx.doi.org/10.1016/j.bioorg.2019.103119] [PMID: 31349117]

[69]   Korcz, M.; Sączewski, F.; Bednarski, P.J.; Kornicka, A. Synthesis, Structure, chemical stability, and in vitro cytotoxic properties of novel quinoline-3-carbaldehyde hydrazones bearing a 1,2,4-triazole or benzotriazole moiety. *Molecules,* **2018**, *23*(6), 1497.
[http://dx.doi.org/10.3390/molecules23061497] [PMID: 29925826]

[70]   Gayam, A.T.V.; Ravi, S. Synthesis, anticancer activity and molecular docking studies of some novel quinoline hydrazide derivatives of substituted benzaldehydes. *Rasayan J. Chem.,* **2019**, *12*, 880-890.
[http://dx.doi.org/10.31788/RJC.2019.1225137]

[71]   Katariya, K.D.; Shah, S.R.; Reddy, D. Anticancer, antimicrobial activities of quinoline based hydrazone analogues: Synthesis, characterization and molecular docking. *Bioorg. Chem.,* **2020**, *94*, 103406.
[http://dx.doi.org/10.1016/j.bioorg.2019.103406] [PMID: 31718889]

[72]   Kornienko, A.; Magedov, I. V.; Rogelj, S. Pyrano [3,2-c] pyridones and related heterocyclic compounds as pharmaceutical agents for treating disorders responsive to apoptosis, antiproliferation or vascular disruption, and the use thereof. **2013**.

[73]   Upadhyay, K.D.; Dodia, N.M.; Khunt, R.C.; Chaniara, R.S.; Shah, A.K. Synthesis and biological screening of pyrano[3,2-c]quinoline analogues as anti-inflammatory and anticancer agents. *ACS Med. Chem. Lett.,* **2018**, *9*(3), 283-288.
[http://dx.doi.org/10.1021/acsmedchemlett.7b00545] [PMID: 29541375]

[74]   Azéma, J.; Guidetti, B.; Korolyov, A.; Kiss, R.; Roques, C.; Constant, P.; Daffé, M.; Malet-Martino, M. Synthesis of lipophilic dimeric C-7/C-7-linked ciprofloxacin and C-6/C-6-linked levofloxacin derivatives. Versatile in vitro biological evaluations of monomeric and dimeric fluoroquinolone derivatives as potential antitumor, antibacterial or antimycobacterial agents. *Eur. J. Med. Chem.,* **2011**, *46*(12), 6025-6038.
       [http://dx.doi.org/10.1016/j.ejmech.2011.10.014] [PMID: 22036229]

[75]   Kassab, A.E.; Gedawy, E.M. Novel ciprofloxacin hybrids using biology oriented drug synthesis (BIODS) approach: Anticancer activity, effects on cell cycle profile, caspase-3 mediated apoptosis, topoisomerase II inhibition, and antibacterial activity. *Eur. J. Med. Chem.,* **2018**, *150*, 403-418.
       [http://dx.doi.org/10.1016/j.ejmech.2018.03.026] [PMID: 29547830]

[76]   Kuang, W-B.; Huang, R-Z.; Qin, J-L.; Lu, X.; Qin, Q-P.; Zou, B-Q.; Chen, Z-F.; Liang, H.; Zhang, Y. Design, synthesis and pharmacological evaluation of new 3-(1*H*-benzimidazol-2-yl)quinolin-2(1*H*)-one derivatives as potential antitumor agents. *Eur. J. Med. Chem.,* **2018**, *157*, 139-150.
       [http://dx.doi.org/10.1016/j.ejmech.2018.07.066] [PMID: 30092368]

[77]   Buriez, O.; Heldt, J.M.; Labbé, E.; Vessières, A.; Jaouen, G.; Amatore, C.; Amatore, C. Reactivity and antiproliferative activity of ferrocenyl-tamoxifen adducts with cyclodextrins against hormone-independent breast-cancer cell lines. *Chemistry,* **2008**, *14*(27), 8195-8203.
       [http://dx.doi.org/10.1002/chem.200800507] [PMID: 18668496]

[78]   Pejović, A.; Drabowicz, J.; Cieslak, M.; Kazmierczak-Baranska, J.; Królewska-Golińska, K. Synthesis, characterization and anticancer activity of novel ferrocene containing quinolinones: 1-ally-2-ferrocenyl-2,3-dihydroquinolin-4(1*H*)-ones   and   1-allyl-2-ferrocenylquinolin-4(1*H*)-ones. *J. Organomet. Chem.,* **2018**, *873*, 78-85.
       [http://dx.doi.org/10.1016/j.jorganchem.2018.08.004]

[79]   Magedov, I.V.; Manpadi, M.; Ogasawara, M.A.; Dhawan, A.S.; Rogelj, S.; Van Slambrouck, S.; Steelant, W.F.; Evdokimov, N.M.; Uglinskii, P.Y.; Elias, E.M.; Knee, E.J.; Tongwa, P.; Antipin, M.Y.; Kornienko, A. Structural simplification of bioactive natural products with multicomponent synthesis. 2. antiproliferative and antitubulin activities of pyrano[3,2-c]pyridones and pyrano[3,2-c]quinolones. *J. Med. Chem.,* **2008**, *51*(8), 2561-2570.
       [http://dx.doi.org/10.1021/jm701499n] [PMID: 18361483]

[80]   Kumari, P.; Narayana, C.; Dubey, S.; Gupta, A.; Sagar, R. Stereoselective synthesis of natural product inspired carbohydrate fused pyrano[3,2-c]quinolones as antiproliferative agents. *Org. Biomol. Chem.,* **2018**, *16*(12), 2049-2059.
       [http://dx.doi.org/10.1039/C7OB03186F] [PMID: 29411817]

[81]   Gollner, A.; Rudolph, D.; Arnhof, H.; Bauer, M.; Blake, S.M.; Boehmelt, G.; Cockroft, X.L.; Dahmann, G.; Ettmayer, P.; Gerstberger, T.; Karolyi-Oezguer, J.; Kessler, D.; Kofink, C.; Ramharter, J.; Rinnenthal, J.; Savchenko, A.; Schnitzer, R.; Weinstabl, H.; Weyer-Czernilofsky, U.; Wunberg, T.; McConnell, D.B. WeyerCzernilofsky, U.; Wunberg, T.; McConnell, D. B. Discovery of novel spiro[3H-indole-3,2-pyrrolidin]-2(1H)-one compounds as chemically stable and orally active inhibitors of the MDM2–p53 interaction. *J. Med. Chem.,* **2016**, *59*(22), 10147-10162.
       [http://dx.doi.org/10.1021/acs.jmedchem.6b00900] [PMID: 27775892]

[82]   Shyamsivappan, S.; Vivek, R.; Saravanan, A.; Arasakumar, T.; Subashini, G.; Suresh, T.; Shankar, R.; Mohan, P.S. Synthesis and X-ray study of dispiro 8-nitroquinolone analogues and their cytotoxic properties against human cervical cancer HeLa cells. *MedChemComm,* **2019**, *10*(3), 439-449.
       [http://dx.doi.org/10.1039/C8MD00482J] [PMID: 31015907]

[83]   Turel, I. Special issue: practical applications of metal complexes. *Molecules,* **2015**, *20*(5), 7951-7956.
       [http://dx.doi.org/10.3390/molecules20057951] [PMID: 26007166]

[84]   Hernández-López, H.; Sánchez-Miranda, G.; Araujo-Huitrado, J.G.; Granados-López, A.J.; López, J.A.; Leyva-Ramos, S.; Chacón-García, L. Hern'andez-L' opez, H.; S'anchez-Miranda, G.; Huitrado, J. G. A.; Granados-L'opez, A. J.; Adri'an L'opez, J.; Leyva-Ramos, S.; Chac'on-Garc'ıa, L. Synthesis of hybrid fluoroquinolone-boron complexes and their evaluation in cervical cancer cell lines. *J. Chem.,*

**2019**, *2019*, 1-6.
[http://dx.doi.org/10.1155/2019/5608652]

[85]  Kumar, S.; Deep, A.; Narasimhan, B. A review on synthesis, anticancer and antiviral potentials of pyrimidine derivatives. *Curr. Bioact. Compd.,* **2019**, *15*(3), 289-303.
[http://dx.doi.org/10.2174/1573407214666180124160405]

[86]  Ngoc Toan, D.; Thanh, N.D.; Truong, M.X.; Van, D.T. Quinoline-pyrimidine hybrid compounds from 3-acetyl-4-hydroxy-1-methylquinolin-2(1*H*)-one: Study on synthesis, cytotoxicity, ADMET and molecular docking. *Arab. J. Chem.,* **2020**, *13*(11), 7860-7874.
[http://dx.doi.org/10.1016/j.arabjc.2020.09.018]

[87]  Noolvi, M.N.; Patel, H.M.; Kaur, M. Benzothiazoles: search for anticancer agents. *Eur. J. Med. Chem.,* **2012**, *54*, 447-462.
[http://dx.doi.org/10.1016/j.ejmech.2012.05.028] [PMID: 22703845]

[88]  Bolakatti, G.; Palkar, M.; Katagi, M.; Hampannavar, G.; Karpoormath, R.V.; Ninganagouda, S.; Badiger, A. Novel series of benzo[*d* ]thiazolyl substituted-2-quinolone hybrids: Design, synthesis, biological evaluation and *in-silico* insights. *J. Mol. Struct.,* **2020**, *10*, 129413.

[89]  Shyamsivappan, S.; Arjunan, S.; Vivek, R.; Suresh, T.; Ramasamy, S.; Gothandam, K.M.; Mohan, P.S. A novel phenyl and thiophene dispiro indenoquinoxaline pyrrolidine quinolones induced apoptosis *via* G1/S and G2/M phase cell cycle arrest in MCF-7 cells. *New J. Chem.,* **2020**, *44*(35), 15031-15045.
[http://dx.doi.org/10.1039/D0NJ02588G]

[90]  Saha, D.; Jain, G.; Sharma, A. Benzothiazepines: chemistry of a privileged scaffold. *RSC Advances,* **2015**, *5*(86), 70619-70639.
[http://dx.doi.org/10.1039/C5RA12422K]

[91]  Toan, D.N.; Nguyen, D.T.; Bang, D.N.; Thanh Nga, M.; Mai, X.T.; Nguyen, T.T.H. Synthesis, cytotoxic activity, ADMET and molecular docking study of quinoline-based hybrid compounds of 1,5-benzothiazepines. *New J. Chem.,* **2020**, *44*(47), 20715-20725.
[http://dx.doi.org/10.1039/D0NJ04295A]

# CHAPTER 5

# Tetrazoles: Structure and Activity Relationship as Anticancer Agents

**M.V. Basavanag Unnamatla[1,2], Fazlur-Rahman Nawaz Khan[3]** and **Erick Cuevas Yañez[1,2,*]**

[1] *Centro Conjunto de Investigación en Química Sustentable UAEM-UNAM. Carretera Toluca-Atlacomulco Km 14.5, Toluca, Estado de México, 50200, México. Universidad Autónoma del Estado de México*

[2] *Facultad de Química, Universidad Autónoma del Estado de México, Carretera Toluca-Atlacomulco Km 14.5, Unidad San Cayetano, Toluca, Estado de México, C. P. 50200 México*

[3] *Organic and Medicinal Chemistry Research Laboratory, School of Advanced Sciences, Vellore Institute of Technology, Vellore-632 014, Tamil Nadu, India*

**Abstract:** Heterocyclic compounds play an important role in drug design and discovery, and they have been used to treat a variety of diseases, including cancer. Cancer is one of the leading causes of death in the world. However, various drugs and therapies are available on the market. The novel synthetic drugs show promising in-vitro activity, but the route to clinical trials is hampered by their low bioavailability and rapid metabolism. Tetrazoles have gained a lot of attention in recent years because they have the broadest biological activity spectrum of any heterocycle. Tetrazoles are a type of nitrogen heterocycle that has been found to be active in a variety of natural products as well as the biologically active nucleus. A vast number of studies have demonstrated the importance of this moiety in medicinal chemistry. The tetrazole ring has a similar structure to carboxylic acids and functions as a bioisostere analogue. A bioisostere is a group of molecules that have similar physiological properties, including biological activity. Tetrazole derivatives have been shown to have anti-hypertension, anti-fungal, anti-malarial, anti-leishmaniasis, anti-diabetic, anti-cancer, and a variety of other biological activities. The tetrazole moiety functions as a good pharmacophore in the drug design and discovery fields, particularly in terms of rational drug design with high efficiency with structure and anti-cancer activity.

**Keywords:** Bioavailability, Bioisosteres, SAR, Synthesis, Tetrazole.

* **Corresponding author Erick Cuevas Yañez:** Centro Conjunto de Investigación en Química Sustentable UAEM-UNAM. Carretera Toluca-Atlacomulco Km 14.5, Toluca, Estado de México, 50200, México. Universidad Autónoma del Estado de México and Facultad de Química, Universidad Autónoma del Estado de México, Carretera Toluca-Atlacomulco Km 14.5, Unidad San Cayetano, Toluca, Estado de México, C. P. 50200 México; Tel: +527224114234; E-mail: ecuevasy@uaemex.mx

# INTRODUCTION

Cancer is one of the world's leading causes of death [1]. Cancer is caused by uncontrolled cell proliferation and the spread of cancer to other parts of the body. According to a global survey, new cases and more than half of cancer deaths worldwide in 2018 were estimated in Asian countries. There will be a rise of over 21.4 million new cases per year with 13.2 million deaths by 2030.

Breast, lung, and colorectal cancers are the most common cancer types, accounting for one-third of all cancer-related deaths worldwide [1, 2]. However, scientific progress has focused on understanding the exact pathophysiology of the disease, and as a result, significant progress in cancer early detection has been made, resulting in a lower mortality rate. Furthermore, in some developing countries, the survival rate is extremely low. This is because of the late stage of detection and the limited availability of qualitative treatment [3]. The primary methods of cancer treatment are radiotherapy, surgery, and chemotherapy [4]. Among these treatments, chemotherapy is regarded as an effective first-line strategy for suppressing tumour prognosis and eradication.

Chemotherapy drugs work on cellular mechanisms by inhibiting cell division, preventing cancer cell multiplication. Current clinically approved cancer drugs act on metabolically active or rapidly replicating cancer cells, but they also have drawbacks such as selectivity between cancer and healthy cells [5].

These cancer cells generally disrupt the cell signalling pathways and tissue morphogenesis that support the neoplastic tumours. The therapeutic approach for these targeted cell pathways involves the use of cytotoxic agents that have been shown to inhibit tumour growth and disease progression. However, the current chemotherapeutic drugs' higher toxic profiles and poor tolerance are major barriers to effective cancer treatment [6, 7]. As a result, while new drugs are being developed for this purpose, they are still insufficient to control this global threat [8, 9].

Heterocycles such as indole, morpholine, thiazolidinedione, benzothiazole, camptothecin, and benzimidazole are all thought to be anti-cancer agents [10, 11]. Tetrazole, as a heterocyclic moiety, has recently received a lot of attention in the field of medicine. There have been numerous publications about biological activity and FDA-approved drugs based on this moiety. It is a five-membered heterocycle that is regarded to be bioisosteric of carboxylic acid. A "bioisoster" is a group of chemical constituents with similar physiological and biological properties. In addition, the five heteroatoms in a heteroaromatic system have an acidic character and are thought to be a bioisosteric replacement for a carboxylic acid group (Fig. **1**). In an *in vivo* study, this system has a similar pka to carboxylic acid and ionised at physiological pH, as well as similar biological activity [12]. Tetrazole is a five-membered heterocycle with one carbon atom and four nitrogen atoms that can function as both a donor and acceptor of multicentre hydrogen bonds [13 - 16].

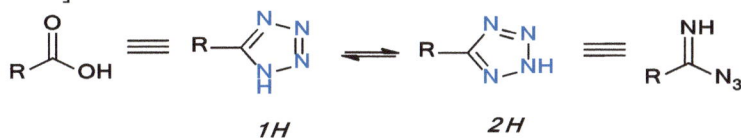

**Fig. (1).** Tetrazole as bioisostere.

Tetrazole derivatives are ten times more lipophilic than carboxylic acid derivatives, which increase drug concentration in the systemic circulation. As a result, when the tetrazole is incorporated into an organic molecule, the potency and bioavailability of the drug may increase. The nitrogen atoms in the heterocycles play an important role in charge delocalization, which is required for binding to the angiotensin II (AII) receptor. Researchers have recently become interested in the aforementioned factors, as well as metabolic stability and the incorporation of the tetrazole moiety into drug molecules [17].

## BIOLOGICAL BACKGROUND OF TETRAZOLE NUCLEUS

Tetrazoles and its derivatives exhibit various biological activities such as antibacterial (1) [18 - 20], antifungal (2) [21, 22], antiviral (3) [23], anti-tubercular (4) [24, 25], antimalarial (5) [26], (Fig. **2**).

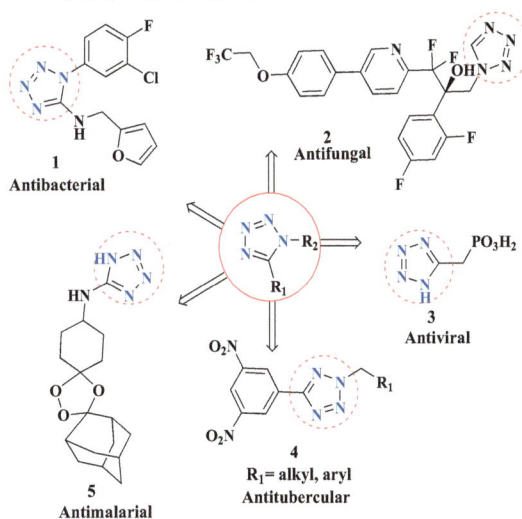

**Fig. (2).** Biologically active tetrazole hybrids.

However, apart from these compounds, the tetrazole moiety in their structure gives them a wide range of biological activity. There has been significant progress in the biological activity of tetrazole incorporated moieties over the last two decades. Aside from these activities, other biological activities such as anti-convulsant, anti-diabetic, anti-hypertensive, and anti-inflammatory antipro liferative activity have been reported in the literature [27]. Among these activities, tetrazoles are being studied for their anti-cancer properties. In this context, we will look at recent findings and the structure-activity relationship of tetrazole-incorporated moieties as anti-cancer agents [17]. One of the most well-known uses of tetrazole is the drug, Losartan 6 (Fig. **3**) and its derivatives. Losartan, a tetrazole-incorporated derivative containing angiotensin II receptor antagonists, has received a lot of attention in the literature [28, 29].

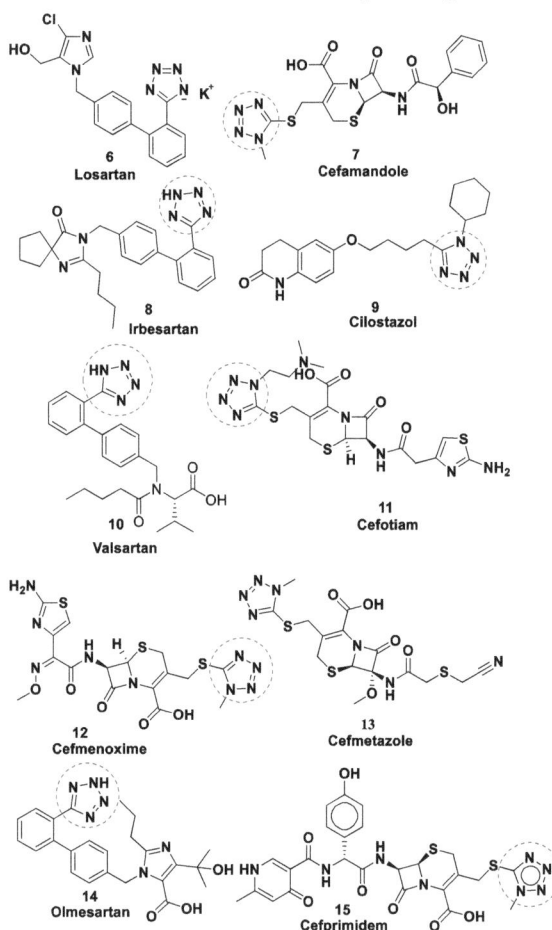

**Fig. (3a).** Chemical Structures and name of drugs based on tetrazole moiety.

Based on the above structure, it is assumed that a Losartan (6) binds to the receptor and blocks the molecule that occupies the receptor's lipophilic pockets *via* lipophilic substituents at the 2nd and 4th positions of the imidazole. Aside from them, there is a basic group in one section of the molecule that requires an acidic function, which is why Losartan has a tetrazole ring. During the development of Losartan, a large number of compounds with various functional groups in the biphenyl part were studied to learn about the structure-activity relationship and the importance of tetrazole incorporation [30].

Moreover, there are many tetrazole-based drugs [31] (Fig. **3a-c**), such as Cefamandole (7), Irbesartan (8) (Angiotensin receptor blocker, ARB, hypertensive agent), Cilostazol (9) [20], (Intermittent claudication in individuals with peripheral vascular disease), Valsartan (10) (DB0177-Antihypertensive agent), Cefotiam (11) (DB00229-antibiotic against both gram-positive and gram-negative microorganisms) Cefmenoxime (12) (DB00267-third-generation antibiotic), Cefmetazole (13) (DB00274-antibiotic against both gram-positive and gram-negative microorganisms), Olmesartan (14) (Antihypertensive agents), Cefprimidem (15) (Antibiotic), Losartan (6) (Antihypertensive agent), Candesartan (16) (Antihypertensive), Alfentanil (17) (anesthetic, and analgesic fentanyl), Pemirolast (18) (antiallergic agent), Ceforanide (19) (second-generation antibiotic), Cefamandole (20) (vast spectrum cephalosporin antibiotic), Cefazolin (21) (antibiotic), Cefonicid (22) (A second-generation cephalosporin), Cefoperazone (23) (semisynthetic cephalosporin), Cefotetan (24) (antibiotic), Tasosartan (25) (A long-acting angiotensin II receptor blocker), Latamoxef (26) (antibiotic), Tedizolid Phosphate (27) (oxazolidinone-class antibiotic prodrug), Fimasartan (28) (nonpeptide angiotensin II receptor antagonist), Pranlukast (29) (A cyteinyl leukotriene receptor-1 antagonist) Nojrimycin tetrazole (30) (Glycogen phosphorylase, muscle form) and Forasartan (31) (angiotensin II antagonist).

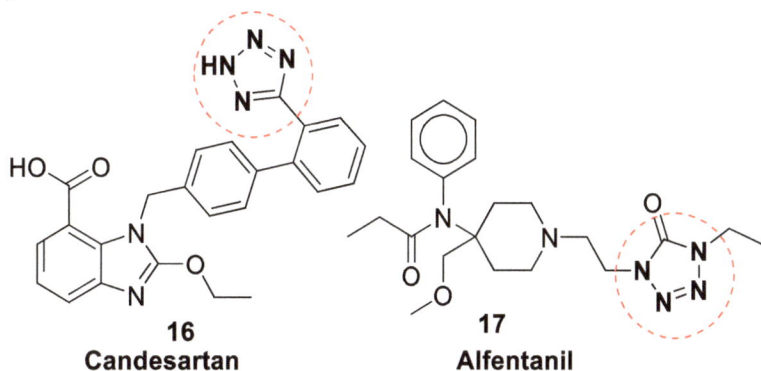

**16**
**Candesartan**

**17**
**Alfentanil**

*(Fig. 3b) contd.....*

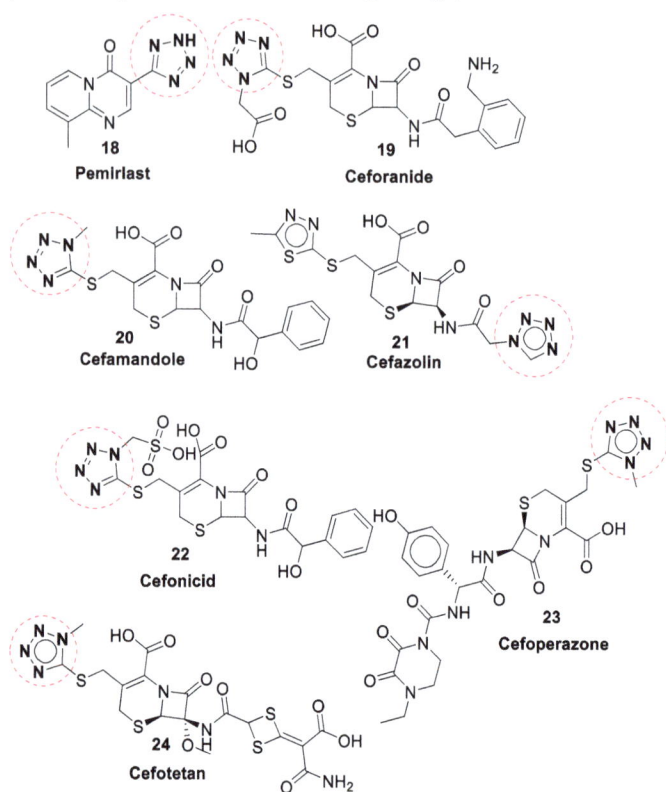

**Fig. (3b).** Chemical Structures and name of drugs based on tetrazole moiety.

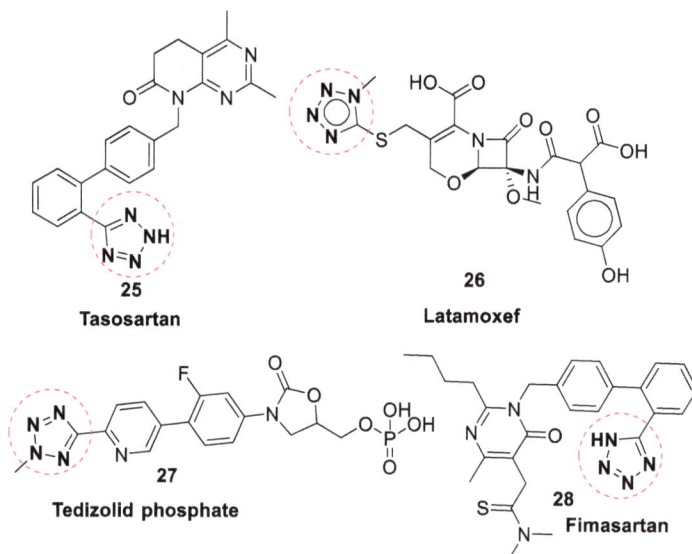

*(Fig. 3c) contd.....*

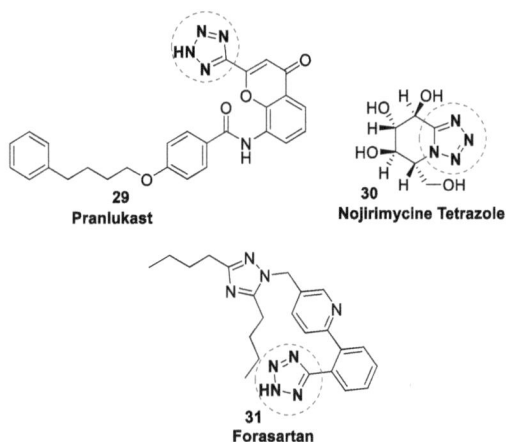

**Fig. (3c).** Chemical Structures and name of drugs based on tetrazole moiety.

In this book chapter, we discuss the synthesis and development of tetrazoles as anti-cancer agents in recent years. Tetrazoles have been found to have higher anti-cancer activity while being less toxic. Because of its appealing biological profile and easy bioavailability with metabolic stability, the incorporation of tetrazole moiety into drug molecules has recently piqued the interest of many researchers [17, 32].

## SYNTHESIS OF TETRAZOLES

The synthesis of tetrazole-containing compounds can be accomplished *via* a variety of approaches. Initially, hydrazoic acid was used to incorporate the tetrazole ring into any structure. Because it was explosive and dangerous, sodium azide was eventually employed instead of hydrazoic acid as an azide source. The first 5-phenyl-1-acyl-1,2,3,4-tetrazoles were synthesised by using sodium azide, which was reported by Finnegan *et al.* in 1958 [33]. However, the reaction conditions were refluxing under high temperatures using solvents like dimethylformamide and dimethyl sulfoxide as these solvents sustain high temperatures due to their high boiling points. These were common solvents used in tetrazole synthesis (Scheme 1).

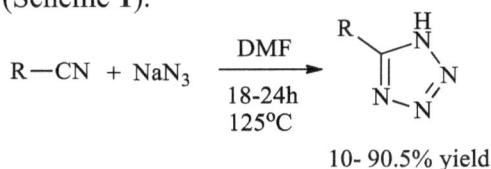

10- 90.5% yield

**Scheme. (1).** Synthesis of 5-substituted aryl tetrazoles.

Researchers have reported a number of methodologies for introducing the tetrazole moiety, but the most convenient method is the 2+3 cycloaddition of nitriles with sodium azide ($NaN_3$) in the presence of a catalyst [34]. Catalyst, particularly Lewis acid catalyst, plays an important role in tetrazole synthesis [35 - 37]. The use of a catalyst has the advantage of avoiding higher reaction temperatures and longer reaction times; however, depending on the reactant, the catalyst may fail to catalyse the reaction [31, 38].

The following section presents examples of various methods and catalysts used to incorporate tetrazoles [39 - 41]. The required amount of catalyst was added to the reaction mixture of nitriles, including sodium azide (Scheme **2**), and stirred vigorously at 120 °C under reflux conditions. To generate 5-substituted-1H tetrazoles, acidification is required to free up the nitrogen N1 position [42].

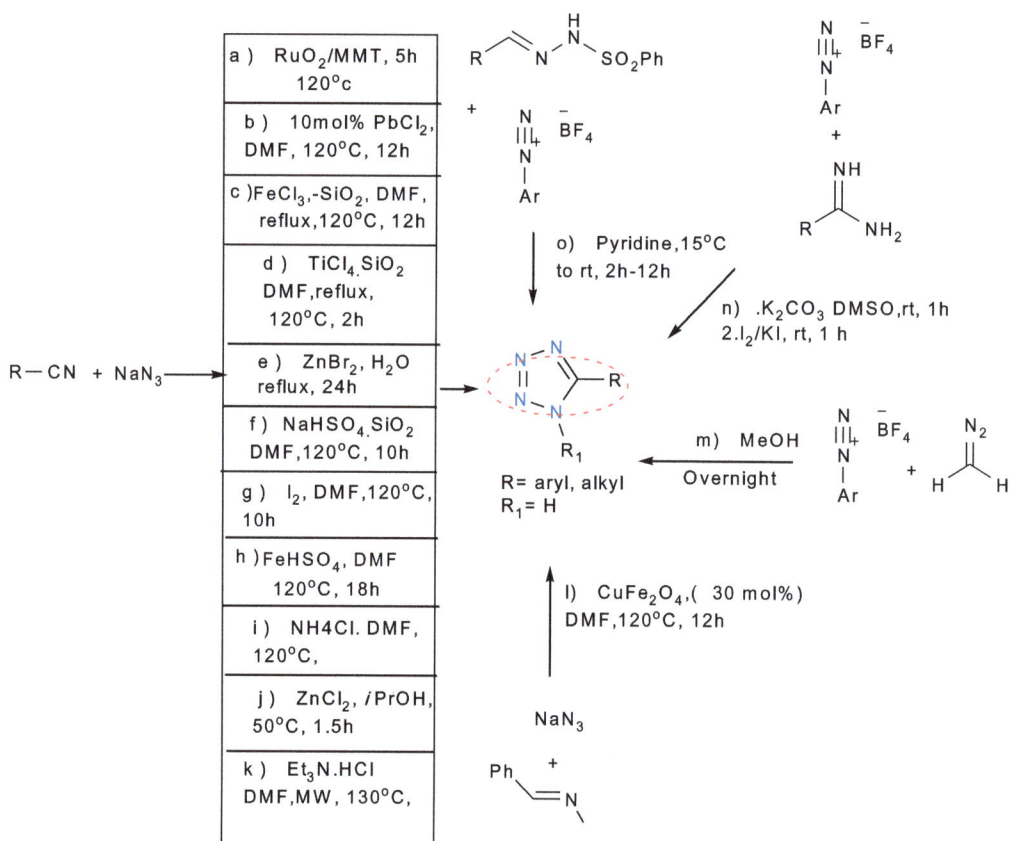

**Scheme. (2).** Different strategies for the synthesis of tetrazoles.

Pawar and co-workers reported a facile, one-pot, three-component method to obtain *N*-substituted tetrazole using $RuO_2$/MMT (**a**) nanocomposite catalytic system. The above catalytic system yields *N*-substituted tetrazoles in good to excellent yields. The catalytic system also has high recyclability up to five cycles, with a 5% reduction in tetrazole yield after the fifth cycle [41].

Kant *et al*. synthesised 5-substituted-1H-tetrazoles using lead salts Pb(II) (b) *via* [3+2] cycloaddition of nitriles and sodium azide. They developed a simple, mild, and efficient method [40].

Nasrollahzadeh *et al*. reported the synthesis of 5-substituted-1H-tetrazoles with a heterogeneous $FeCl_3$: $SiO_2$(c) catalyst [43].The efficiency of the synthesis is determined by the recyclability of the acid catalyst and simple workup procedures. Shaik *et al*. reported the synthesis of tetrazoles using triethylamine using toluene as a solvent, but the drawback of the synthesis was the reaction time was 48 h [44, 45]. Zamani and his co-workers [46] used nano-$TiCL_4.SiO_2$ (**d**) in the synthesis of 5-substituted-1*H*-tetrazole derivatives. They found this nano-supported catalyst extremely efficient for synthesizing tetrazole derivatives. Demko and Sharpless [47] carried out the synthesis in an aqueous medium, despite the fact that water is not a good solvent for organic compounds. Das *et al*. have developed a good synthesis of 5-substituted-1*H*-tetrazole derivatives by using a heterogeneous catalyst such as silica-supported sodium hydrogen sulphate ($NaHSO_4.SiO_2$) (**f**) or iodine (**g**) as a catalyst [48]. In other methodologies for obtaining tetrazoles, they have used Fe $(HSO_4)_3$ (h) [49], ammonium chloride ($NH_4Cl$) (i) [50], $ZnCl_2$ (j) [51] and $Et_3N.HCl$ (k) [52] as catalysts. Apart from the nitriles, aryl diazonium salts play a key role in obtaining the tetrazoles *via* click reaction (m, n, o) [53]. Using (E)-aldoximes and sodium azide under heterogeneous catalysis with copper ferrite nanoparticles (l) as recyclable catalyst, Akula and his colleagues reported a new approach for the synthesis of 5-substituted-1H-tetrazoles [54].

## Other Methodologies of Synthesis

The other methodologies for synthesizing tetrazoles *via* multicomponent reactions are convergent reactions that give very diverse adducts. In that case, the Ugi-Azide reaction (Scheme **3**) is one of the essential methods for obtaining 1,5 disubstituted tetrazoles [31, 55].

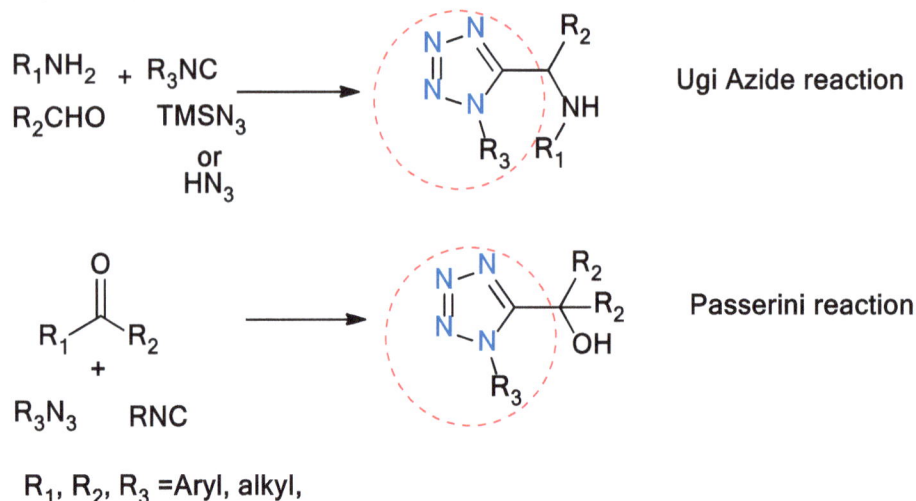

Ugi Azide reaction

Passerini reaction

$R_1, R_2, R_3$ = Aryl, alkyl,

**Scheme. (3).** Synthesis of 1,5 di-substituted tetrazoles *via* Ugi-Azide reaction.

Apart from the Ugi-Azide reaction [56, 57], the Passerini three-component reaction is another well-studied method for producing 1,5 disubstituted tetrazoles (Scheme **3**) [58, 59]. These reactions are mainly based on isocyanide-based multicomponent reactions.

## TETRAZOLE CONTAINING COMPOUNDS WITH ANTI-CANCER ACTIVITY

Tetrazole-based anti-cancer drug candidates have demonstrated their anti-cancer [60] potency by several mechanisms. In that, PRMT (Protein Arginine Methyltransferases) inhibition [61], COX-2 (Cyclooxygenase-2) [62, 63], angiogenesis [64, 65], efflux pump, HIF- and tubulin polymerization [66, 67] are included. The analogues of tetrazoles are reported to regulate the expression of Ki-62, Bcl-2, and caspases by stopping the cell cycle, which promotes apoptosis (Fig. **4**) [68].

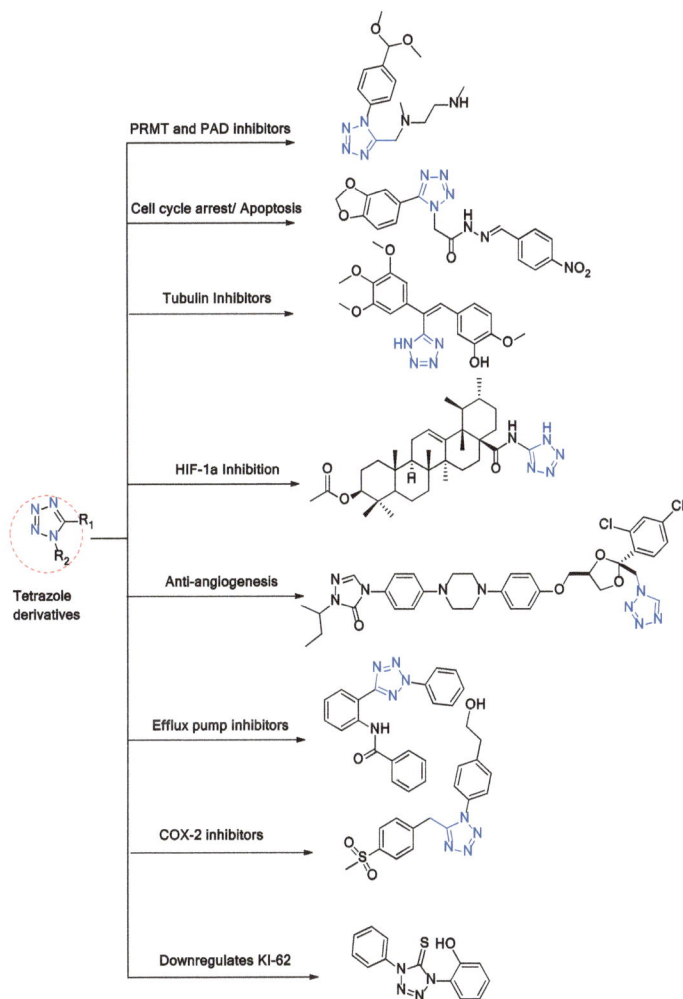

**Fig. (4).** Anti-cancer mechanism of action-oriented tetrazole derivatives.

## STRUCTURE AND ACTIVITY RELATIONSHIP STUDIES

The structure-activity relationship of tetrazole is one of the most important factors in drug discovery. Tetrazoles are considered important ligands because they are metabolically stable and have highly flexible features. Tetrazole scaffolds can operate as pharmacophores for the carboxylate group, adapting to various binding modes and having high bioavailability, which can boost drug efficacy. The bioisosteres of *cis* amides in peptidomimetics are another essential property of 1,5 disubstituted tetrazoles (Fig. **5**) [69]. According to Allen et al., X-ray analysis and theoretical calculations verified that the tetrazolyl fragment is a bioisostere of a carboxylic acid group [70].

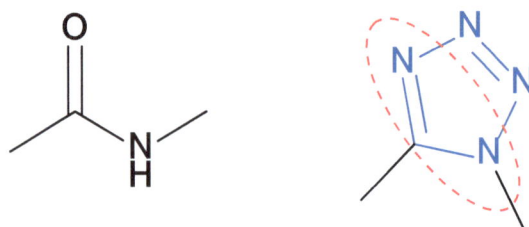

**Fig. (5).** Bioisosterism of *cis* amide bond in 1,5-disubsituted tetrazoles.

Tetrazoles with four nitrogen atoms undergo four hydrogen bonds due to four nitrogen lone pair electrons. However, this tetrazole moiety is an excellent and promising ligand in metal coordination that is like carboxylate [71]. There are literature reports on tetrazole based on metal coordinated compounds as anti-tumour agents [72]. Rosenberg *et al.* discovered cisplatin (*cis*[Pt(NH$_3$)$_2$Cl$_2$]) in 1965, and it is one of the most effective anti-cancer medications. However, there are certain disadvantages, such as severe neurotoxicity and mutagenesis activities. Because of these limitations, it was suggested that platinum (II)-based medications be developed in order to eliminate adverse effects and increase efficiency. This can be accomplished through the use of heterocycles. Tetrazole has been identified as a promising species for use in this drug design. Serebryanskaya *et al.* prepared a series of tetrazole based platinum (II) chloride complexes (Scheme 4) [73, 74]. They enhanced the activity of both *cis* and *trans*-platinum complexes.

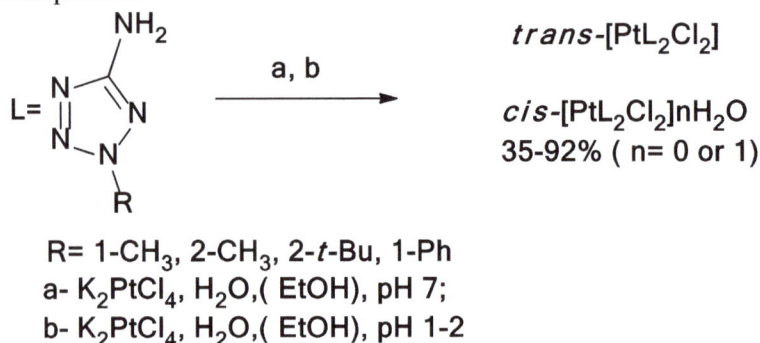

**Scheme. (4).** Synthesis of tetrazole based platinum complexes.

The antiproliferative activity of these platinum complexes was considerable, and the cytotoxicity was dependent on the geometry and hydrophobicity of the carrier ligands. The cytotoxicity activity of cis-[PtL$_2$Cl$_2$] against the Hela cell line (trypan blue assay) is Based on the results of cytotoxicity activity against Hela cell line (trypan blue assay) is considered, *cis*-[PtL$_2$Cl$_2$]. H$_2$O complexes where the ligand is L = 5-amino-1-phenyl-tetrazole (IC$_{50}$=1.3 µM) and L=5-amino-2-*tert*-butyltetrazole (IC$_{50}$ = 0.9 µM) are more promising. The *trans*-[PtL$_2$Cl$_2$] complex with L=-amino-2-*tert*-butyltetrazole has shown promising activity against HeLa cells with an IC$_{50}$ of 5.6 µM. This value corresponds to an intermediate value between cisplatin and carboplatin [75].

Bekhit and colleagues [76] reported the synthesis of platinum(II) cis-complexes with ligands tetrazolo[1,5-a] quinolone Schiff bases and their anti-tumor activity. They evaluated these complexes' cytotoxicity against HL-60 (human promyelocytic leukemia) cells, and the authors found that these complexes have higher efficiency than cisplatin.

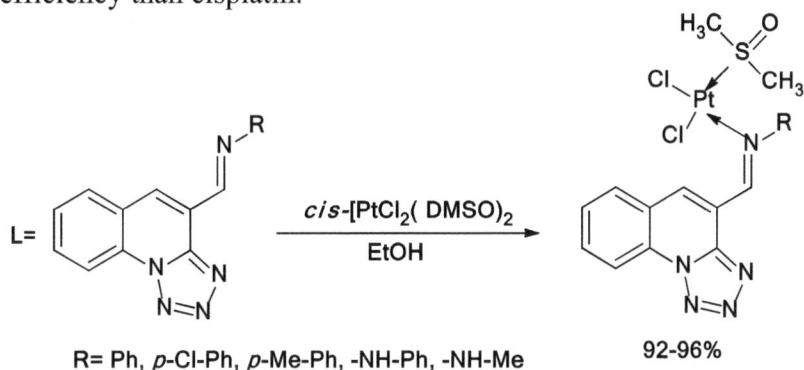

R= Ph, *p*-Cl-Ph, *p*-Me-Ph, -NH-Ph, -NH-Me          92-96%

**Scheme. (5).** Synthesis of platinum complexes with tetrazolo[1,5-*a*]quinoline based Schiff bases.

Seiji Komeda*et al,* reported tetrazolato-bridged dinuclear platinum(II) complexes (Fig. **6**) and demonstrated antitumor activity against pancreatic cancer [77].

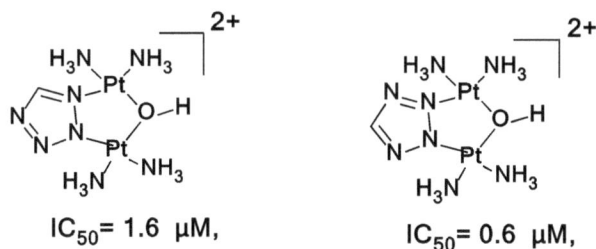

IC$_{50}$= 1.6 µM,          IC$_{50}$= 0.6 µM,

**Fig. (6).** *In vitro* cytotoxicity of azolato-bridged dinuclear platinum (II), complexes and cisplatin towards H460 human NSCLC cell line.

The same authors presented a few literature reports and explained their anti-cancer study on tetrazolato bridged dinuclear platinum compounds [78 - 80].

Zhang and his co-workers have briefly explained the structure and activity relationship of tetrazole substituted hybrids [81]. The review explored various tetrazole hybrid structures and their structure-activity relationships towards anti-cancer activity. The anti-cancer potency is increased by the hybridization of the tetrazole moiety with pharmacophores. These overcome drug resistance and side effects. They found in their review three compounds that have promising potency against drug-resistant, susceptible cancer cell lines: pipemidic acid-tetrazole conjugate **(32)**, tetrazole-steriod **(33)**, and tetrazole-reservatrol **(34)**. These compounds have an $IC_{50}$ nanomolar level, demonstrating the potential anti-cancer candidates (Fig. **7**).

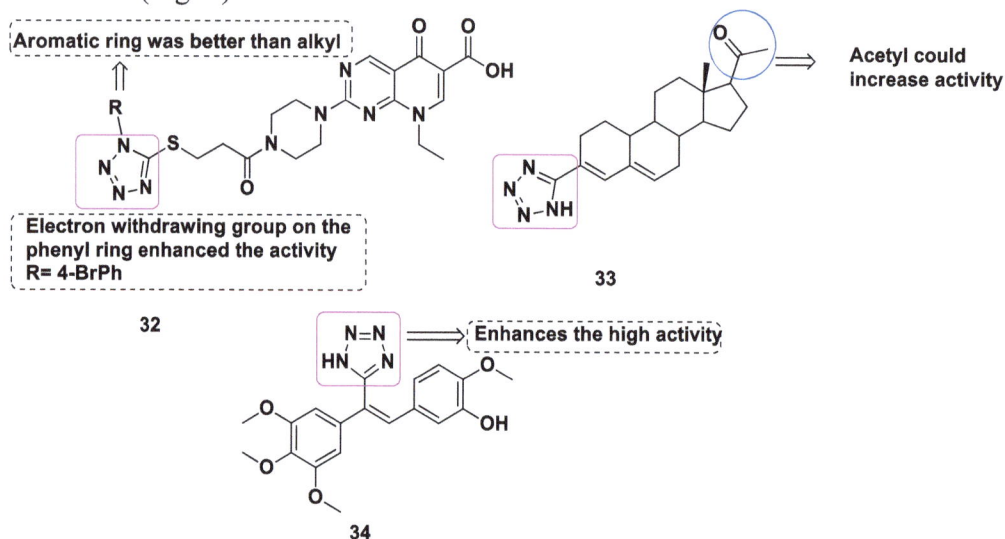

**Fig. (7).** Potential anticancer tetrazole hybrids structures.

## MECHANISM OF ACTION

Tetrazole-based drug candidates can acquire target-oriented anti-cancer potency in a variety of ways. (Fig. **4**). Here we describe and highlight the comparison of SAR with the target-specific mechanism.

## Protein Arginine Methyl Transferase 1 Inhibitors

Protein arginine methyltransferase was found in mammalian cells to be involved in the formation of MMA (-NG-mono-methylarginine), ADMA (NG-asymmetric dimethylarginine), and SDMA (NG-symmetric dimethylarginine).The addition of the methyl group to an arginine residue replaces the potential hydrogen bond donor and its shape. This can affect the bulkiness and hydrophobicity of a protein and cause protein-protein interactions in the form of positive and negative feedback. The main reason is that methylation does not neutralise the cationic charge of the arginine residue [61]. These are generally expressed and control essential cellular processes that can affect cell growth, proliferation, and differentiation. The overexpression of these enzymes may probably be involved in the pathogenesis of many diseases, including cancer [82, 83]. Tetrazole-based PRMT inhibitors are more potent than furan-incorporated PRMT inhibitors (stillbamidine, allantodapsone) previously developed by Yang and colleagues [84, 85]. Herein, they mentioned the results of tetrazole containing PRMT1 inhibitors (35), which showed initial screening effects at 9 µM and increased from 32% to 51% (Fig. **8**). The structure and activity of PRMT1, a detailed study, were described from the homology modelling study. They found two aromatic amino acids (Tyr47 and Tyr156) at the arginine binding site, and also amino acid negatively charged residues (Glu 152 and Glu 161) created strong interactions with arginine.

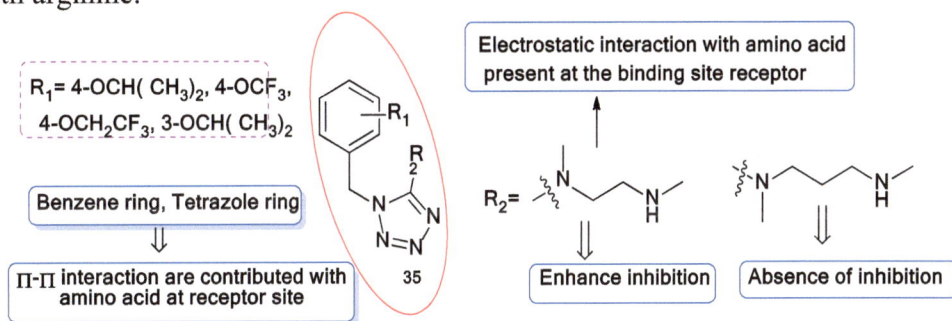

**Fig. (8).** SAR of tetrazole base PRMT1 inhibitors.

| Compound | $R_1$ | $R_2$ | PRMT1 $IC_{50}(\mu m)$ |
|---|---|---|---|
| 1 | 4-OCH(CH$_3$)$_2$ | | 3.5 |
| 2 | 4-OCF$_3$ | | 23.8 |
| 3 | 4-OCH$_2$F$_3$ | | 19.9 |
| 4 | 3- OCH(CH$_3$)$_2$ | | - |

(Table 8) cont.....

| Compound | $R_1$ | $R_2$ | PRMT1 $IC_{50}(\mu m)$ |
|---|---|---|---|
| 5 | 4-OCH(CH$_3$)$_2$ | | - |
| 6 | 4-OCH(CH$_3$)$_2$ | | 10 |
| 7 | 4-OCH(CH$_3$)$_2$ | | 29 |

An aromatic ring and two positively charged nitrogen atoms make up the structure of the tetrazole substituted pharmacophore. The results reflected the inhibitory activity of *para*-substituted compounds **1-3** better when compared with *meta*-substitution **4**. The ethylenediamine side-chain plays a key role in binding with the amino acids (Tyr47, Tyr156, Asp84, Glu108, and Glu152) at the receptor site. They found that replacing the amine side chain with propylenediamine **5** resulted in the absence of activity. The moderate activity was found in compounds 6-7 with an $IC_{50}$ of 30 μM after replacing the side chain. According to the findings, compound 1 has occupied the substrate arginine binding site of PRMT1 without competition, and there is no clear evidence for this [86].

## PAD (Protein Arginine Deiminases) Inhibitors

Another enzyme family that catalyses PTM from arginine that results from citrulline is the protein arginine deiminases (PAD). Changes in the position of the charged residue may have an effect on the protein structure [87]. PAD regulate gene transcription, apoptosis, cell differentiation, and other processes. PAD upregulation is linked to a variety of diseases, including cancer. The amidine is effective against cancer by inhibiting PADs, and various variants have been developed to improve bioavailability, selectivity, and biological potency issues [88, 89]. Subramanian and colleagues created Cl-amidine analogues by incorporating tetrazoles, which act as bioisosteres of an amide bond. They discovered that having a t-butyl group on the tetrazole ring increases PAD-2 selectivity (Fig. **9**) [90].

HN
X
NH    X= Cl, F

X= F ,
Cellviability % at 20µM= 50
$EC_{50}$= 45 ± 1.2

X= Cl ,
Cellviability % at 20µM= 0
$EC_{50}$= 10 ± 2.5

O

N
H

$R_1$= *t*-Bu

selective toward PAD2

Cl-Amidine ( Standard) 160 ± 20

Increases hydrophobicity

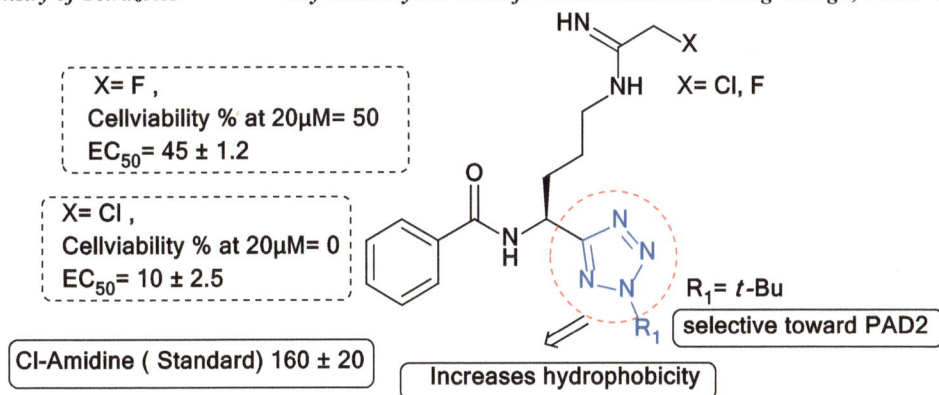

**Fig. (9).** PAD inhibition and SAR of Cl-amidine tetrazole analogues.

## Ki-67 Expression Suppression

Ki-67 is an antigen discovered in the 1980s to be related to nuclear antigens. This was used as a cell proliferation indicator. Increased expression in human cancer cells usually indicates an aggressive nature [91]. Ki-67 is found in all cell cycle phases (G1, S, G2, and M), but not in resting cells (G0) [92, 93]. As a panel of genes that define the risk of recurrence for a given subtype of cancer, this can be used as a prognosis marker in breast cancer and other malignancies [94]. It is an excellent marker in the study of antiproliferative activity in this context [95].

| Compound | X | $R_1$ | $IC_{50}(\mu M)$ | |
|----------|---|-------|------|------|
| | | | Day1 | Day4 |
| 36g | O | OH | 12.0±0.3 | 7.1±0.2 |
| 37g | S | OH | 3.8±0.1 | 2.5±0.1 |
| 36f | O | | 16.1±0.4 | 12.9±0.3 |

Gundugola and his co-workers synthesised a series of 1,4-diaryl tetrazolyl-5-ones with oxo and thio derivatives. They evaluated these compounds against L1210 (leukemia cancer cells) and SK-BR-3 (human breast adenocarcinoma) tumour cells. According to their findings, the compounds 36g, 37g, and 36f are more potent against L1210. They reduced the expression of the cell proliferation marker Ki-67 in SR-BR-3 cells as well as the rate of DNA synthesis in L1210 cells (Fig. **10**) [96].

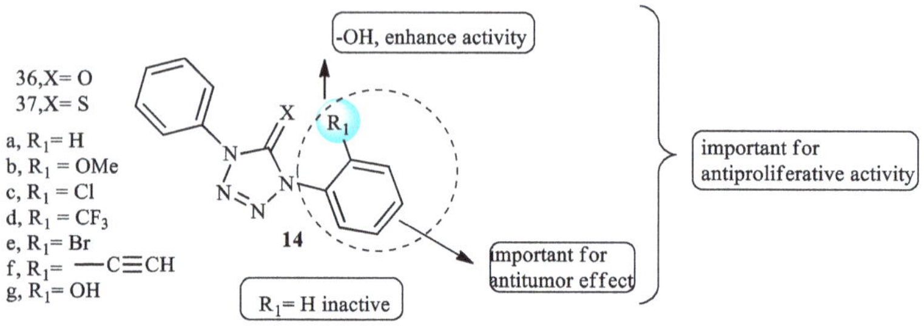

36,X= O
37,X= S

a, $R_1$= H
b, $R_1$ = OMe
c, $R_1$ = Cl
d, $R_1$ = $CF_3$
e, $R_1$= Br
f, $R_1$= —C≡CH
g, $R_1$= OH

**14**

-OH, enhance activity

important for antiproliferative activity

important for antitumor effect

$R_1$= H inactive

| Compound | X | $R_1$ | $IC_{50}(\mu M)$ | |
|---|---|---|---|---|
| | | | Day1 | Day4 |
| 36g | O | OH | 12.0±0.3 | 7.1±0.2 |
| 37g | S | OH | 3.8±0.1 | 2.5±0.1 |
| 36f | O | —C≡CH | 16.1±0.4 | 12.9±0.3 |

**Fig. (10).** Ki-67 inhibitors, SAR of tetrazole-based compounds.

## Efflux Pump Inhibiton

Inhibiting efflux pumps is linked to multidrug resistance chemotherapy in human cancer cells [97 - 99]. The efflux pump is linked to the removal of cell-damaging P-gp (P-glycoprotein). Many human ATP-binding cassette proteins are efflux transporters from a larger protein family. P-glycoprotein (MRP1 gene symbol ABCC1) and breast cancer resistance protein (BCRP gene symbol ABCG2), in particular, are thought to be major efflux transporters responsible for MDR cancer cells. BCRP overexpression in cancer cells, crucially, subsidizes MDR, rendering chemotherapy ineffective.

Gujarati and colleagues synthesized phenyl tetrazole derivatives **38** (Fig. **11**) and tested them for cytotoxicity against the H460 small lung cancer cell line and the H460/MX20 mitoxantrone resistant cell line using the MTT assay. These derivatives were found to serve as potential BCRP inhibitors [100].

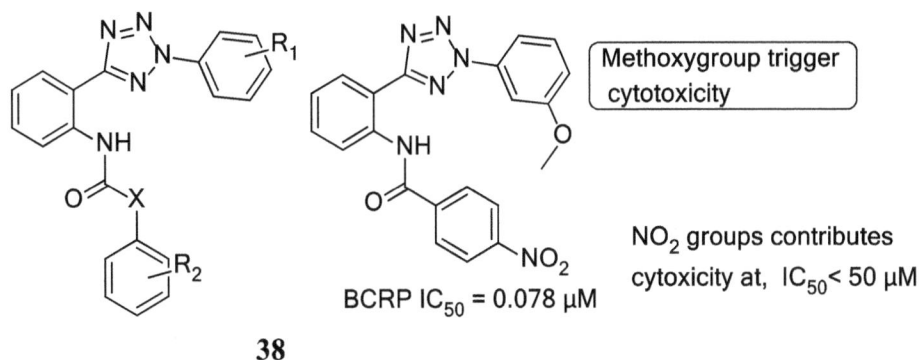

**38**

**Fig. (11).** SAR of selective BCRP inhibitor – phenyl tetrazole derivatives.

## CONCLUSION

This book chapter discusses a number of tetrazole substrates, each with its own mode of action against cancer. Cancer treatment relies heavily on anti-cancer drugs. Drug-resistant cancers have become more common in recent decades, but generic drugs to treat them are now available. Tetrazole scaffold is a significant pharmacophore. Because of their unique properties such as bioisosterism, which improves solubility, metabolism, and bioavailability, these tetrazole analogues are essential pharmacophores for a variety of anti-cancer therapeutic candidates. The incorporation of tetrazole into a variety of antineoplastic compounds and derivatives is one of the promising anti-cancer drug options. The various tetrazole moiety structures and their inhibitory activities for PRMT1, PADs, Ki-67, and efflux pump inhibition are discussed in this chapter of the book. The various tetrazole moiety structures and their inhibitory activities for PRMT1, PADs, Ki-67, and efflux pump inhibition are discussed in this chapter of the book. The SAR studies discussed here could pave the way for the development of tetrazole derivatives with promising activity, optimum bioavailability and reduced toxicity *via* a variety of pathways.

## CONSENT FOR PUBLICATION

All authors have given their consent for the publication of this manuscript.

## CONFLICT OF INTEREST

The authors declare no conflict of interest, financial or otherwise.

## ACKNOWLEDGEMENTS

Declared none.

# REFERENCES

[1]     Bray, F.; Ferlay, J.; Soerjomataram, I.; Siegel, R.L.; Torre, L.A.; Jemal, A. Global cancer statistics 2018: GLOBOCAN estimates of incidence and mortality worldwide for 36 cancers in 185 countries. *CA Cancer J. Clin.,* **2018**, *68*(6), 394-424.https://doi.org/https://doi.org/10.3322/caac.21492
[http://dx.doi.org/10.3322/caac.21492] [PMID: 30207593]

[2]     DeSantis, C.E.; Ma, J.; Gaudet, M.M.; Newman, L.A.; Miller, K.D.; Goding Sauer, A.; Jemal, A.; Siegel, R.L. Breast cancer statistics, 2019. *CA Cancer J. Clin.,* **2019**, *69*(6), 438-451.https://doi.org/https://doi.org/10.3322/caac.21583
[http://dx.doi.org/10.3322/caac.21583] [PMID: 31577379]

[3]     Siegel, R.L.; Miller, K.D.; Jemal, A. Cancer statistics, 2019. *CA Cancer J. Clin.,* **2019**, *69*(1), 7-34.https://doi.org/https://doi.org/10.3322/caac.21551
[http://dx.doi.org/10.3322/caac.21551] [PMID: 30620402]

[4]     Arruebo, M.; Vilaboa, N.; Sáez-Gutierrez, B.; Lambea, J.; Tres, A.; Valladares, M.; González-Fernández, A. Assessment of the evolution of cancer treatment therapies. *Cancers (Basel),* **2011**, *3*(3), 3279-3330.
[http://dx.doi.org/10.3390/cancers3033279] [PMID: 24212956]

[5]     Bayat Mokhtari, R.; Homayouni, T.S.; Baluch, N.; Morgatskaya, E.; Kumar, S.; Das, B.; Yeger, H. Combination therapy in combating cancer. *Oncotarget,* **2017**, *8*(23), 38022-38043.https://www.oncotarget.com/article/16723/text/
[http://dx.doi.org/10.18632/oncotarget.16723] [PMID: 28410237]

[6]     Padma, V.V. An overview of targeted cancer therapy. *Biomedicine (Taipei),* **2015**, *5*(4), 19.
[http://dx.doi.org/10.7603/s40681-015-0019-4] [PMID: 26613930]

[7]     Housman, G.; Byler, S.; Heerboth, S.; Lapinska, K.; Longacre, M.; Snyder, N.; Sarkar, S. Drug resistance in cancer: an overview. *Cancers (Basel),* **2014**, *6*(3), 1769-1792.
[http://dx.doi.org/10.3390/cancers6031769] [PMID: 25198391]

[8]     Rashid, H.U.; Xu, Y.; Muhammad, Y.; Wang, L.; Jiang, J. Research advances on anticancer activities of matrine and its derivatives: An updated overview. *Eur. J. Med. Chem.,* **2019**, *161*, 205-238.https://doi.org/https://doi.org/10.1016/j.ejmech.2018.10.037
[http://dx.doi.org/10.1016/j.ejmech.2018.10.037] [PMID: 30359819]

[9]     Counihan, J.L.; Grossman, E.A.; Nomura, D.K. Cancer Metabolism: Current Understanding and Therapies. *Chem. Rev.,* **2018**, *118*(14), 6893-6923.
[http://dx.doi.org/10.1021/acs.chemrev.7b00775] [PMID: 29939018]

[10]    Kumari, A.; Singh, R.K. Medicinal chemistry of indole derivatives: Current to future therapeutic prospectives. *Bioorg. Chem.,* **2019**, *89*, 103021.
[http://dx.doi.org/10.1016/j.bioorg.2019.103021] [PMID: 31176854]

[11]    Kumari, A.; Singh, R.K. Morpholine as ubiquitous pharmacophore in medicinal chemistry: Deep insight into the structure-activity relationship (SAR). *Bioorg. Chem.,* **2020**, *96*, 103578.
[http://dx.doi.org/10.1016/j.bioorg.2020.103578] [PMID: 31978684]

[12]    Ostrovskii, V.A.; Trifonov, R.E.; Popova, E.A. Medicinal chemistry of tetrazoles. *Russ. Chem. Bull.,* **2012**, *61*, 768-780.
[http://dx.doi.org/10.1007/s11172-012-0108-4]

[13]    Malik, M.A.; Wani, M.Y.; Al-Thabaiti, S.A.; Shiekh, R.A. Tetrazoles as carboxylic acid isosteres: chemistry and biology. *J. Incl. Phenom. Macrocycl. Chem.,* **2014**, *78*, 15-37.
[http://dx.doi.org/10.1007/s10847-013-0334-x]

[14]    Zou, Y.; Liu, L.; Liu, J.; Liu, G. Bioisosteres in drug discovery: focus on tetrazole. *Future Med. Chem.,* **2020**, *12*(2), 91-93.
[http://dx.doi.org/10.4155/fmc-2019-0288] [PMID: 31762337]

[15]   Biot, C.; Bauer, H.; Schirmer, R.H.; Davioud-Charvet, E. 5-substituted tetrazoles as bioisosteres of carboxylic acids. Bioisosterism and mechanistic studies on glutathione reductase inhibitors as antimalarials. *J. Med. Chem.,* **2004**, *47*(24), 5972-5983.
[http://dx.doi.org/10.1021/jm0497545] [PMID: 15537352]

[16]   Herr, R.J. 5-Substituted-1H-tetrazoles as carboxylic acid isosteres: medicinal chemistry and synthetic methods. *Bioorg. Med. Chem.,* **2002**, *10*(11), 3379-3393.https://doi.org/https://doi.org/10.10 16/S0968-0896(02)00239-0
[http://dx.doi.org/10.1016/S0968-0896(02)00239-0] [PMID: 12213451]

[17]   Popova, E.A.; Protas, A.V.; Trifonov, R.E. Tetrazole Derivatives as Promising Anticancer Agents. *Anticancer. Agents Med. Chem.,* **2018**, *17*(14), 1856-1868.https://doi.org/http://dx.doi.org/10.2174 /1871520617666170327143148
[http://dx.doi.org/10.2174/1871520617666170327143148] [PMID: 28356016]

[18]   Méndez, Y.; De Armas, G.; Pérez, I.; Rojas, T.; Valdés-Tresanco, M.E.; Izquierdo, M.; Alonso Del Rivero, M.; Álvarez-Ginarte, Y.M.; Valiente, P.A.; Soto, C.; de León, L.; Vasco, A.V.; Scott, W.L.; Westermann, B.; González-Bacerio, J.; Rivera, D.G. Discovery of potent and selective inhibitors of the *Escherichia coli* M1-aminopeptidase via multicomponent solid-phase synthesis of tetrazole-peptidomimetics. *Eur. J. Med. Chem.,* **2019**, *163*, 481-499.https://doi.org/https://doi.org/10.1016 /j.ejmech.2018.11.074
[http://dx.doi.org/10.1016/j.ejmech.2018.11.074] [PMID: 30544037]

[19]   Gao, F.; Xiao, J.; Huang, G. Current scenario of tetrazole hybrids for antibacterial activity. *Eur. J. Med. Chem.,* **2019**, *184*, 111744.https://doi.org/https://doi.org/10.1016/j.ejmech.2019.111744
[http://dx.doi.org/10.1016/j.ejmech.2019.111744] [PMID: 31605865]

[20]   Szulczyk, D.; Dobrowolski, M.A.; Roszkowski, P.; Bielenica, A.; Stefańska, J.; Koliński, M.; Kmiecik, S.; Jóźwiak, M.; Wrzosek, M.; Olejarz, W.; Struga, M. Design and synthesis of novel 1H-tetrazol-5-amine based potent antimicrobial agents: DNA topoisomerase IV and gyrase affinity evaluation supported by molecular docking studies. *Eur. J. Med. Chem.,* **2018**, *156*, 631-640.https://doi.org/https://doi.org/10.1016/j.ejmech.2018.07.041
[http://dx.doi.org/10.1016/j.ejmech.2018.07.041] [PMID: 30031974]

[21]   Wang, S-Q.; Wang, Y-F.; Xu, Z. Tetrazole hybrids and their antifungal activities. *Eur. J. Med. Chem.,* **2019**, *170*, 225-234.https://doi.org/https://doi.org/10.1016/j.ejmech.2019.03.023
[http://dx.doi.org/10.1016/j.ejmech.2019.03.023] [PMID: 30904780]

[22]   Gonzalez-Lara, M.F.; Sifuentes-Osornio, J.; Ostrosky-Zeichner, L. Drugs in Clinical Development for Fungal Infections. *Drugs,* **2017**, *77*(14), 1505-1518.
[http://dx.doi.org/10.1007/s40265-017-0805-2] [PMID: 28840541]

[23]   Hutchinson, D.W.; Naylor, M. The antiviral activity of tetrazole phosphonic acids and their analogues. *Nucleic Acids Res.,* **1985**, *13*(23), 8519-8530.
[http://dx.doi.org/10.1093/nar/13.23.8519] [PMID: 2417198]

[24]   Gao, C.; Chang, L.; Xu, Z.; Yan, X.F.; Ding, C.; Zhao, F.; Wu, X.; Feng, L.S. Recent advances of tetrazole derivatives as potential anti-tubercular and anti-malarial agents. *Eur. J. Med. Chem.,* **2019**, *163*, 404-412.https://doi.org/https://doi.org/10.1016/j.ejmech.2018.12.001
[http://dx.doi.org/10.1016/j.ejmech.2018.12.001] [PMID: 30530192]

[25]   Kalaria, P.N.; Karad, S.C.; Raval, D.K. A review on diverse heterocyclic compounds as the privileged scaffolds in antimalarial drug discovery. *Eur. J. Med. Chem.,* **2018**, *158*, 917-936.https://doi.org/https://doi.org/10.1016/j.ejmech.2018.08.040
[http://dx.doi.org/10.1016/j.ejmech.2018.08.040] [PMID: 30261467]

[26]   Karabanovich, G.; Němeček, J.; Valášková, L.; Carazo, A.; Konečná, K.; Stolaříková, J.; Hrabálek, A.; Pavliš, O.; Pávek, P.; Vávrová, K.; Roh, J.; Klimešová, V. S-substituted 3,5-dinitrophenyl 1,3,4-oxadiazole-2-thiols and tetrazole-5-thiols as highly efficient antitubercular agents. *Eur. J. Med. Chem.,* **2017**, *126*, 369-383.https://doi.org/https://doi.org/10.1016/j.ejmech.2016.11.041

[http://dx.doi.org/10.1016/j.ejmech.2016.11.041] [PMID: 27907875]

[27]   Asif, M. Biological Potentials of Substituted Tetrazole Compounds. *Pharm. Methods,* **2014**, *5*, 39-46.
       [http://dx.doi.org/10.5530/phm.2014.2.1]

[28]   Myznikov, L.V.; Hrabalek, A.; Koldobskii, G.I. Drugs in the tetrazole series. *Chem. Heterocycl. Compd.,* **2007**, *43*, 1-9. [Review].
       [http://dx.doi.org/10.1007/s10593-007-0001-5]

[29]   Wexler, R.R.; Greenlee, W.J.; Irvin, J.D.; Goldberg, M.R.; Prendergast, K.; Smith, R.D.; Timmermans, P.B. Nonpeptide angiotensin II receptor antagonists: the next generation in antihypertensive therapy. *J. Med. Chem.,* **1996**, *39*(3), 625-656.
       [http://dx.doi.org/10.1021/jm9504722] [PMID: 8576904]

[30]   Le Bourdonnec, B.; Meulon, E.; Yous, S.; Goossens, J.F.; Houssin, R.; Hénichart, J.P. Synthesis and pharmacological evaluation of new pyrazolidine-3, 5-diones as AT(1) angiotensin II receptor antagonists. *J. Med. Chem.,* **2000**, *43*(14), 2685-2697.
       [http://dx.doi.org/10.1021/jm9904147] [PMID: 10893306]

[31]   Neochoritis, C.G.; Zhao, T.; Dömling, A. Tetrazoles *via* Multicomponent Reactions. *Chem. Rev.,* **2019**, *119*(3), 1970-2042.
       [http://dx.doi.org/10.1021/acs.chemrev.8b00564] [PMID: 30707567]

[32]   Singh, H.; Singh Chawla, A. 4 Medicinal Chemistry of Tetrazoles. **1980**.
       https://doi.org/https://doi.org/10.1016/S0079-6468(08)70159-0

[33]   Finnegan, W.G.; Henry, R.A.; Lofquist, R. An Improved Synthesis of 5-Substituted Tetrazoles. *J. Am. Chem. Soc.,* **1958**, *80*, 3908-3911.
       [http://dx.doi.org/10.1021/ja01548a028]

[34]   Manafi Khajeh Pasha, A.; Raoufi, S.; Ghobadi, M.; Kazemi, M. Biologically active tetrazole scaffolds: Catalysis in magnetic nanocomposites. *Synth. Commun.,* **2020**, *50*, 3685-3716.
       [http://dx.doi.org/10.1080/00397911.2020.1811872]

[35]   Oklješa, A.M.; Klisurić, O.R. Synthesis, structural and computational studies of new tetrazole derivatives. *J. Mol. Struct.,* **2021**, *1226*, 129341.https://doi.org/https://doi.org/10.1016/j.molstruc.2020.129341
       [http://dx.doi.org/10.1016/j.molstruc.2020.129341]

[36]   Selvarasu, S.; Srinivasan, P. Synthesis, characterization, *in silico* molecular modeling, anti-diabetic and antimicrobial screening of novel 1-aryl-N-tosyl-1H-tetrazole-5-carboxamide derivatives. *Chem. Data Collect,* **2021**.https://doi.org/https://doi.org/10.1016/j.cdc.2021.100648

[37]   Varala, R. A Click Chemistry Approach to Tetrazoles: Recent Advances. , **2018**.
       [http://dx.doi.org/10.5772/intechopen.75720]

[38]   Chandgude, A.L. Convergent Three-Component Tetrazole Synthesis. *European J. Org. Chem,* **2016**.https://doi.org/https://doi.org/10.1002/ejoc.201600317

[39]   Patil, D.R.; Wagh, Y.B.; Ingole, P.G.; Singh, K.; Dalal, D.S. β-Cyclodextrin-mediated highly efficient [2+3] cycloaddition reactions for the synthesis of 5-substituted 1H-tetrazoles. *New J. Chem.,* **2013**, *37*, 3261-3266.
       [http://dx.doi.org/10.1039/c3nj00569k]

[40]   Kant, R.; Singh, V.; Agarwal, A. An efficient and economical synthesis of 5-substituted 1H-tetrazoles *via* Pb(II) salt catalyzed [3+2] cycloaddition of nitriles and sodium azide. *C. R. Chim.,* **2016**, *19*, 306-313.https://doi.org/https://doi.org/10.1016/j.crci.2015.11.016
       [http://dx.doi.org/10.1016/j.crci.2015.11.016]

[41]   Pawar, H.R.; Chikate, R.C. One pot three-component solvent-free synthesis of N-substituted tetrazoles using $RuO_2$/MMT catalyst. *J. Mol. Struct.,* **2021**, *1225*, 128985.https://doi.org/https://doi.org/10.1016/j.molstruc.2020.128985
       [http://dx.doi.org/10.1016/j.molstruc.2020.128985]

[42]    Tamoradi, T.; Ghorbani-Choghamarani, A.; Ghadermazi, M. $Fe_3O_4$–adenine–Zn: a novel, green, and magnetically recoverable catalyst for the synthesis of 5-substituted tetrazoles and oxidation of sulfur containing compounds. *New J. Chem.,* **2017**, *41*, 11714-11721.
[http://dx.doi.org/10.1039/C7NJ02337E]

[43]    Nasrollahzadeh, M.; Bayat, Y.; Habibi, D.; Moshaee, S. $FeCl_3$–$SiO_2$ as a reusable heterogeneous catalyst for the synthesis of 5-substituted 1H-tetrazoles *via* [2+3] cycloaddition of nitriles and sodium azide. *Tetrahedron Lett.,* **2009**, *50*, 4435-4438.
https://doi.org/https://doi.org/10.1016/j.tetlet.2009.05.048
[http://dx.doi.org/10.1016/j.tetlet.2009.05.048]

[44]    Shaikh, S.K.J.; Kamble, R.R.; Somagond, S.M.; Devarajegowda, H.C.; Dixit, S.R.; Joshi, S.D. Tetrazolylmethyl quinolines: Design, docking studies, synthesis, anticancer and antifungal analyses. *Eur. J. Med. Chem.,* **2017**, *128*, 258-273.https://doi.org/https://doi.org/10.1016/j.ejmech.2017.01.043
[http://dx.doi.org/10.1016/j.ejmech.2017.01.043] [PMID: 28192709]

[45]    Patouret, R.; Kamenecka, T. M, Synthesis of 2-aryl-2H-tetrazoles *via* a regioselective [3+2] cycloaddition reaction. *Tetrahedron Lett.,* *1597–1599*, *2016*, 57.
[http://dx.doi.org/10.1016/j.tetlet.2016.02.102] [PMID: 27041776]

[46]    Zamani, L.; Mirjalili, B.B.F.; Zomorodian, K.; Zomorodian, S. Synthesis and characterization of 5-substituted 1H-tetrazoles in the presence of nano-TiCl4.SiO2. *S. Afr. J. Chem.,* **2015**, *68*, 133-137.
[http://dx.doi.org/10.17159/0379-4350/2015/v68a19]

[47]    Demko, Z.P; Sharpless, K.B Preparation of 5-Substituted 1H-Tetrazoles from Nitriles in Water. *J. Org. Chem,* **2001**, *66*, 7945-7950.
[http://dx.doi.org/10.1021/jo010635w]

[48]    Das, B.; Reddy, C. R; Kumar D.N; Krishnaiah M; Narender R; A Simple, Advantageous Synthesis of 5-Substituted 1H-Tetrazoles. *Synlett,* **2010**, *2010*, 391-394.
[http://dx.doi.org/10.1055/s-0029-1219150]

[49]    Eshghi, H.; Seyedi, S.M.; Zarei, E.R. Ferric Hydrogensulfate [Fe(HSO4)3] As a Reusable Heterogeneous Catalyst for the Synthesis of 5-Substituted-1H-Tetrazoles and Amides. *ISRN Org. Chem.,* **2011**, *2011*, 195850.
[http://dx.doi.org/10.5402/2011/195850] [PMID: 24052817]

[50]    Bhaskar, M.P.V. Synthesis, characterization and evaluation of anti-cancer activity of some tetrazole derivatives. *J. Optoelectron. Biomed. Mater.,* **2010**, *2*, 249-259.

[51]    Vorona, S.; Artamonova, T.; Zevatskii, Y.; Myznikov, L. An Improved Protocol for the Preparation of 5-Substituted Tetrazoles from Organic Thiocyanates and Nitriles. *Synthesis,* **2014**, *46*, 781-786.
[http://dx.doi.org/10.1055/s-0033-1340616]

[52]    Yoneyama, H.; Usami, Y.; Komeda, S.; Harusawa, S. Efficient Transformation of Inactive Nitriles into 5-Substituted 1H-Tetrazoles Using Microwave Irradiation and Their Applications. *Synthesis,* **2013**, *45*, 1051-1059.
[http://dx.doi.org/10.1055/s-0032-1318476]

[53]    Zhang, F.G.; Chen, Z.; Cheung, C.W.; Ma, J.A. Aryl Diazonium Salt-Triggered Cyclization and Cycloaddition Reactions: Past, Present, and Future. *Chin. J. Chem.,* **2020**, *38*, 1132-1152.https://doi.org/https://doi.org/10.1002/cjoc.202000270
[http://dx.doi.org/10.1002/cjoc.202000270]

[54]    Akula, R.K.; Adimulam, C.S.; Gangaram, S.; Kengiri, R.; Pamulaparthy, N.B.S.R. $CuFe_2O_4$ Nanoparticle Mediated Method for the Synthesis of 5-Substituted 1H-Tetrazoles from (E)-Aldoximes. *Lett. Org. Chem.,* **2014**, *11*, 440-445.https://doi.org/http://dx.doi.org/10.2174/1570178611666140210213157
[http://dx.doi.org/10.2174/1570178611666140210213157]

[55]    Unnamatla, M.V.; Islas-Jácome, A.; Quezada-Soto, A.; Ramírez-López, S.C.; Flores-Álamo, M.;

Gámez-Montaño, R. Alejandro IJ; Andrea Q.S; Sandra C. R.-L.; Marcos F.-Á.; Rocio G.M., Multicomponent one pot synthesis of 3-tetrazolyl and 3-imidazo[1,2-a]pyridin tetrazolo[1,5-*a*]quinolines. *J. Org. Chem.,* **2016**, *81*(21), 10576-10583.
[http://dx.doi.org/10.1021/acs.joc.6b01576] [PMID: 27560617]

[56]    Mohammadkhani, L.; Heravi, M.M. Synthesis of N-heterocycles containing 1,5-disubstituted--H-tetrazole *via* post-Ugi-azide reaction. *Mol. Divers.,* **2020**, *24*(3), 841-853.
[http://dx.doi.org/10.1007/s11030-019-09972-1] [PMID: 31222498]

[57]    Abdelraheem, E.M.M.; Goodwin, I.; Shaabani, S.; de Haan, M.P.; Kurpiewska, K.; Kalinowska-Tłuścik, J.; Dömling, A. 'Atypical Ugi' tetrazoles. *Chem. Commun. (Camb.),* **2020**, *56*(12), 1799-1802.
[http://dx.doi.org/10.1039/C9CC09194G] [PMID: 31950120]

[58]    Chandgude, A.L.; Dömling, A. An efficient Passerini tetrazole reaction (PT-3CR). *Green Chem.,* **2016**, *18*(13), 3718-3721.
[http://dx.doi.org/10.1039/C6GC00910G] [PMID: 27840590]

[59]    Marquarding, D.; Gokel, G. The Passerini Reaction and Related Reactions, in: I.B.T.-O.C. Ugi (Ed.), **1971**https://doi.org/https://doi.org/10.1016/B978-0-12-706150-4.50012-5**1971**, 133-143.

[60]    Bommagani, S.; Penthala, N.R.; Balasubramaniam, M.; Kuravi, S.; Caldas-Lopes, E.; Guzman, M.L.; Balusu, R.; Crooks, P.A. A novel tetrazole analogue of resveratrol is a potent anticancer agent. *Bioorg. Med. Chem. Lett.,* **2019**, *29*(2), 172-178.https://doi.org/https://doi.org/10.1016/j.bmcl.2018.12.006
[http://dx.doi.org/10.1016/j.bmcl.2018.12.006] [PMID: 30528695]

[61]    Yang, Y.; Bedford, M.T. Protein arginine methyltransferases and cancer. *Nat. Rev. Cancer,* **2013**, *13*(1), 37-50.
[http://dx.doi.org/10.1038/nrc3409] [PMID: 23235912]

[62]    Swetha, K.S.; Parameshwar, R.; Reddy, B.M. babu V.H, Synthesis of novel pyrazolyl tetrazoles as selective COX-2 inhibitors. *Med. Chem. Res.,* **2013**, *22*, 4886-4892.
[http://dx.doi.org/10.1007/s00044-013-0500-0]

[63]    Labib, M.B.; Fayez, A.M.; El-Nahass, E.S.; Awadallah, M.; Halim, P.A. Novel tetrazole-based selective COX-2 inhibitors: Design, synthesis, anti-inflammatory activity, evaluation of PGE$_2$, TNF-α, IL-6 and histopathological study. *Bioorg. Chem.,* **2020**, *104*, 104308.https://doi.org/https://doi.org/10.1016/j.bioorg.2020.104308
[http://dx.doi.org/10.1016/j.bioorg.2020.104308] [PMID: 33011534]

[64]    Li, Y.; Pasunooti, K.K.; Peng, H.; Li, R.J.; Shi, W.Q.; Liu, W.; Cheng, Z.; Head, S.A.; Liu, J.O. Design and Synthesis of Tetrazole- and Pyridine-Containing Itraconazole Analogs as Potent Angiogenesis Inhibitors. *ACS Med. Chem. Lett.,* **2020**, *11*(6), 1111-1117.
[http://dx.doi.org/10.1021/acsmedchemlett.9b00438] [PMID: 32550989]

[65]    Ionescu, C.; Sippelli, S.; Toupet, L.; Barragan-Montero, V. New mannose derivatives: The tetrazole analogue of mannose-6-phosphate as angiogenesis inhibitor. *Bioorg. Med. Chem. Lett.,* **2016**, *26*(2), 636-639.https://doi.org/https://doi.org/10.1016/j.bmcl.2015.11.059
[http://dx.doi.org/10.1016/j.bmcl.2015.11.059] [PMID: 26631320]

[66]    Kamal, A.; Viswanath, A.; Ramaiah, M.J. Murty J.N.S.R.C; Sultana F; Ramakrishna G; Tamboli J.R; Pushpavalli S.N.C.V.L; pal D; Kishor C; Addlagatta A; pal Bhadra M, Synthesis of tetrazole–isoxazoline hybrids as a new class of tubulin polymerization inhibitors. *MedChemComm,* **2012**, *3*, 1386-1392.
[http://dx.doi.org/10.1039/c2md20085f]

[67]    Jedhe, G.S.; Paul, D.; Gonnade, R.G.; Santra, M.K.; Hamel, E.; Nguyen, T.L.; Sanjayan, G.J. Correlation of hydrogen-bonding propensity and anticancer profile of tetrazole-tethered combretastatin analogues. *Bioorg. Med. Chem. Lett.,* **2013**, *23*(16), 4680-4684.https://doi.org/https://doi.org/10.1016/j.bmcl.2013.06.004
[http://dx.doi.org/10.1016/j.bmcl.2013.06.004] [PMID: 23809851]

[68]   Subba Rao, A.V.; Swapna, K.; Shaik, S.P.; Lakshma Nayak, V.; Srinivasa Reddy, T.; Sunkari, S.; Shaik, T.B.; Bagul, C.; Kamal, A. Synthesis and biological evaluation of cis-restricted triazole/tetrazole mimics of combretastatin-benzothiazole hybrids as tubulin polymerization inhibitors and apoptosis inducers. *Bioorg. Med. Chem.,* **2017,** *25*(3), 977-999.https://doi.org/https://doi.org/10.1016/j.bmc.2016.12.010
       [http://dx.doi.org/10.1016/j.bmc.2016.12.010] [PMID: 28034647]

[69]   Choudhary, A.; Raines, R.T. An evaluation of peptide-bond isosteres. *ChemBioChem,* **2011,** *12*(12), 1801-1807.
       [http://dx.doi.org/10.1002/cbic.201100272] [PMID: 21751326]

[70]   Allen, F.H.; Groom, C.R.; Liebeschuetz, J.W.; Bardwell, D.A.; Olsson, T.S.; Wood, P.A. The hydrogen bond environments of 1H-tetrazole and tetrazolate rings: the structural basis for tetrazole-carboxylic acid bioisosterism. *J. Chem. Inf. Model.,* **2012,** *52*(3), 857-866.
       [http://dx.doi.org/10.1021/ci200521k] [PMID: 22303876]

[71]   Toney, J.H.; Fitzgerald, P.M.; Grover-Sharma, N.; Olson, S.H.; May, W.J.; Sundelof, J.G.; Vanderwall, D.E.; Cleary, K.A.; Grant, S.K.; Wu, J.K.; Kozarich, J.W.; Pompliano, D.L.; Hammond, G.G. Antibiotic sensitization using biphenyl tetrazoles as potent inhibitors of Bacteroides fragilis metallo-beta-lactamase. *Chem. Biol.,* **1998,** *5*(4), 185-196.
       [http://dx.doi.org/10.1016/S1074-5521(98)90632-9] [PMID: 9545432]

[72]   Gaponik, P.N.; Voitekhovich, S.V.; Ivashkevich, O.A. Metal derivatives of tetrazoles. *Russ. Chem. Rev.,* **2006,** *75*, 507-539.
       [http://dx.doi.org/10.1070/RC2006v075n06ABEH003601]

[73]   Serebryanskaya, T.V.; Yung, T.; Bogdanov, A.A.; Shchebet, A.; Johnsen, S.A.; Lyakhov, A.S.; Ivashkevich, L.S.; Ibrahimava, Z.A.; Garbuzenco, T.S.; Kolesnikova, T.S.; Melnova, N.I.; Gaponik, P.N.; Ivashkevich, O.A. Synthesis, characterization, and biological evaluation of new tetrazole-based platinum(II) and palladium(II) chlorido complexes--potent cisplatin analogues and their trans isomers. *J. Inorg. Biochem.,* **2013,** *120*, 44-53.https://doi.org/https://doi.org/10.1016/j.jinorgbio.2012.12.001
       [http://dx.doi.org/10.1016/j.jinorgbio.2012.12.001] [PMID: 23305964]

[74]   Jonassen, H.B.; Nelson, J.H.; Schmitt, D.L.; Henry, R.A.; Moore, D.W. Platinum- and palladium-tetrazole complexes. *Inorg. Chem.,* **1970,** *9*, 2678-2681.
       [http://dx.doi.org/10.1021/ic50094a011]

[75]   Voitekhovich, S.V.; Serebryanskaya, T.V.; Lyakhov, A.S.; Gaponik, P.N.; Ivashkevich, O.A. Copper(II), palladium(II) and platinum(II) chloride complexes with 5-amino-2-tert-butyltetrazole: Synthesis, characterization and cytotoxicity. *Polyhedron,* **2009,** *28*, 3614-3620.https://doi.org/https://doi.org/10.1016/j.poly.2009.07.054
       [http://dx.doi.org/10.1016/j.poly.2009.07.054]

[76]   Bekhit, A.A.; El-Sayed, O.A.; Al-Allaf, T.A.K.; Aboul-Enein, H.Y.; Kunhi, M.; Pulicat, S.M.; Al-Hussain, K.; Al-Khodairy, F.; Arif, J. Synthesis, characterization and cytotoxicity evaluation of some new platinum(II) complexes of tetrazolo[1,5-a]quinolines. *Eur. J. Med. Chem,* **2004,** *39*(6), 499-505.https://doi.org/https://doi.org/10.1016/j.ejmech.2004.03.003

[77]   Komeda, S. A Tetrazolato-Bridged Dinuclear Platinum(II) Complex Exhibits Markedly High *in vivo* Antitumor Activity against Pancreatic Cancer. *Chem.Med.Chem,* **2011,** *6*, 987-990.https://doi.org/https://doi.org/10. 1002/cmdc.201100141

[78]   Komeda, S.; Takayama, H.; Suzuki, T.; Odani, A.; Yamori, T.; Chikuma, M. Synthesis of antitumor azolato-bridged dinuclear platinum(ii) complexes with *in vivo* antitumor efficacy and unique *in vitro* cytotoxicity profiles. *Metallomics,* **2013,** *5*(5), 461-468.
       [http://dx.doi.org/10.1039/c3mt00040k] [PMID: 23608770]

[79]   Uemura, M.; Yoshikawa, Y.; Yoshikawa, K.; Sato, T.; Mino, Y.; Chikuma, M.; Komeda, S. Second- and higher-order structural changes of DNA induced by antitumor-active tetrazolato-bridged dinuclear platinum(II) complexes with different types of 5-substituent. *J. Inorg. Biochem.,* **2013,** *127*,

169-174.https://doi.org/https://doi.org/10.1016/j.jinorgbio.2013.05.004
[http://dx.doi.org/10.1016/j.jinorgbio.2013.05.004] [PMID: 23725767]

[80]   Uemura, M.; Suzuki, T.; Nishio, K.; Chikuma, M.; Komeda, S. An *in vivo* highly antitumor-active tetrazolato-bridged dinuclear platinum(II) complex largely circumvents *in vitro* cisplatin resistance: two linkage isomers yield the same product upon reaction with 9-ethylguanine but exhibit different cytotoxic profiles. *Metallomics,* **2012**, *4*(7), 686-692.
[http://dx.doi.org/10.1039/c2mt20026k] [PMID: 22473092]

[81]   Zhang, J.; Wang, S.; Ba, Y.; Xu, Z. Tetrazole hybrids with potential anticancer activity. *Eur. J. Med. Chem.,* **2019**, *178*, 341-351.https://doi.org/https://doi.org/10.1016/j.ejmech.2019.05.071
[http://dx.doi.org/10.1016/j.ejmech.2019.05.071] [PMID: 31200236]

[82]   Deng, X.; Von Keudell, G.; Suzuki, T.; Dohmae, N.; Nakakido, M.; Piao, L.; Yoshioka, Y.; Nakamura, Y.; Hamamoto, R. PRMT1 promotes mitosis of cancer cells through arginine methylation of INCENP. *Oncotarget,* **2015**, *6*(34), 35173-35182.https://www.oncotarget.com/article/6050/text/
[http://dx.doi.org/10.18632/oncotarget.6050] [PMID: 26460953]

[83]   Mathioudaki, K.; Papadokostopoulou, A.; Scorilas, A.; Xynopoulos, D.; Agnanti, N.; Talieri, M. The PRMT1 gene expression pattern in colon cancer. *Br. J. Cancer,* **2008**, *99*(12), 2094-2099.
[http://dx.doi.org/10.1038/sj.bjc.6604807] [PMID: 19078953]

[84]   Yang, H.; Ouyang, Y.; Ma, H. Design and synthesis of novel PRMT1 inhibitors and investigation of their binding preferences using molecular modelling. *Bioorg. Med. Chem. Lett,* **2017**, *27*(20), 4635-4642.https://doi.org/https://doi.org/10.1016/j.bmcl.2017.09.016

[85]   Spannhoff, A.; Heinke, R.; Bauer, I.; Trojer, P.; Metzger, E.; Gust, R.; Schüle, R.; Brosch, G.; Sippl, W.; Jung, M. Target-based approach to inhibitors of histone arginine methyltransferases. *J. Med. Chem.,* **2007**, *50*(10), 2319-2325.
[http://dx.doi.org/10.1021/jm061250e] [PMID: 17432842]

[86]   Sun, Y.; Wang, Z.; Yang, H.; Zhu, X.; Wu, H.; Ma, L.; Xu, F.; Hong, W.; Wang, H. The Development of Tetrazole Derivatives as Protein Arginine Methyltransferase I (PRMT I) Inhibitors. *Int. J. Mol. Sci.,* **2019**, *20*(15), E3840.
[http://dx.doi.org/10.3390/ijms20153840] [PMID: 31390828]

[87]   Witalison, E.E.; Cui, X.; Causey, C.P.; Thompson, P.R.; Hofseth, L.J. Molecular targeting of protein arginine deiminases to suppress colitis and prevent colon cancer. *Oncotarget,* **2015**, *6*(34), 36053-36062.https://www.oncotarget.com/article/5937/
[http://dx.doi.org/10.18632/oncotarget.5937] [PMID: 26440311]

[88]   Slack, J.L.; Causey, C.P.; Thompson, P.R. Protein arginine deiminase 4: a target for an epigenetic cancer therapy. *Cell. Mol. Life Sci.,* **2011**, *68*(4), 709-720.
[http://dx.doi.org/10.1007/s00018-010-0480-x] [PMID: 20706768]

[89]   Chumanevich, A.A.; Causey, C.P.; Knuckley, B.A.; Jones, J.E.; Poudyal, D.; Chumanevich, A.P.; Davis, T.; Matesic, L.E.; Thompson, P.R.; Hofseth, L.J. Suppression of colitis in mice by Cl-amidine: a novel peptidylarginine deiminase inhibitor. *Am. J. Physiol. Gastrointest. Liver Physiol.,* **2011**, *300*(6), G929-G938.
[http://dx.doi.org/10.1152/ajpgi.00435.2010] [PMID: 21415415]

[90]   Subramanian, V.; Knight, J.S.; Parelkar, S.; Anguish, L.; Coonrod, S.A.; Kaplan, M.J.; Thompson, P.R. Design, synthesis, and biological evaluation of tetrazole analogs of Cl-amidine as protein arginine deiminase inhibitors. *J. Med. Chem.,* **2015**, *58*(3), 1337-1344.
[http://dx.doi.org/10.1021/jm501636x] [PMID: 25559347]

[91]   Li Tao, L.; Jiang, G.; Chen, Q. Zheng Nian J; Ki67 is a promising molecular target in the diagnosis of cancer. *Mol. Med. Rep.,* **2015**, *11*, 1566-1572. [Review].
[http://dx.doi.org/10.3892/mmr.2014.2914] [PMID: 25384676]

[92]   Hooghe, B.; Hulpiau, P.; van Roy, F.; De Bleser, P. ConTra: a promoter alignment analysis tool for identification of transcription factor binding sites across species. *Nucleic Acids Res.,* **2008**, *36*(Web

Server issue), W128-32.
[http://dx.doi.org/10.1093/nar/gkn195] [PMID: 18453628]

[93]    Shirendeb, U.; Hishikawa, Y.; Moriyama, S.; Win, N.; Thu, M.M.M.; Mar, K.S.; Khatanbaatar, G.; Masuzaki, H.; Koji, T. Human papillomavirus infection and its possible correlation with p63 expression in cervical cancer in Japan, Mongolia, and Myanmar. *Acta Histochem. Cytochem.,* **2009**, *42*(6), 181-190.
[http://dx.doi.org/10.1267/ahc.09030] [PMID: 20126571]

[94]    Cidado, J.; Wong, H.Y.; Rosen, D.M.; Cimino-Mathews, A.; Garay, J.P.; Fessler, A.G.; Rasheed, Z.A.; Hicks, J.; Cochran, R.L.; Croessmann, S.; Zabransky, D.J.; Mohseni, M.; Beaver, J.A.; Chu, D.; Cravero, K.; Christenson, E.S.; Medford, A.; Mattox, A.; De Marzo, A.M.; Argani, P.; Chawla, A.; Hurley, P.J.; Lauring, J.; Park, B.H. Ki-67 is required for maintenance of cancer stem cells but not cell proliferation. *Oncotarget,* **2016**, *7*(5), 6281-6293.
[http://dx.doi.org/10.18632/oncotarget.7057] [PMID: 26823390]

[95]    Sun, X.; Kaufman, P.D. Ki-67: more than a proliferation marker. *Chromosoma,* **2018**, *127*(2), 175-186.
[http://dx.doi.org/10.1007/s00412-018-0659-8] [PMID: 29322240]

[96]    Gundugola, A.S.; Chandra, K.L.; Perchellet, E.M.; Waters, A.M.; Perchellet, J-P.H.; Rayat, S. Synthesis and antiproliferative evaluation of 5-oxo and 5-thio derivatives of 1,4-diaryl tetrazoles. *Bioorg. Med. Chem. Lett.,* **2010**, *20*(13), 3920-3924.
https://doi.org/https://doi.org/10.1016/j.bmcl.2010.05.012
[http://dx.doi.org/10.1016/j.bmcl.2010.05.012] [PMID: 20627565]

[97]    Ughachukwu, P.; Unekwe, P. Efflux pump-mediated resistance in chemotherapy. *Ann. Med. Health Sci. Res.,* **2012**, *2*(2), 191-198.
[http://dx.doi.org/10.4103/2141-9248.105671] [PMID: 23439914]

[98]    Mao, Q.; Unadkat, J.D. Role of the breast cancer resistance protein (BCRP/ABCG2) in drug transport--an update. *AAPS J.,* **2015**, *17*(1), 65-82.
[http://dx.doi.org/10.1208/s12248-014-9668-6] [PMID: 25236865]

[99]    Gottesman, M.M.; Pastan, I.H. The Role of Multidrug Resistance Efflux Pumps in Cancer: Revisiting a JNCI Publication Exploring Expression of the MDR1 (P-glycoprotein) Gene. *J. Natl. Cancer Inst.,* **2015**, *107*(9), djv222.
[http://dx.doi.org/10.1093/jnci/djv222] [PMID: 26286731]

[100]   Gujarati, N.A.; Zeng, L.; Gupta, P.; Chen, Z-S.; Korlipara, V.L. Design, synthesis and biological evaluation of benzamide and phenyltetrazole derivatives with amide and urea linkers as BCRP inhibitors. *Bioorg. Med. Chem. Lett.,* **2017**, *27*(20), 4698-4704.
https://doi.org/https://doi.org/10.1016/j.bmcl.2017.09.009
[http://dx.doi.org/10.1016/j.bmcl.2017.09.009] [PMID: 28916341]

# CHAPTER 6

# Progress in Nitrogen and Oxygen-based Heterocyclic Compounds for their Anticancer Activity: An Updates (2017-2020)

**Sakshi Choudhary[1], Archana Kumari[2], Rajesh Kumar[1], Sahil Kumar[3] and Rajesh K. Singh[1,*]**

[1] *Department of Pharmaceutical Chemistry, Shivalik College of Pharmacy, Nangal, Dist. Rupnagar, 140126, Punjab, India*

[2] *School of Pharmaceutical Sciences, Lovely Professional University, Phagwara - 144411, Punjab, India*

[3] *Delhi Institute of Pharmaceutical Sciences and Research (DIPSAR)-Delhi Pharmaceutical Sciences and Research University (DPSRU), New Delhi, 110017, India*

**Abstract:** Cancer, which is spreading throughout the world, is quickly becoming the leading cause of major fatalities. The most difficult task for global researchers today is to develop anticancer leads with minimal side effects. Heterocyclic chemistry is an important and unique class of medicinal chemistry as a large number of drugs being used in chemotherapy have a heterocyclic ring as their basic structure, in spite of various side effects. Because of the presence of heteroatoms such as oxygen, nitrogen, and sulphur, heterocyclic compounds can be used as hydrogen bond donors and acceptors. As a result, they can more effectively bind to pharmacological targets and receptors *via* intermolecular hydrogen bonds, resulting in pharmacological effects. They can also change the liposolubility and thus the aqueous solubility of drug molecules, resulting in remarkable pharmacotherapeutic properties. Medicinal chemists are concentrating on anticancer agents based on heterocyclic compounds. The goal of this chapter is to attempt to compile a dataset of advances in various nitrogen and oxygen-containing heterocyclic rings with anticancer activities from 2017 to 2020. The chapter covered the most recent research on novel anticancer heterocyclic derivatives, as well as the structure-activity relationship (SAR). The chapter provides the reader with advanced knowledge of the strategies required for designing nitrogen- and oxygen-containing heterocyclic compounds as anticancer agents.

**Keywords:** Anticancer drugs, Cancer, Heterocyclic, Nitrogen, Oxygen, SAR.

* **Corresponding author Rajesh K. Singh:** Department of Pharmaceutical Chemistry, Shivalik College of Pharmacy, Nangal, Dist. Rupnagar, 140126, Punjab, India; E-mail: rksingh244@gmail.com

# INTRODUCTION

Heterocyclic compounds contain five or six-membered cyclic structures with one or more heteroatoms other than carbon, *i.e.*, nitrogen (N), oxygen (O), or sulphur (S) in the ring. They can be aromatic or non-aromatic, such as pyridine, pyrrole, furan, indole, quinoline, oxadiazole, azole, benzimidazole, and thiophene. They are found to be a central part of nature. Pyrimidine and purine are heterocyclics that are parts of DNA, vitamins, enzymes, information carriers, and neurotransmitters, and thus important for human survival [1].

Heterocyclic compounds have been critical in the development of anticancer drug design [2]. *N*-heterocyclic compounds, in particular, are essential molecules found in many vitamins, nucleic acids, pharmaceuticals, antibiotics and natural alkaloids. They are pharmacologically active molecules with anticancer, anti-HIV, anti-malarial, anti-tubercular, anti-microbial, diabetic activities, and so on. N-heterocyclic anticancer drugs include vincristine, vinblastine, and indolocarbazole [3 - 5].

With the advancement of the N-heterocyclic compound, researchers' focus has shifted to O-based heterocyclic compounds. Since 2010, approximately 8% of all heterocycles approved by the FDA have been oxygen-based heterocycles with anticancer activity. In 2010, the FDA approved approximately 8% of O-heterocyclic compounds with anticancer properties. Cabazitaxel and eribulin are two potent O-heterocyclic drugs recently approved by the FDA for anticancer effects *via* microtubule inhibition mechanims [6]. Two-thirds of all anticancer drugs approved by the FDA between 2010 and 2015 contain a heterocyclic moiety [7].

Their great therapeutic effect is attributed to their involvement in cellular processes, metabolic pathways, and cancer pathology. At the molecular level, they show a high prevalence in receptor/enzyme interactions through Van der Waals, hydrophobic, and hydrogen bonding interactions. Because of their variety in geometry, shape, and size, heterocyclic rings are very flexible moieties, allowing proper interaction with the active site of the receptor or enzyme. Furthermore, due to changes in their physicochemical properties, different substitutions alter the efficacy and activity of heterocyclic drugs [8 - 11]. A variety of heterocyclic compounds are currently available on the market as anticancer agents, but patients face issues such as multi-drug resistance, poor therapeutic efficacy, adverse side effects, poor bioavailability, and so on. This necessitates and motivates researchers to progress and develop anticancer drug therapy. The importance of heterocyclic moieties as anticancer agents is discussed in this chapter. Among the numerous heterocyclic moieties, a few important ones are highlighted here, along with their important anticancer activities with structure-activity relationships (SAR).

## ACRIDINE

### Chemistry of Acridine

Acridine is a nitrogen-containing heterocyclic aromatic compound with the molecular formula $C_{13}H_9N$. As shown in Fig. (1), the structure of acridine is related to the anthracene ring, in which central CH groups are replaced by nitrogen. Due to its acrid smell and irritating action on the skin, the compound is referred to as "acridine". Because of its intercalating properties, acridine and its oxidised form, acridone, are used as potential drug targets for cancer treatment. Intercalation is the insertion of molecules between the bases of DNA [12].

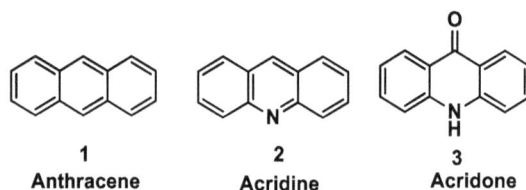

|        1        |    2     |      3      |
|:---------------:|:--------:|:-----------:|
| **Anthracene**  | **Acridine** | **Acridone** |

**Fig. (1).** Chemical structures of various types of acridines.

### Anticancer Activity of Acridine Derivatives

Histone deacetylases (HDACs) are a type of enzyme that removes acetyl groups from histone N-acetyl lysine amino acids [13]. The main protein components of chromatin are histones. Histone protein more tightly binds to DNA, allowing acetylation and deacetylation to control DNA expression. Histone acetylation is crucial in the regulation of gene expression [14]. Chen Jiwei *et al.* worked on acridine-hydroxamic acid derivatives as topo and HDAC inhibitors. In their study, vorinostat and m-AMSA, *i.e.*, HDAC and topo inhibitors, respectively, were joined by the linker to design new compounds that have both topo and HDAC inhibitory activity. All the synthesized compounds were evaluated against lymphoma U937 cells. Compound **4** (Fig. **2**) ($R_1$=H, $R_2$=H, n=2) exhibits the most potent antiproliferation against HDAC1, HDAC6, and lymphoma U937 cell lines, with ($IC_{50}$=3.9 nM, 2.9 nM, 0.90±0.01 μM) [15].

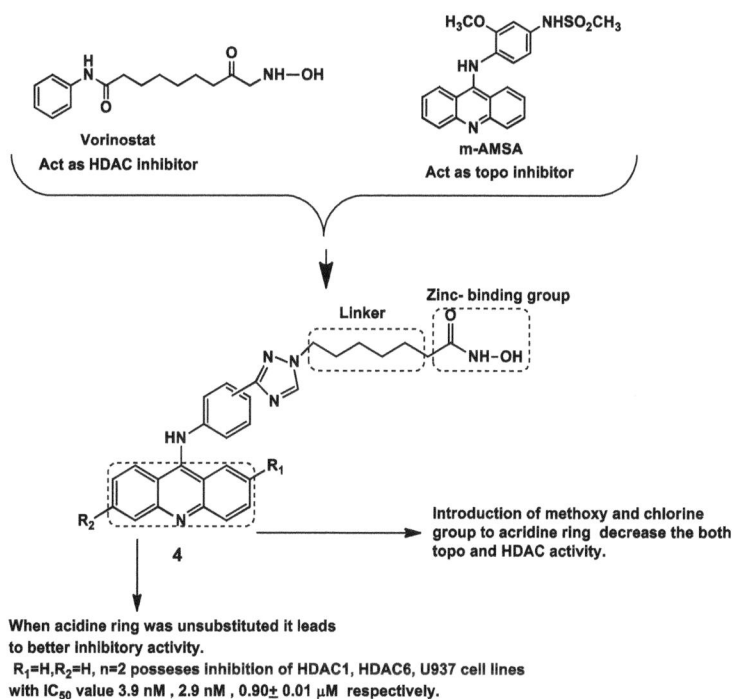

**Fig. (2).** SAR study of acridine-hydroxamic acid derivatives showing anticancer activity through dual topo and HDAC inhibition.

Mahanti *et al.* 2019, reported the design, synthesis, and evaluation of 1,2,4-triazole-substituted acridine derivatives. Derivatives were subjected to anticancer activity against four cancer cell lines: A549 (Lung), MCF7 (Breast), A375 (Melanoma) and HT-29 (Colon). Among the synthesized compounds, **5**, **6**, **7**, **8**, **9**, and **10** were found to be the most potent, with $IC_{50}$ values ranging from 0.11±0.02 to 13.8±0.99 µM as compared to the standard drug combretastatin-4, with $IC_{50}$ values of 0.11±0.02 to 0.93±0.056 µM. Docking studies were also conducted to explain that intercalation between the active sites of DNA targets was the mechanism of action. Studies highlight the maximum interaction of compounds **8** and **10**. SAR studies concluded that 3, 4, 5, trimethoxy, 4-chloro, and 4-trifluoromethyl groups at the *para* position of the phenyl ring are required for the activity, as shown in Fig. (**3**) [16].

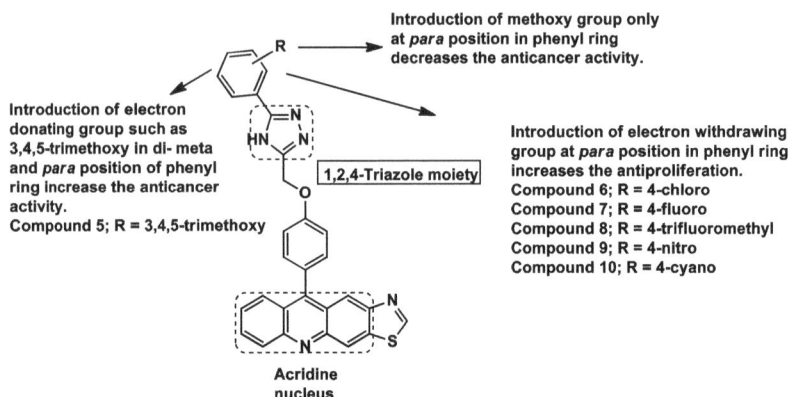

**Fig. (3).** SAR study of fused 1,2,4-triazole-acridine derivatives having anticancer activity.

Chen *et al.* (2019) mentioned data on the synthesis and evaluation of thiosemicarbazide derivatives of acridine. Among all the compounds, the most potent were **11** ($IC_{50}$ =18.42 ± 1.18 μM) (Fig. **4**), **12** ($IC_{50}$ =15.73 ± 0.90 μM) (Fig. **4**), **13** ($IC_{50}$ =10.96 ± 0.62 μM) (Fig. **4**), and **14** ($IC_{50}$ =11.63 ± 0.11 μM) (Fig. **4**), as compared with reference drug Cisplatin ($IC_{50}$ = 5.99 ± 0.12 μM) against the MT-4 cell lines. Topo I inhibitory activity and apoptosis were the mechanisms of action involved. Molecular docking studies showed that planar naphtho-fused rings and flexible thiourea groups are required for better interaction with enzymes [17].

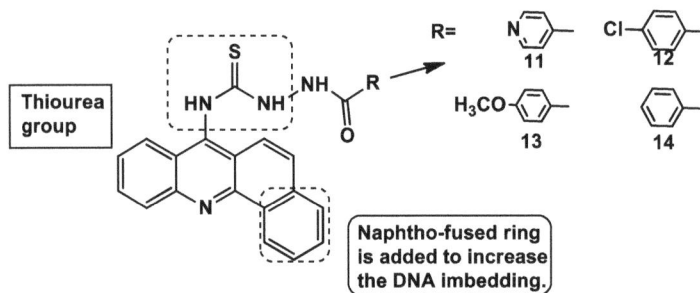

**Fig. (4).** SAR study of thiosemicarbazide derivatives of acridine having anticancer activity.

Lisboa *et al.* worked on thiophene and acridine hybrids which show antitumour effects against various cancer cell lines such as human colon carcinoma cells, human cervical cancer cells, *etc.* in *in vitro* and *in vivo* models. Compound 15 (Fig. **5**) was created by molecularly modifying two compounds: 6,9-dichloro-2-methoxyacridine and 2-amino-5,6,7,8-tetrahydro[b]-cyclohepta[b]-thiophene-3-carbonitrile. The compound shows a minimum inhibitory concentration ($IC_{50}$ value = 23.11±1.03 μM) against human colon carcinoma cells [18].

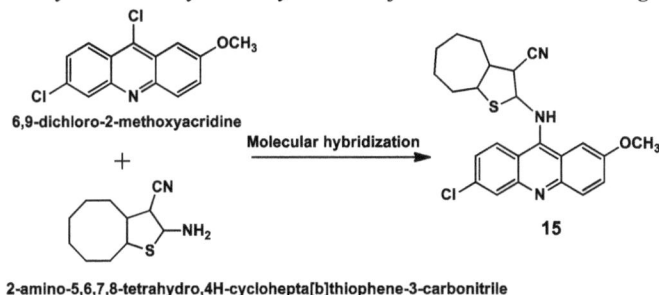

6,9-dichloro-2-methoxyacridine

+

2-amino-5,6,7,8-tetrahydro,4H-cyclohepta[b]thiophene-3-carbonitrile

Molecular hybridization

**15**

**Fig. (5).** SAR study of acridine and thiphene hybrid having anticancer activity.

Ismail *et al.* (2018) studied N-(3, 5-dimethoxy phenyl) acridin-9-amine **16** (Fig. **6**) against normal cells (WRL 68, $IC_{50}$= 49 ± 0.05 µg/mL) and cancer cell lines MCF-7($IC_{50}$= 22 ± 0.04 µg/mL), HT29 ($IC_{50}$= 17.5 ± 0.02 µg/mL) and HL60 ($IC_{50}$= 15 ± 0.03 µg/mL). No toxic effects were observed in mice, even at high doses [19].

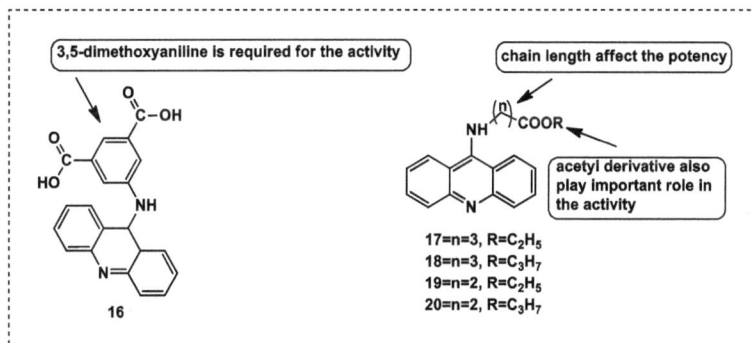

**16**

17=n=3, R=$C_2H_5$
18=n=3, R=$C_3H_7$
19=n=2, R=$C_2H_5$
20=n=2, R=$C_3H_7$

**Fig. (6).** Structure and SAR studies of anticancer acridine containing compounds.

Rupar *et al.* (2019) provided a detailed description of amino acid substituted acridine derivatives. Evaluation of compounds was conducted against K562 and A549 cancer cell lines and the normal diploid cell line MRC5 using the MTT assay. Compounds **17, 18, 19, 20** (Fig. **6**) demonstrated potent antiproliferative activity against K562 ($IC_{50}$ =11.2 ± 0.4 µM, 21.8 ± 5.4 µM, 19.2 ± 2.4 µM, 16.4 ± 2.5 µM), MRC5 ($IC_{50}$ =15.8 ± 3.2 µM, 16.9 ± 1.7 µM, 12.1 ± 1.6 µM, 11.6 ± 1.3 µM) and A549 ($IC_{50}$ = 9.5 ± 0.9 µM, 19.3 ± 4.0 µM, 6.15 ± 0.6 µM, 6.3 ± 0.2 µM) cancer cell lines when compared with Amsacrine ($IC_{50}$ = 13.8 ± 8.0 µM, 15.4 ± 2.6 µM, 22.2 ± 2.8 µM. Versatility can be seen in the mechanism of action. Compounds **17, 18, 19, and 20** showed topoisomerase inhibition, whereas compound **18** also showed an intercalation process [20].

Veligeti *et al.* 2020 designed, synthesized, and evaluated the acridone derivatives against HT29, MDAMB231, and HEK293T cancer cell lines using the MTT assay. According to SAR studies, substitution of cyclopropyl-acetyl, benzoyl, *p*-hydroxybenzoyl, *p*-(trifluoromethyl) benzoyl, *p*-fluorobenzoyl, *m*-fluorobenzoyl, picolinoyl, 6-methylpicolinoyl, and 3-nicotinoyl groups was best for activity. Molecular docking was also conducted against HT29, MDAMB231, and HEK293T cancer cell lines. Drug properties were also ascertained by ASMET, QSAR, protein binding, and bioactivity studies. A few compounds, **21** (IC$_{50}$ = 49.020.12 µg/mL), **22** (IC$_{50}$ = 50.860.39 µg/mL) (Fig. **7**), were found to have good potency as compared with doxorubicin (IC$_{50}$ = 54.380.49 µg/mL). Molecular docking studies also suggested that compounds showed good interactions with glycine and lysine (neutral amino acid) residues of enzymatic proteins 4N5Y, 1IGT, and 2VWD [21].

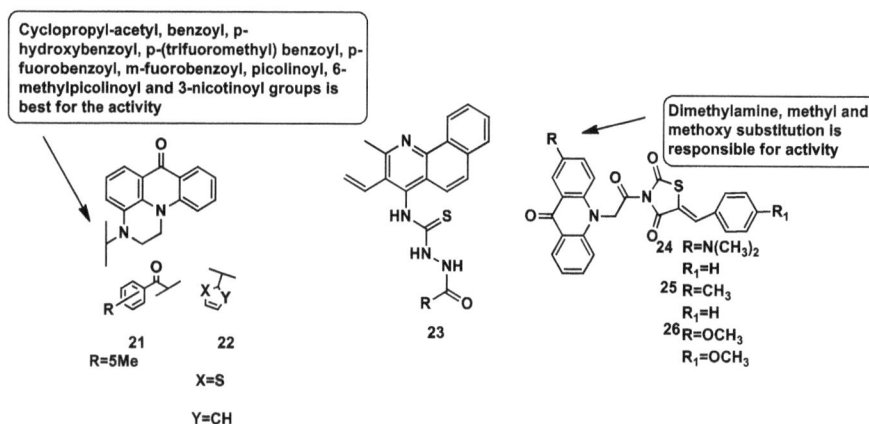

**Fig. (7).** Chemical structures and SAR studies of anticancer acridine-containing compounds.

Kozurkova *et al.* in 2020 conducted studies on 9-substituted acridines with various biological activities. Derivatives 23 (Fig. **7**) were discovered to inhibit topoisomerase enzyme activity and interfere with normal DNA biological functions [22]. In the same year, Padigela *et al.* designed, synthesized, and evaluated novel thiazolidine substituted acridine derivatives. All the compounds were evaluated against MCF-7 and SKVO3 cancer cell lines by the MTT assay. Among all the compounds, **24, 25, and 26** (Fig. **7**), were found to be the most potent against MCF7 (IC$_{50}$ = 17.98, 21.88, 23.21, and 10.8 µg/mL) and also against SKVO3 (IC$_{50}$ = 18.12, 35.12, 28.03, and 09.7 µg/mL) respectively, as compared with doxorubicin. SAR studies concluded that dimethylamine, methyl, and methoxy substitutions are critical for activity [23].

# BENZIMIDAZOLE

## Chemistry of Benzimidazole

Benzimidazole is an important heterocyclic organic compound. The combination of benzene and imidazole ring gives the fused bicyclic compound "benzimidazole". Many pharmaceutical drugs, including omeprazole, pantoprazole, rabeprazole, and others, contain the benzimidazole skeleton [24]. Benzimidazole is weakly basic in nature. They are slightly less basic than imidazoles. The proton at 1-position, *i.e.*, the imide nitrogen, is usually readily soluble in polar solvents and less soluble in organic solvents. Thus, benzimidazole is readily soluble in hot water, is poorly soluble in ether, and is insoluble in benzene [25].

## Anticancer Activity of Benzimidazole Derivatives

Cheong *et al.* (2017) reported the anticancer activity of novel water-soluble benzimidazole carbamates. Anthelmintic benzimidazole drugs such as albendazole, mebendazole, and others were clinically safe drugs used to treat GIT infections in past decades. The cytotoxicity profiles reported that anthelmintic benzimidazoles have anticancer activity in prostate and lung cancer cell lines based on their phenotypical screening approaches. As a result, they described **27** (Fig. **8**), a novel water-soluble oxetane-containing benzimidazole carbamate compound that can increase drug solubility while maintaining anticancer activity. Mebendazole was used as a control drug. Herein, docking studies suggest that benzimidazole anthelmintic drugs bind to the colchicine-binding domain of tubulin. The oxetanyl group takes part in electrostatic interactions with Lys352. Both phenyl and benzimidazole moieties occupy a hydrophobic pocket, and the carbamate moiety participates in H-bond interactions with Asn167, Tyr202, and Val238. Interestingly, this H-bond network is essential for the affinity of the benzimidazole compounds to the tubulin protein [26].

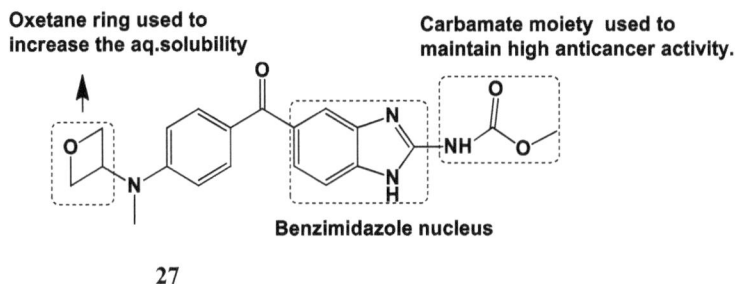

Oxetane ring used to increase the aq.solubility

Carbamate moiety used to maintain high anticancer activity.

Benzimidazole nucleus

27

**Fig. (8).** Structure and SAR of water-soluble benzimidazole carbamate derivatives having anticancer activity.

Akhtar *et al.* 2017, mentioned the designing, synthesis, docking, and QSAR study of substituted benzimidazole-linked oxadiazole as cytotoxic agents, EGFR and erbB2 receptor inhibitors. All the compounds were evaluated against EGFR and erbB2 receptors and MCF-7, HaCaT, MDA-MB231, HepG2, and A549 cancer cell lines. Studies concluded that *p*-substituted chloro/methoxy phenyl at the fifth position of oxadiazole is responsible for the activity. Compound **28** (Fig. **9**) was found to have significant $IC_{50}$ values of 5.0 and 2.55 µM against EGFR and erbB2 receptors as compared with 5-fluorouracil ($IC_{50}$ = 7.12 µM), which was found to be the most potent. MCF-7 was potently inhibited by **28** ($IC_{50}$ = 5.0 µM) (Fig. **9**) and **29** (**$IC_{50}$ = 2.55 µM**) (Fig. **9**), and both also inhibit MDA-MB231 ($IC_{50}$ = 0.131-14.5 µM) potently. A molecular docking study was also conducted where compounds **28** and **29** were found to show a similar binding pattern with the EGFR receptor as that of the standard drug erlotinib [27].

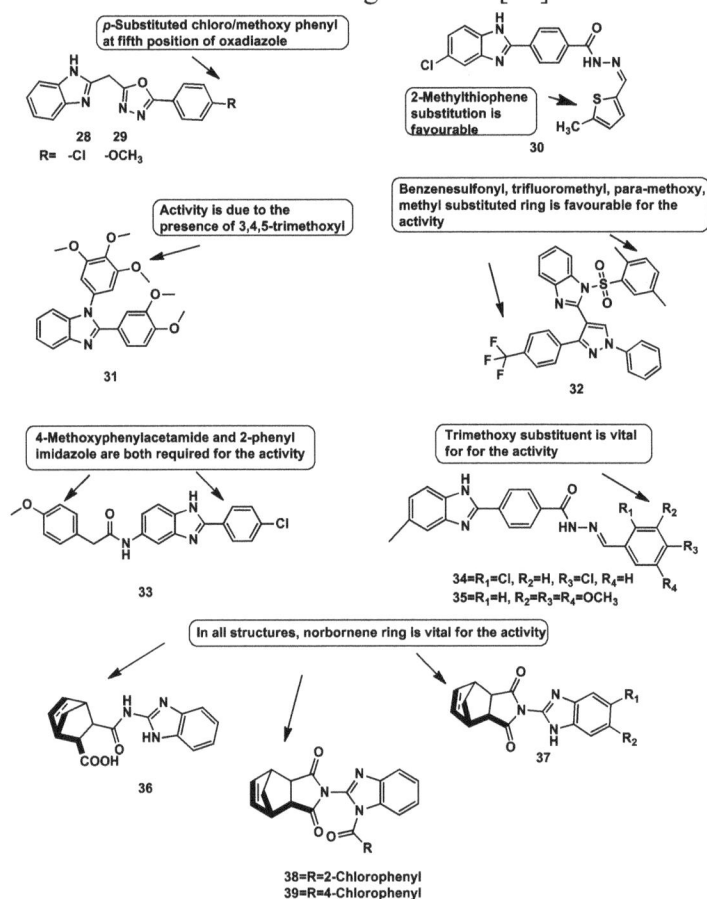

**Fig. (9).** Chemical structures and SAR studies of anticancer benzimidazole containing compounds.

In 2018, Cevik and colleagues mentioned the synthesis and evaluation of hydrazone substituted benzimidazole derivatives as anticancer agents against A549, MCF-7, and NIH/3T3 cell lines, which were evaluated by the MTT assay. Compound **30** ($IC_{50}$ = 0.0316 µM) (Fig. **9**) showed maximum activity against MCF-7 human breast cancer cells and lower cytotoxicity against the healthy cell line, NIH/3T3 as compared with standard cisplatin ($IC_{50}$ = 0.052 µM). According to SAR studies, 2-methyl thiophene substitution is favourable [28]. In the same year, Zang and colleagues reported anticancer studies using molecular docking on 1,2-diarylbenzimidazole analogues. All of the derivatives function by inhibiting microtubule assembly. According to the SAR studies, the presence of 3,4,5-trimethoxyl is required for the activity. When compared to the standard ($GI_{50}$ = 0.65±0.09-2.12±0.61), compound **31** (Fig. **9**) demonstrated the highest anti-tumor activity ($GI_{50}$ = 0.71-2.41 µM against HeLa, HepG2, A549, and MCF-7 cells) and the lowest toxicity to normal cells ($CC_{50}$ > 100 µM against L02 cells). Compound **31** also showed potent inhibition of microtubule polymerization ($IC_{50}$ = 8.47 M). Docking interactions showed that compound **31** has good binding interactions with colchicine, the same as that of a reference drug [29].

Wang mentioned the synthesis and evaluation of benzimidazole-attached benzsulfamide-pyrazole ring derivatives. All derivatives were evaluated for their potential tubulin polymerization inhibition against A549, Hela, HepG2 and MCF-7. SAR highlighted the importance of benzenesulfonyl, trifluoromethyl, *para-methoxy, and* methyl-substituted rings for anticancer activity. Tubulin-targeting drugs have increasingly become the focus of anticancer drug research. Twenty-five novel benzimidazole grafted benzsulfamide-containing pyrazole ring derivatives were synthesized and evaluated for bioactivity as potential tubulin polymerization inhibitors. Among all the twenty five derivatives, compound **32** (Fig. **9**) showed the maximum inhibition of tubulin assembly ($IC_{50}$ = 1.52 µM). The provided *in vitro* studies demonstrated that compound **32** (Fig. **9**) is potent against four human cancer cell lines ($IC_{50}$ = 0.15, 0.21, 0.33, and 0.17 µM, respectively for A549, Hela, HepG2, and MCF-7) when compared to standard drugs colchicine with $IC_{50}$ = 22±0.12, 0.36±0.07, 0.44±0.18, 2.26±0.25, and CA-4 with $IC_{50=}$ 0.16 ± 0.04, 0.24 ± 0.08, 0.33 ± 0.12, 0.18 ± 0.17, 1.61 ± 0.31 µM [30].

The recent development of small-molecule kinase inhibitors for the treatment of various types of cancer has been clinically successful. Yuan and workers synthesized the 6-amide-2-aryl benzoxazole/benzimidazole derivatives in 2019. The assessment was based on binding in the active site of the enzymes VEGFR-2 kinase, EGFR, HUVEC, HepG2, A549, and MDA-MB-231 cancer cell lines. Among all, compound **33** (Fig. **9**), showed the most potent anti-angiogenesis ability (79% inhibition) and cytotoxic activities (*in vitro* against the HUVEC ($IC_{50}$ = 1.47 µM) and HepG2 ($IC_{50}$ = 2.57 µM) cell lines as well as potent VEGFR-2 kinase inhibition (IC50 = 0.051 M). The molecular docking studies also highlight the maximum potency of compound **33** (Fig. **9**) against VEGFR-2 kinase. SAR studies highlight the importance of 4-methoxyphenylacetamide and 2-phenyl imidazole for binding with an enzyme that is almost similar to standard YQY-26 and Sorafenib [31].

Morcoss*et al* 2020, synthesized hydrazone-linked benzimidazole derivatives and evaluated them on a large pool of different cancer cell lines. Compounds **34** and **35** (Fig. **9**) were the most potent, showing 50–84% activity. Molecular docking studies were also performed on the active site of VEGFR-2. Compound **36** showed good binding affinity as compared to compound **34**. It showed that electron-donating groups, *i.e.*, tri-methoxy substituents, are vital for the activity [32]. Recently, Capan with colleagues mentioned the designing and evaluation of benzimidazole derivatives with norbornene or dibenzobarrelene skeletons. Evaluation involves various cancer cell lines, *i.e.*, MDA-MB-231 (human breast cancer), A549 (lung cancer), Ovcar3 (Human Ovarian cancer), and Panc1 (human pancreas cancer) cell lines using the MTT assay test. According to the SAR study, the activity of the synthesized derivatives was due to the norbornene skeleton. Compounds **36** ($IC_{50}$ = 26-59 µM), **37** ($IC_{50}$ = 21-29 µM), **38** ($IC_{50}$ = 31-118 µM) and **39** ($IC_{50}$ = 10–54 µM) (Fig. **9**), were found to be the most potent against all cancer cell lines. Among these compounds, **39** ($IC_{50}$=10 µM) (Fig. **9**) was found to be the most potent against A549 [33].

Huynh *et al.* 2020 synthesized 2-substituted benzimidazole derivatives to check the antiproliferation against various cancer cell lines such as human lung cancer cells, breast cancer cells, and prostate cancer cells. The SAR and potent compounds **40** and **41** with $IC_{50}$ values are listed below in Fig. (**10**) [34]. In the same year, Sireesha *et al.* 2020, designed, synthesized, and evaluated β-carbolin-benzimidazole/benzoxazole linked derivatives. The standard MTT assay was applied to MCF-7 (breast), A549 (lung), Colo-205 (colon) and A2780 (ovarian) for evaluation. SAR studies concluded that β-carboline substituted with methoxy, nitro, cyano, and methyl groups are promising groups for the activity. Benzimidazole derivatives **42** ($IC_{50}$= 0.34±0.071-1.23±0.55 µM) (Fig. **11**), and **43** ($IC_{50}$= 0.41±0.12-1.90±0.88 µM) (Fig. **11**) were found to be most potent as compared with standard drug Etoposide ($IC_{50}$= 0.13 ± 0.017-3.08 ± 0.135 µM). Molecular interaction studies showed that the interaction of benzimidazole derivatives is due to the presence of β-carbolines with various enzymes, *i.e.*, CDC-like kinase (CLK-1 to CLK-4), epidermal growth factor reductase (EGFR) kinase, protein (ATR) kinase, and APC-Asef interface. It highlights the importance of the β-carboline moiety [35].

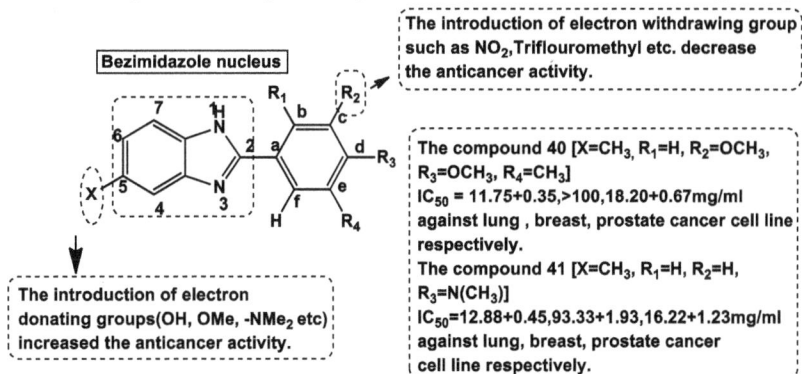

The introduction of electron withdrawing group such as $NO_2$, Triflouromethyl etc. decrease the anticancer activity.

The compound 40 [X=$CH_3$, $R_1$=H, $R_2$=$OCH_3$, $R_3$=$OCH_3$, $R_4$=$CH_3$] $IC_{50}$ = 11.75+0.35,>100,18.20+0.67mg/ml against lung , breast, prostate cancer cell line respectively.
The compound 41 [X=$CH_3$, $R_1$=H, $R_2$=H, $R_3$=N($CH_3$)] $IC_{50}$=12.88+0.45,93.33+1.93,16.22+1.23mg/ml against lung, breast, prostate cancer cell line respectively.

The introduction of electron donating groups(OH, OMe, -$NMe_2$ etc) increased the anticancer activity.

**Fig. (10).** Structure and SAR of benzimidazole derivative having anticancer activity.

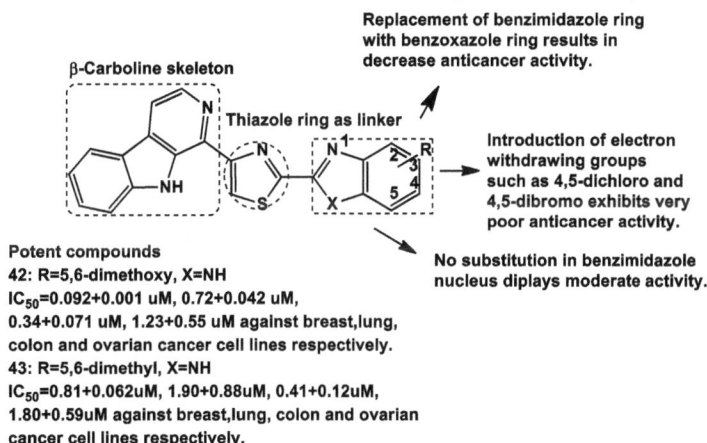

Replacement of benzimidazole ring with benzoxazole ring results in decrease anticancer activity.

Introduction of electron withdrawing groups such as 4,5-dichloro and 4,5-dibromo exhibits very poor anticancer activity.

No substitution in benzimidazole nucleus diplays moderate activity.

Potent compounds
42: R=5,6-dimethoxy, X=NH
$IC_{50}$=0.092+0.001 uM, 0.72+0.042 uM, 0.34+0.071 uM, 1.23+0.55 uM against breast,lung, colon and ovarian cancer cell lines respectively.
43: R=5,6-dimethyl, X=NH
$IC_{50}$=0.81+0.062uM, 1.90+0.88uM, 0.41+0.12uM, 1.80+0.59uM against breast,lung, colon and ovarian cancer cell lines respectively.

**Fig. (11).** Structure and SAR profile of benzimidazole derivatives having anticancer activity.

# OXADIAZOLE

## Chemistry of Oxadizole

Oxadiazole is an azole class of five-membered heterocyclic aromatic compounds. Its molecular formula is $C_2H_2N_2O$ [36]. The ring system of oxadiazole exists in the form of structural isomers, *i.e.*, **44** (1,2,3-oxadiazole), **45** (1,2,4-oxadiazole), **46** (1,2,5-oxadiazole), and **47** (1,3,4-oxadiazole). From these four isomers of oxadiazole **44,** one is unstable due to the formation of a diazoketone tautomer after tautomerization, as shown in Fig. **(12)**. The other oxadiazole isomers, *i.e.*, **45**, **46**, **47,** are versatile compounds found in many drugs, such as oxolamine, furamizole, butalamine, *etc.* [37]. In recent years, 1, 3, and 4-oxadiazole have become major lead molecules for drug discovery and the development of new potent anticancer drugs due to the presence of toxophoric-N=C-O-linkage [38].

**45,46,47 isomers are active due the presence of -N=C-O linkage**

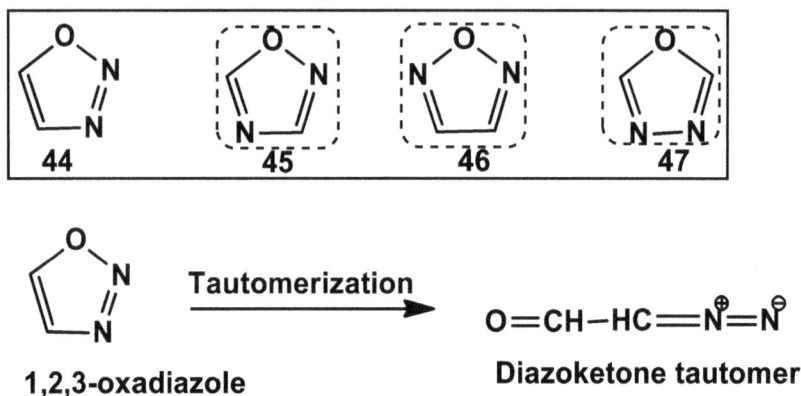

**1,2,3-oxadiazole**   **Tautomerization**   **Diazoketone tautomer**

$$O=CH-HC=\overset{\oplus}{N}=\overset{\ominus}{N}$$

**Fig. (12).** Isomeric forms of oxadiazole and modification of unstable ring 1, 2, 3-oxadiazole.

## Anticancer Activity of Oxadiazole Derivatives

The bark of *Combretum caffrum* contains combretastatin, a highly effective natural anticancer agent. Combretastatin **48** contains two substituted benzene rings and an ethylene bridge, and its structure-activity relationship is shown in Fig. (**13**) [39].

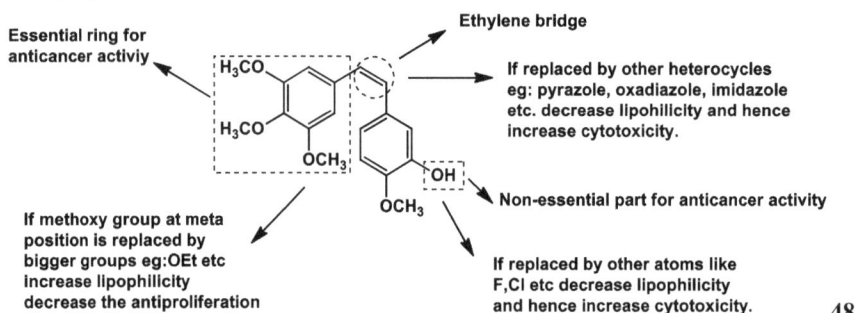

**Fig. (13).** Structure and SAR profile of combretastatin.

Due to the unstable ethylene bridge, a 1,3,4-oxadiazole ring is introduced, which shows lower lipophilicity and high metabolic stability. This strategy is useful for both cytotoxicity and anti-tubulin activity. Kamal Ahmed *et al.* (2016) studied combretastatin linked to 1,3,4-oxadiazole against various cancer cell lines such as human breast adenocarcinoma, human prostate cancer *etc*. Based on their cytotoxicity data, compound **49** (Fig. **14**) having a trimethoxy substituent on the oxadiazole ring exhibits potent anticancer activity with an IC$_{50}$ value of 0.118 µM [40].

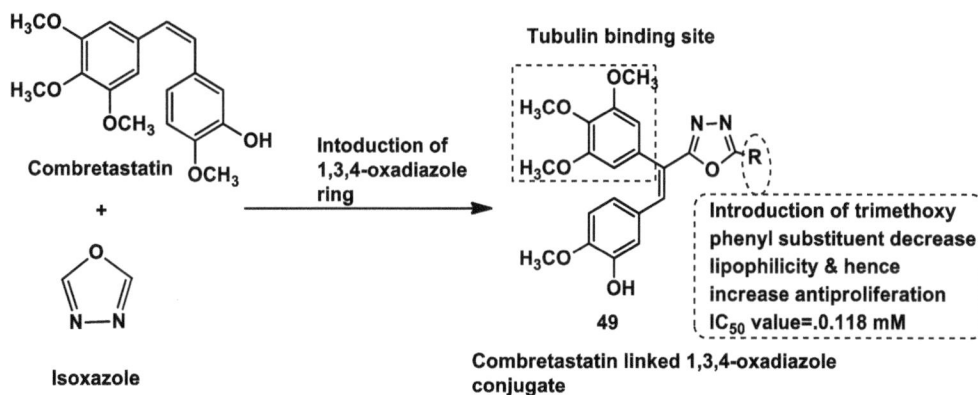

**Fig. (14).** Combretastatin-isoxazole hybrid formation having anticancer activity.

Sun *et al*. 2017 worked on 1,3,4-oxadiazole derivatives as FAK inhibitors. The research work includes several phenylpiperazine derivatives of 1,3,4-oxadiazole derivatives. Based on their cytotoxicity data, the compound having 3-trifluoromethyl piperazine linked with 1,3,4-oxadiazole is the most effective for FAK inhibition. The compound **50** (Fig. **15**) inhibits the growth of liver cancer cells with an IC$_{50}$ value of 0.78 µM [41].

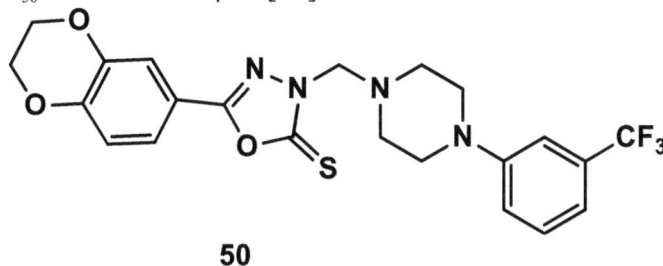

**50**

**Fig. (15).** Structure of phenylpiperazine-1,3,4-oxadiazole derivative having anticancer activity.

In 2018, Altintop *et al*. worked on thiazole and benzothiazole derivatives of 1,3,4-oxadiazole as FAK inhibitors. Several compounds were tested on cancer cell lines such as human lung cancer, rat glioma, *etc*. The compound **51** (Fig. **16**) linked with the 1,3,4-oxadiazole ring shows an effective anti-proliferative effect as a FAK inhibitor with an IC$_{50}$ value of 19.50±2.12 µM [42].

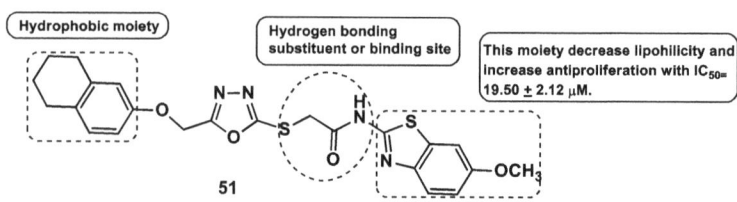

**Fig. (16).** Structure and SAR of benzothiazole-1,3,4-oxadiazole derivative having anticancer activity.

Ehrsam *et al.* (2019) provide the data aimed at studying oxadiazole derivatives as potent topoisomerase II inhibitors. According to the SAR study, the *p*-CF$_3$ and *p*-Cl substituted phenyl rings are favourable for the activity. Compound **52** (Fig. **17**) was found to be most potent against HCT-116 (GI$_{50}$ = 0.95±0.02 µM), HeLa (GI$_{50}$ = 1.48±0.3 M), MCF7 (GI$_{50}$ = 8.50 µM), MDAMB 468 (GI$_{50}$ = 10.59 µM), and MeT-5A (GI$_{50}$ = 7.3 µM) cancer cell lines. From the above study, it was suggested that the compounds act through the mechanism of inhibition of topoisomerase II *via* interacting with microtubules [43].

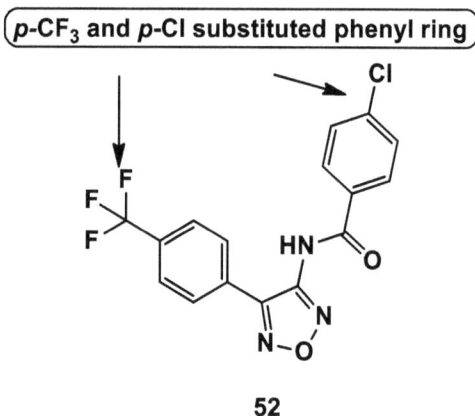

**Fig. (17).** Structure and SAR of oxadiazole derivative having anticancer activity.

Han *et al.* in 2020 worked on 2-phenyl-4*H*-chromone derivatives containing a 1,3,4-oxadiazole moiety as a telomerase inhibitory activity. In their work, 2-phenyl-4H-chromone is used as a basic scaffold. According to their findings, compound **53** (Fig. **18**) with a methoxy group at R$_1$ has telomerase inhibitory and antiproliferative activity with an IC$_{50}$ value of 0.44±0.09 µM [44].

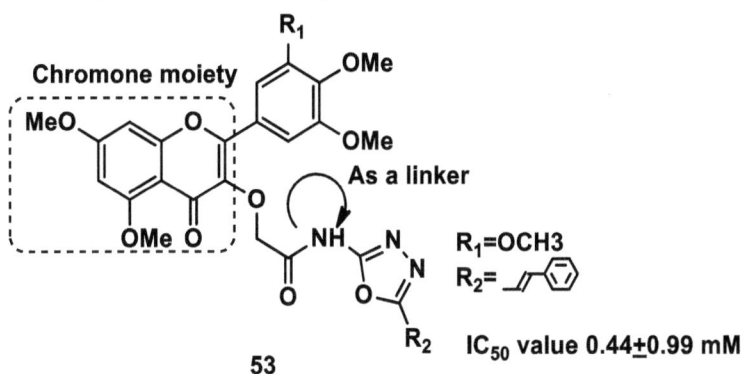

**Fig. (18).** Structure and SAR of Chromone-1,3,4-oxadiazole derivative having anticancer activity.

Srinivas *et al.* 2019, studied 1,2,4-oxadiazole-isoxazole linked quinazoline derivatives against four human cancer cell lines, including MCF-7 (breast), A549 (lung), DU145 (prostate), and MDA MB-231 (breast) by using the MTT assay. The SAR study concluded that the presence of 3,4,5-trimethoxy group is required for the activity against four cancer cell lines. Compound **54** ($IC_{50}$= 0.011±0.001-0.76±0.0033 µM) (Fig. **19**) was most potent as compared with standard Etoposide ($IC_{50}$= 1.97±0.45-3.08±0.135 µM) against all four cancer cell lines [45]. Alderawy *et al.* 2020, synthesized and evaluated ibuprofen-1,3,4-oxadiazole derivatives. Compounds were evaluated against the MCF-7 cell line by the MTT assay. Among all the compounds, **55** (% inhibition = 85.1%) (Fig. **19**) was found to be the most potent. It was observed that the increase in the effectiveness of ibuprofen was due to the presence of oxadiazole, 4-$NO_2$ and 4-fluoro moieties [46].

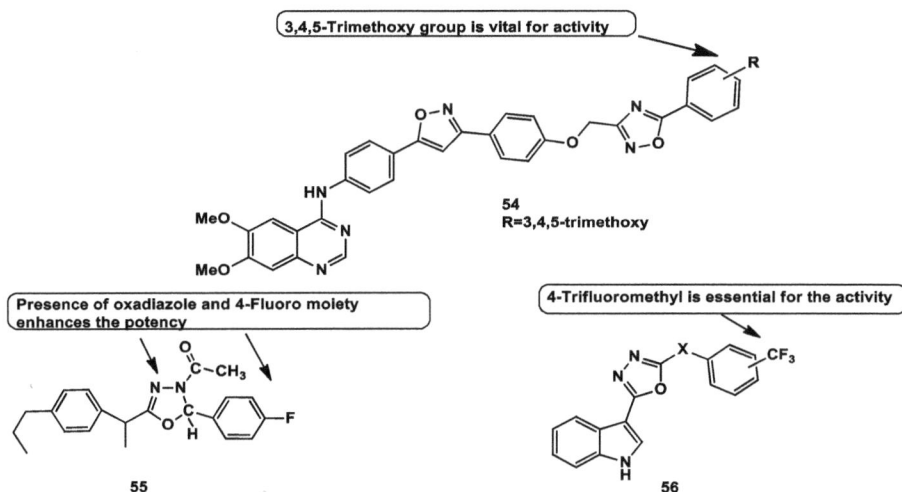

*(Fig. 19) contd.....*

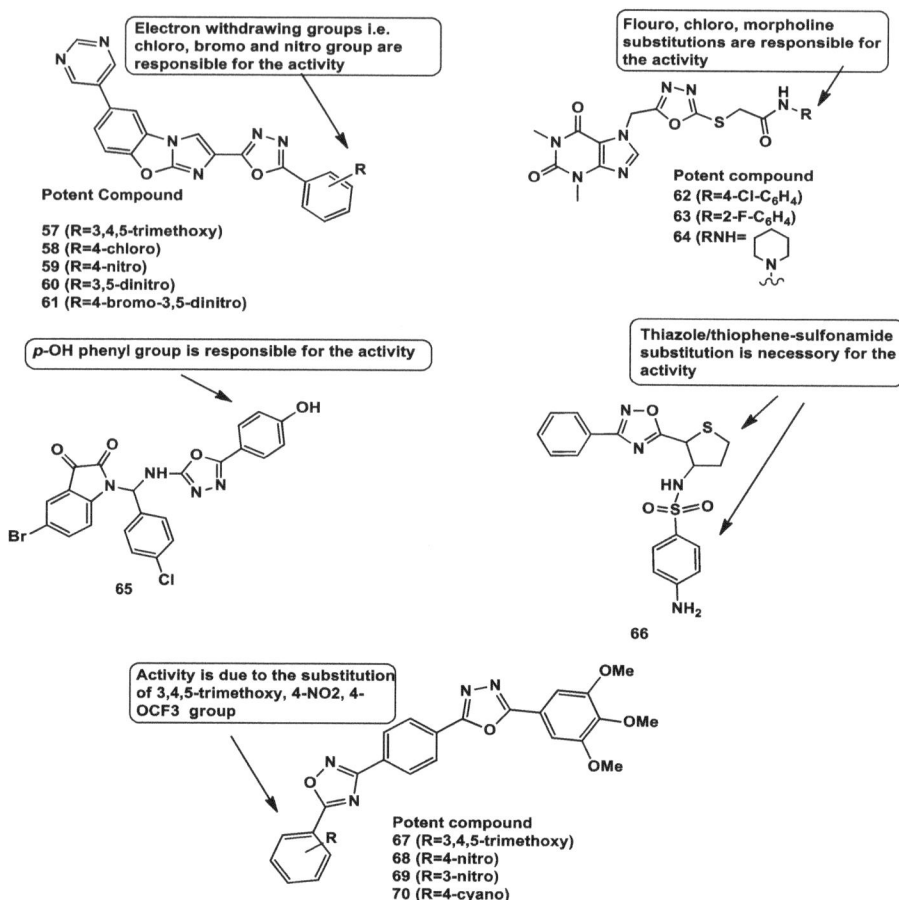

**Fig. (19).** Chemical structures and SAR studies of anticancer oxadiazole containing compounds.

Hamdy *et al.* 2020, designed, synthesized and evaluated a novel indole substituted 1,3,4-oxadiazole and checked it against pro-apoptotic Bcl-2 inhibitory anticancer agents. Compound **56** ($IC_{50}$ = 0.52–0.88 μM) was the most effective against MDA-MB-231, HeLa, KG1a, and Jurkat (Fig. **19**). SAR studies concluded that the presence of 4-trifluoromethyl is required for the activity. An ELISA assay was performed to evaluate Bcl-2 binding where compound **56** ($IC_{50}$ = 0.33±0.05 μM) (Fig. **19**) was found to be the most potent as compared with positive control Gossypol ($IC_{50}$ = 0.60±0.09 μM) [47]. Pragathi *et al.* 2020, reported a novel series of pyrimidin-oxazole derivatives and evaluated them against a panel of human cancer cell lines such as MCF-7 (breast cancer), A549 (lung cancer), Colo-205 (colon cancer), and A2780 (ovarian cancer) using the MTT assay. SAR studies concluded that the presence of electron-withdrawing groups, *i.e.*, chloro, bromo, and nitro groups, are required for the activity. Among all, five compounds, *i.e.*,

**57**, **58**, **59**, **60**, and **61** (Fig. **19**), were found to be the most potent, with $IC_{50}$ values ranging from 00.011±0.0093 to 19.4±6.59 µM, as compared with the $IC_{50}$ values of 0.13±0.017 to 3.08±0.135 µM of the reference drug etoposide [48].

Shahzadi 2020 *et al* reported the study of 1, 3, and 4-oxadiazole-purine derivatives as potent anticancer agents. As a result of the SAR studies, higher activity is due to the flouro, chloro, and morpholine substitutions. The *in silico* study suggested that compound **62** (Fig. **19**) was found to be a better derivative against human liver cancer cell lines (Huh7) (cell *via*bility 53.58±1.28) than that of the standard drug acefylline (86.32±11.75). Hemolytic and thrombolytic activities also showed that the compound is less toxic and more potent. Whereas compound **63** (Fig. **19**) was found to be least toxic with 0.1% hemolysis as compared to ABTS (95.5%) and **64** (Fig. **19**) had potent clot lysis activity (90%) relative to negative control DMSO (0.57%) [49].

Bhatt 2020 *et al*. mentioned the data of indoline substituted 1,3,4-oxadiazol derivatives. SAR demonstrated that the *p*-OH phenyl group is required for the activity. According to the MTT assay, **65** (Fig. **19**) displayed maximum potency against three human cancer cell lines: breast cancer cell line MCF-7 ($IC_{50}$ = 0.86±0.47 µM), colorectal cancer cell line HT-29 ($IC_{50}$ = 0.78±0.19 µM) and liver cancer cell line Hep G2 ($IC_{50}$ = 0.26±0.15 µM). The molecular docking study was also conducted using autodock, showing that **65** displayed good interaction with two enzymes-EGFR and CDK2 kinases [50]. Shamsi *et al*., 2020, designed, synthesized and evaluated novel 1,2,4-oxadiazole-sulfonamide based compounds. AAll of the synthesised compounds were tested for their ability to inhibit carbonic anhydrase IX (CAIX). SAR studies suggested that thiazole/thiophene-sulfonamide substitution is required for the activity. Among all the compounds, 66 (Fig. **19**) (IC50 = 6.0 µM) (Fig. **17**) was found to be most potent and also effectively inhibited CAIX (IC50 = 0.74 µM) as compared with acetazolamide (IC50 = 0.034 ± 0.002 µM). Apoptosis, ROS generation, colony formation inhibition, and colon cancer cell migration have all been proposed as mechanisms of action [51]. In the same year, Polothi *et al*. published a paper on the synthesis of 1,2,4-oxadiazole linked 1,3,4-oxadiazole derivatives in three human cancer cell lines (lung, breast).According to the SAR study, substitution of 3,4,5-trimethoxy, 4-NO$_2$, and 4-OCF$_3$ groups is required for the activity. The evaluation was conducted against three human cancer cell lines. Compounds **67**, **68**, **69**, and **70** are the most potent ($IC_{50}$=0.34 ± 0.025 to 2.45 ± 0.23 µM) as compared with Doxorubicin ($IC_{50}$= 2.10 ± 0.14 to 3.41 ± 0.23µM) against three human cancer cell lines: MCF-7, A549, and MDA MB-231. A docking study was also conducted where compound **69** (Fig. **19**) displayed strong binding affinity with the target protein EGFR [52].

# ISOXAZOLE

## Chemistry of Isoxazole

Isoxazole is an azole class of five-membered heterocyclic compounds with an oxygen atom next to the nitrogen. The structural features of isoxazole make it possible for multiple interactions: 1) Hydrogen bonds 2) pi-pi stacking, as illustrated in Fig. (**20**) [53].

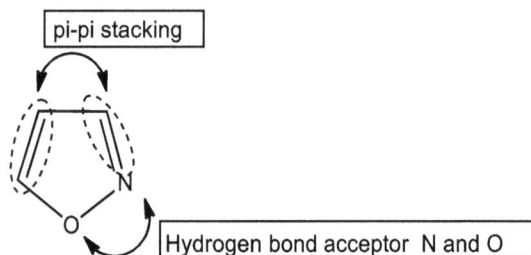

**Fig. (20).** Chemistry of isoxazole.

## Anticancer Activity of Isoxazole Derivatives

There are different targets of isoxazole as anticancer agents, such as HSP90, microtubules, and topoisomerase. HSP90 is a heat shock protein, and 90 signifies that it weighs roughly 90 kilos. As its name implies, it stabilizes proteins against heat stress. It also allows other proteins to fold properly [54]. Hence, in the last ten years, HSP90 has become a major therapeutic target for cancer due to its ATPase, ATP binding, and hydrolysis properties. Many isoxazole-based HSP90 inhibitors have been developed by researchers. In 2016, Zhang *et al.* incorporated amino acid derivatives into the 3-amido motif of the isoxazole scaffold based on **71**, NYPAUY922. It is an experimental drug candidate. In the NYPAUY922 drug, the isoxazole plays a core role in the binding site. The terminal valine moiety and ethylene-glycol linker formed an apolar and polar interaction network. Compound **72** (Fig. **21**) was identified to have high Hsp90 binding potency (14 nM) [55].

In the last two decades, hybrid molecules have been synthesized by the combination of different biologically active moieties to achieve therapeutic activities. They can potentially overcome pharmacokinetic drawbacks [56].

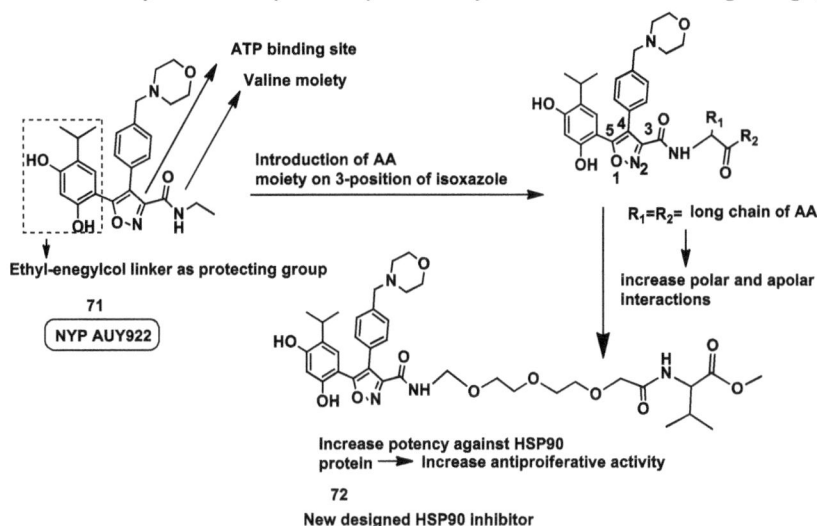

**Fig. (21).** Structure, synthesis and SAR of isoxazole derivative having anticancer activity.

In 2019, Vidhya *et al.* worked on the synthesis of hybrid molecules of isoxazole derivatives in search of new anticancer drugs. Compounds were evaluated for their anti-cancer activity in selected human cancer cell lines like prostate cancer (DU145), breast cancer (MDA MB-231, MCF-7) and non-small cell lung cancer cell lines (A549) by using the sulforhodamine B (SRB) method, using trimethoxy chalcone (TMC) as positive control (Fig. **22**) [57].

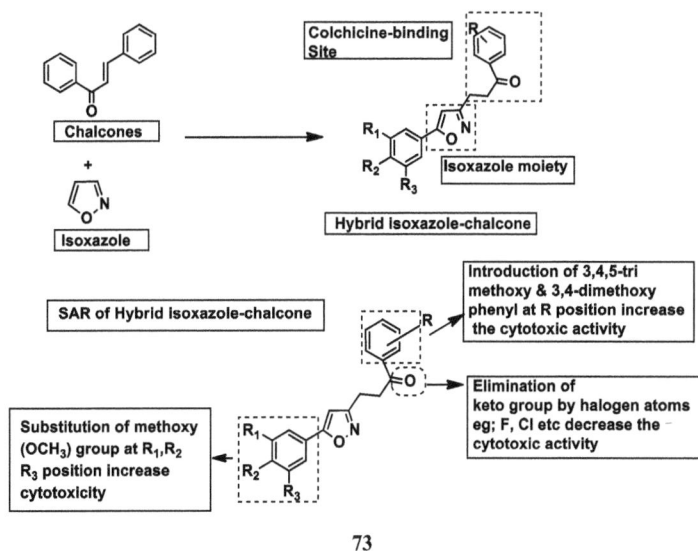

73

**Fig. (22).** Structure, synthesis and SAR of hybrid isoxazole derivatives having anticancer activity.

Thiriveedhi *et al.* mentioned the synthesis of chalcone-isoxazole derivatives using Claisen-Schmidt condensation. According to the SAR study, the presence of electron donating groups, *i.e.*, methoxy, dimethoxy or trimethoxy substituted phenyl rings, were important for the activity. The evaluation was conducted against human cancer cell lines DU-145, MDA MB-231, MCF-7, A-549, **74**, **75**, **76**, **77**, **78**, and **79** (Fig. **23**) against prostate DU-145 (IC$_{50}$=0.96-1.93 µM) as compared to trimethoxy chalcone (IC$_{50}$=4.10 µM) [58]. Calskana *et al.* (2018) mentioned the synthesis of a novel series of isoxazole-arylpiperazine derivatives and evaluated them against human liver (Huh7 and Mahlavu) and breast (MCF-7) cancer cell lines. Derivatives act by inducing oxidative stress in the PTEN protein, inhibition of the cell survival pathway, apoptosis, and cell cycle arrest. SAR studies highlighted that prenyl and 1,3-dimethylpyrazol-5-ylmethyl groups increased the activity. Compounds **80** (IC$_{50}$ = 0.3–2.7 µM) (Fig. **24**) and **81 (IC$_{50}$** = 0.3–3.7 **µM)** (Fig. **23**) were found to be active against all three cancer cell lines, specifically the liver cancer cell line [59].

Presence of electron donating groups i.e., methoxy, dimethoxy or trimethoxy substituted phenyl ring is necessary for the activity

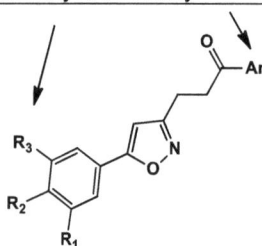

74 R$_1$=R$_2$=R$_3$-OCH$_3$, Ar=3,4,5-trimethoxyphenyl
75 R$_1$=R$_2$=R$_3$-OCH$_3$, Ar=3,4-dimethoxyphenyl
76 R$_1$=H R$_2$=R$_3$-OCH$_3$, Ar=3,4,5-trimethoxyphenyl
77 R$_1$=H R$_2$=OCH$_3$, R$_3$-H, Ar=3,4,5-trimethoxyphenyl
78 R$_1$=H R$_2$=OCH$_3$, R$_3$-H, Ar=3,4-dimethoxyphenyl
79 R$_1$=H R$_2$=OCH$_3$, R$_3$-H, Ar=4-methoxyphenyl

Prenyl and 1,3-dimethylpyrazol-5-ylmethyl groups are favourable for the activity

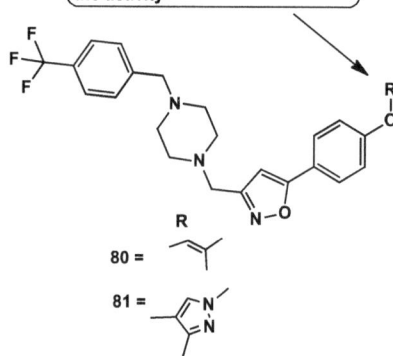

80 =

81 =

Pyrazoline ring is important for activity

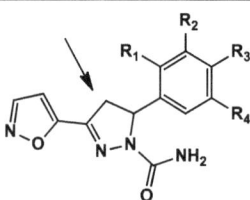

3,4,5-Trimethoxy, 4-nitro are favourable substitutions are vital substitutions

|    | R$_1$ | R$_2$ | R$_3$ | R$_4$ |
|----|----|----|----|----|
| 82 | F | OCH$_3$ | OCH$_3$ | H |
| 83 | H | H | OCH$_3$ | OCH$_3$ |

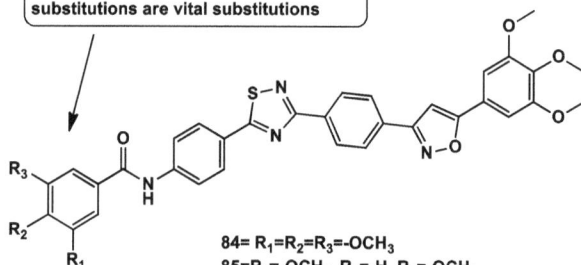

84= R$_1$=R$_2$=R$_3$=-OCH$_3$
85=R$_1$=-OCH$_3$, R$_2$=-H, R$_3$=-OCH$_3$
86=R$_1$=-H, R$_2$=-OCH$_3$, R$_3$=-H
87=R$_1$=-H, R$_2$=-Cl, R$_3$=-H
88=R$_1$=-H, R$_2$=-NO$_2$, R$_3$=-H
89=R$_1$=-H, R$_2$=-CH$_3$, R$_3$=-H

*(Fig. 23) contd.....*

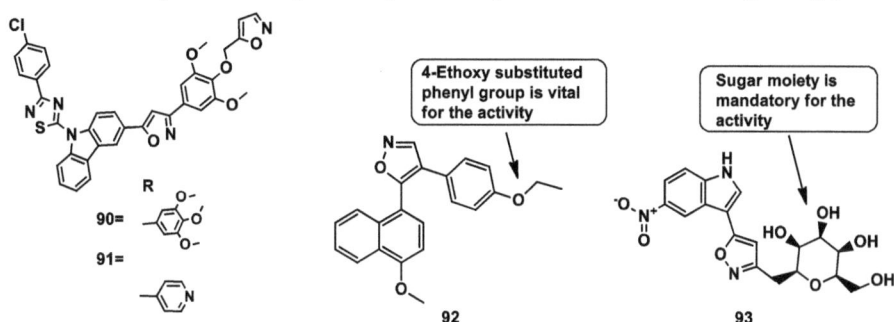

**Fig. (23).** Chemical structures and SAR studies of isoxazole bearing compounds having anticancer activity.

Shaik *et al.* 2019, synthesized chalcones and dihydropyrazoles bearing isoxazole scaffolds. Synthesized derivatives were evaluated against the prostate cancer cell line (DU-145). Compounds were found to be non-toxic when tested on normal human cell lines (LO2). SAR features highlighted that the heterocyclic pyrazoline ring is important for activity. According to the MTT assay, dihydropyrazole derivatives **82** ($IC_{50}$ = 2±1 µg/mL) (Fig. **23**) and **83** ($IC_{50}$ = 4±1 µg/mL) (Fig. **23**) were found to be the most potent as compared with docetaxel ($IC_{50}$ = 5 1 µg/mL) [60]. Shahinshavali *et al.* (2019) reported the synthesis of amide derivatives of 1,2-isoxazole combined with 1,2,4-thiadiazole. Synthesized compounds were evaluated against four cancer cell lines: MCF-7 (breast), A549 (lung), Colo-205 (colon), and A2780 (ovarian) using the MTT assay. According to SAR studies, the 3,4,5-trimethoxy and 4-nitro are favourable substitutions. The compounds **84**, **85**, **86**, **87**, **88**, and **89** (Fig. **23**) were found to be most active ($IC_{50}$=0.011±0.001-2.43±1.880 µM) [61].

Isoxazole-thiadiazole-linked carbazole derivatives were given by Rao *et al* in 2019. All the compounds were evaluated against human cancer cell lines: MCF-7 (breast), A549 (lung), DU-145 (prostate), and MDA MB-231 (breast) by using MTT assay. Among all, **90** ($IC_{50}$=0.021±0.0076-0.11±0.055 µM) (Fig. **23**) and **91** ($IC_{50}$=0.01±0.0025-0.087±0.0048 µM) (Fig. **23**) showed highest activity as compared with reference drug etoposide ($IC_{50}$=1.97±0.45-3.08±0.135 µM) [62]. Similarly, Wang 2020 *et al.* evaluated synthesized isoxazole-naphthalene derivatives for tubulin inhibition. Compound **92** (Fig. **23**) was the most potent ($IC_{50}$<10.0 µM) as compared to cisplatin (15.24±1.27 µM) against the human breast cancer cell line MCF-7. SAR studies highlighted that the 4-ethoxy substituted phenyl group is critical for the activity. At the molecular level, **92** stops the cell cycle at the G2/M phase and induces apoptosis. Molecular docking and *in vitro* studies proved that compound **92** ($IC_{50}$ = 3.4 µM) showed better tubulin polymerization inhibition as compared with Colchicine ($IC_{50}$ = 7.5 µM) [63]. Kumari *et al.* 2020 mentioned the designing and synthesis of pyrazoline-isoxazole bridged indole derivatives. Three cancer lines were used for further evaluation: MCF-7, MDA-MB-453, and MCF-10A. All derivatives showed nontoxicity towards the normal cell line (MCF-10A). Compound **93** (Fig. **23**) (cell *via*bility = 43.40±0.26%) was found to be the most potent as compared with standard menadione and YM155. Among the three cancer cell lines, all derivatives were most active against the MCF-7 cancer cell line. A docking study with the COX-2 enzyme revealed that the activity of derivatives is due to the presence of a carbohydrate moiety showing hydrogen bonding with the COX-2 enzyme [64].

## CONCLUSION

The discovery of new heterocyclic moieties with novel pharmacological effects in pharmacy, medicine, agriculture, plastics, polymers, and other fields speeds up organic chemistry research. Because they can be found in both natural and synthetic materials, heterocyclic moieties are very appealing and a hot topic these days. These compounds have been the subject of numerous studies due to their versatile nature and widespread prevalence. However, as a result of drug resistance and side effects, new challenges in drug discovery have emerged. This is another important reason that encourages research on heterocyclic compounds by introducing structural variations. Many studies have been conducted on heterocyclic moieties as anticancer agents, such as acridine, isoxazole, oxadiazole, and benzimidazole. A variety of synthetic strategies can be used to create these ring derivatives. The pharmacokinetic and pharmacodynamic properties of heterocyclic drugs are also influenced by structural changes that increase solubility and lipophilicity. All of these elements combine to make these rings extremely promising for further investigation. This chapter compiled the most recent research on novel heterocyclic ring derivatives with superior anticancer activity to standard drugs. In addition, significant structural modifications are discussed in the context of the structure-activity relationship (SAR), which encourages medicinal chemists to develop more potent anticancer drugs.

## CONSENT FOR PUBLICATION

All authors have given their consent for the publication of this manuscript.

## CONFLICT OF INTEREST

The authors declare no conflict of interest, financial, or otherwise.

## ACKNOWLEDGEMENT

The author wishes to acknowledge the Management, Shivalik College of Pharmacy, Nangal and Management, Lovely Professional University, Phagwara for the constant encouragement and support.

## REFERENCES

[1]     Sabir, S.; Alhazza, M.I.; Ibrahim, A.A. A review on heterocyclic moieties and their applications. *Catal. Sustain. Energy,* **2015**, *2*, 99-115.
[http://dx.doi.org/10.1515/cse-2015-0009]

[2]     Kumar, S.; Singh, R.K.; Patial, B.; Goyal, S.; Bhardwaj, T.R. Recent advances in novel heterocyclic scaffolds for the treatment of drug-resistant malaria. *J. Enzyme Inhib. Med. Chem.,* **2016**, *31*(2), 173-186.
[http://dx.doi.org/10.3109/14756366.2015.1016513] [PMID: 25775094]

[3]     Kumari, A.; Singh, R.K. Medicinal chemistry of indole derivatives: Current to future therapeutic prospectives. *Bioorg. Chem.,* **2019**, *89*, 103021.
[http://dx.doi.org/10.1016/j.bioorg.2019.103021] [PMID: 31176854]

[4]     Kumari, A.; Singh, R.K. Morpholine as ubiquitous pharmacophore in medicinal chemistry: Deep insight into the structure-activity relationship (SAR). *Bioorg. Chem.,* **2020**, *96*, 103578.
[http://dx.doi.org/10.1016/j.bioorg.2020.103578] [PMID: 31978684]

[5]     Martins, P.; Jesus, J.; Santos, S.; Raposo, L.R.; Roma-Rodrigues, C.; Baptista, P.V.; Fernandes, A.R. Heterocyclic Anticancer Compounds: Recent Advances and the Paradigm Shift towards the Use of Nanomedicine's Tool Box. *Molecules,* **2015**, *20*(9), 16852-16891.
[http://dx.doi.org/10.3390/molecules200916852] [PMID: 26389876]

[6]     Research, C. Research, C. for D.E. and New Drugs at FDA: CDER's New Molecular Entities and New Therapeutic Biological Products. http://www.fda.gov/Drugs/DevelopmentApprovalProcess/DrugInnovation/default.htm

[7]     https://www.ddw-online.com/media/32/(8)-the-importance-of-heterocyclic.pdf

[8]     Sethi, N.S.; Prasad, D.N.; Singh, R.K. An insight into the synthesis and SAR of 2,4-thiazolidinediones (2,4-TZD) as multifunctional scaffold: A review. *Mini Rev. Med. Chem.,* **2020**, *20*(4), 308-330.
[http://dx.doi.org/10.2174/1389557519666191029102838] [PMID: 31660809]

[9]     Sethi, N.S.; Prasad, D.N.; Singh, R.K. Synthesis, anticancer and antibacterial studies of benzylidene bearing 5-substituted and 3,5-disubstituted-2,4-thiazolidinedione derivatives. *Med. Chem.,* **2021**, *17*(4), 369-379.
[http://dx.doi.org/10.2174/1573406416666200512073640] [PMID: 32394843]

[10]    Komeilizadeth, H. Does Nature Prefer Heterocycles? *Iran. J. Pharm. Res.,* **2006**, *4*, 229-230.

[11]    Andreas Schmidt, A.; Liu, M. Recent Advances in the Chemistry of Acridines. *Adv. Heterocycl. Chem.,* **2015**, *115*, 287-353.
[http://dx.doi.org/10.1016/bs.aihch.2015.04.004]

[12]    Prasher, P.; Sharma, M. Medicinal chemistry of acridine and its analogues. *MedChemComm,* **2018**, *9*(10), 1589-1618.
[http://dx.doi.org/10.1039/C8MD00384J] [PMID: 30429967]

[13]    Sanaei, M.; Kavoosi, F. Histone deacetylases and histone deacetylase inhibitors: molecular mechanisms of action in various cancers. *Adv. Biomed. Res.,* **2019**, *8*, 63.
[http://dx.doi.org/10.4103/abr.abr_142_19] [PMID: 31737580]

[14]    Rajan, P.K.; Udoh, U.A.; Sanabria, J.D.; Banerjee, M.; Smith, G.; Schade, M.S.; Sanabria, J.; Sodhi, K.; Pierre, S.; Xie, Z.; Shapiro, J.I.; Sanabria, J. The Role of Histone Acetylation-/Methylatio-

-Mediated Apoptotic Gene Regulation in Hepatocellular Carcinoma. *Int. J. Mol. Sci.,* **2020**, *21*(23), 8894.
[http://dx.doi.org/10.3390/ijms21238894] [PMID: 33255318]

[15]    Chen, J.; Li, D.; Li, W.; Yin, J.; Zhang, Y.; Yuan, Z.; Gao, C.; Liu, F.; Jiang, Y. Design, synthesis and anticancer evaluation of acridine hydroxamic acid derivatives as dual Topo and HDAC inhibitors. *Bioorg. Med. Chem.,* **2018**, *26*(14), 3958-3966.
[http://dx.doi.org/10.1016/j.bmc.2018.06.016] [PMID: 29954683]

[16]    Mahanti, S.; Sunkara, S.; Bhavani, R. Synthesis, biological evaluation and computational studies of fused acridine containing 1,2,4-triazole derivatives as anticancer agents. *Synth. Commun.,* **2019**, *49*(13), 1729-1740.
[http://dx.doi.org/10.1080/00397911.2019.1608450]

[17]    Chen, R.; Huo, L.; Jaiswal, Y.; Huang, J.; Zhong, Z.; Zhong, J.; Williams, L.; Xia, X.; Liang, Y.; Yan, Z. Design, Synthesis, antimicrobial, and anticancer activities of acridine thiosemicarbazides derivatives. *Molecules,* **2019**, *24*(11), 2065.
[http://dx.doi.org/10.3390/molecules24112065] [PMID: 31151235]

[18]    Lisboa, T.; Silva, D.; Duarte, S.; Ferreira, R.; Andrade, C.; Lopes, A.L.; Ribeiro, J.; Farias, D.; Moura, R.; Reis, M.; Medeiros, K.; Magalhães, H.; Sobral, M. Toxicity and antitumor activity of a thiophene-acridine hybrid. *Molecules,* **2019**, *25*(1), 64.
[http://dx.doi.org/10.3390/molecules25010064] [PMID: 31878135]

[19]    Ismail, N.A.; Salman, A.A.; Yusof, M.S.M.; Soh, S.K.C.; Ali, H.M.; Sarip, R. The synthesis of a novel anticancer compound, *n*-(3,5dimethoxyphenyl) acridin-9-amine and evaluation of its toxicity. *Open Chem. J.,* **2018**, *5*, 32-43.
[http://dx.doi.org/10.2174/1874842201805010032]

[20]    Rupar, J.; Dobričić, V.; Grahovac, J.; Radulović, S.; Skok, Ž.; Ilaš, J.; Aleksić, M.; Brborić, J.; Čudina, O. Synthesis and evaluation of anticancer activity of new 9-acridinyl amino acid derivatives. *RSC Med Chem,* **2020**, *11*(3), 378-386.
[http://dx.doi.org/10.1039/C9MD00597H] [PMID: 33479643]

[21]    Veligeti, R.; Madhu, R.B.; Anireddy, J.; Pasupuleti, V.R.; Avula, V.K.R.; Ethiraj, K.S.; Uppalanchi, S.; Kasturi, S.; Perumal, Y.; Anantaraju, H.S.; Polkam, N.; Guda, M.R.; Vallela, S.; Zyryanov, G.V. Synthesis of novel cytotoxic tetracyclic acridone derivatives and study of their molecular docking, ADMET, QSAR, bioactivity and protein binding properties. *Sci. Rep.,* **2020**, *10*(1), 20720.
[http://dx.doi.org/10.1038/s41598-020-77590-1] [PMID: 33244007]

[22]    Kozurkova, M.; Sabolova, D.; Kristian, P. A new look at 9-substituted acridines with various biological activities. *J. Appl. Toxicol.,* **2021**, *41*(1), 175-189.
[http://dx.doi.org/10.1002/jat.4072] [PMID: 32969520]

[23]    Padigela, S. RMRaju.; Prasad, VVS. Synthesis, characterization, and anticancer activity of some novel acridine derivatives. *Asian J. Pharm. Clin.,* **2020**, *13*, 166-169.
[http://dx.doi.org/10.22159/ajpcr.2020.v13i6.35794]

[24]    Singh, P.K.; Silakar, Om. Benzimidazole: Journey from Single Targeting to Multitargeting Molecule. Ed. Om Silakari in Key Heterocycle Cores from Designing Multitargeting Molecules, Elsevier. , **2018**; pp. 31-52.
[http://dx.doi.org/10.1016/B978-0-08-102083-8.00002-9]

[25]    Goud, Nerella Sridhar; Kumar, Pardeep; Bharath, Rose Dawn Recent Developments of Target-Based Benzimidazole Derivatives as Potential Anticancer Agents, Heterocycles - Synthesis and Biological Activities, B. P. Nandeshwarappa and Sadashiv S. O. *IntechOpen,* **2020**.
[http://dx.doi.org/10.5772/intechopen.90758]

[26]    Cheong, J.E.; Zaffagni, M.; Chung, I.; Xu, Y.; Wang, Y.; Jernigan, F.E.; Zetter, B.R.; Sun, L. Synthesis and anticancer activity of novel water soluble benzimidazole carbamates. *Eur. J. Med. Chem.,* **2018**, *144*, 372-385.

[http://dx.doi.org/10.1016/j.ejmech.2017.11.037] [PMID: 29288939]

[27]　Akhtar, M.J.; Siddiqui, A.A.; Khan, A.A.; Ali, Z.; Dewangan, R.P.; Pasha, S.; Yar, M.S. Design, synthesis, docking and QSAR study of substituted benzimidazole linked oxadiazole as cytotoxic agents, EGFR and erbB2 receptor inhibitors. *Eur. J. Med. Chem.*, **2017**, *126*(126), 853-869.
[http://dx.doi.org/10.1016/j.ejmech.2016.12.014] [PMID: 27987485]

[28]　Çevik, U.A.; Sağlık, B.N.; Ardıç, C.M.; Özkay, Y.; Atlı, O. Synthesis and evaluation of new benzimidazole derivatives with hydrazone moiety as anticancer agents. *Turk. J. Biochem.*, **2018**, *43*(2), 151-158.
[http://dx.doi.org/10.1515/tjb-2017-0167]

[29]　Zhang, Y.L.; Yang, R.; Xia, L.Y.; Man, R.J.; Chu, Y.C.; Jiang, A.Q.; Wang, Z.C.; Zhu, H.L. Synthesis, anticancer activity and molecular docking studies on 1,2-diarylbenzimidazole analogues as anti-tubulin agents. *Bioorg. Chem.*, **2019**, *92*, 103219.
[http://dx.doi.org/10.1016/j.bioorg.2019.103219] [PMID: 31476616]

[30]　Wang, Y.T.; Shi, T.Q.; Zhu, H.L.; Liu, C.H. Synthesis, biological evaluation and molecular docking of benzimidazole grafted benzsulfamide-containing pyrazole ring derivatives as novel tubulin polymerization inhibitors. *Bioorg. Med. Chem.*, **2019**, *27*(3), 502-515.
[http://dx.doi.org/10.1016/j.bmc.2018.12.031] [PMID: 30606674]

[31]　Bhatia, R.; Singh, R.K. Introductory Chapter: Protein Kinases as Promising Targets for Drug Design against Cancer.*Protein Kinases - Promising Targets for Anticancer Drug Research*; Singh, R.K., Ed.; IntechOpen: London, **2021**.
[http://dx.doi.org/10.5772/intechopen.100315] bYuan, X.; Yang, Q.; Liu, T.; Li, K.; Liu, Y.; Zhu, C.; Zhang, Z.; Li, L.; Zhang, C.; Xie, M.; Lin, J.; Zhang, J.; Jin, Y. Design, synthesis and *in vitro* evaluation of 6-amide-2-aryl benzoxazole/benzimidazole derivatives against tumor cells by inhibiting VEGFR-2 kinase. *Eur. J. Med. Chem.*, **2019**, *179*, 147-165.
[http://dx.doi.org/10.1016/j.ejmech.2019.06.054] [PMID: 31252306]

[32]　Morcoss, M.M.; Abdelhafez, E.S.M.N.; Ibrahem, R.A.; Abdel-Rahman, H.M.; Abdel-Aziz, M.; Abou El-Ella, D.A. Design, synthesis, mechanistic studies and in silico ADME predictions of benzimidazole derivatives as novel antifungal agents. *Bioorg. Chem.*, **2020**, *101*, 103956.
[http://dx.doi.org/10.1016/j.bioorg.2020.103956] [PMID: 32512267]

[33]　Çapan, S.; Servi, S.; Dalkılıç, S.; Dalkılıç, L.K. Synthesis and anticancer evaluation of benzimidazole derivatives having norbornene/dibenzobarrelene skeletons and different functional Groups. *ChemistrySelect*, **2020**, *5*, 14393-14398.
[http://dx.doi.org/10.1002/slct.202004034]

[34]　Huynh, T.K.H.; Nguyen, T.H.A.; Tran, N.H.S.; Nguyen, T.D.; Hoang, T.K.D. A facile and efficient synthesis of benzimidazole as potential anticancer agents. *J. Chem. Sci.*, **2020**, *132*, 84.
[http://dx.doi.org/10.1007/s12039-020-01783-4]

[35]　Sireesha, R.; Sreenivasulu, R.; Chandrasekhar, C.; Jadav, S.S.; Pavani, Y.; Rao, M.V.B.; Subbarao, M. Design, synthesis, anticancer and binding mode studies of benzimidazole/benzoxazole linked β-carboline derivatives. *J. Mol. Struct.*, **2021**, *1226*, 129351.
[http://dx.doi.org/10.1016/j.molstruc.2020.129351]

[36]　Revarthy, S.; Amruyha, U.; Sneha, J.; Shalumol, A.; Leena, K. Synthesis, characterization and study some of physical properties of novel 1,3,4-oxadiazole derivatives. *Res. J. Pharm. Biol. Chem. Sci.*, **2017**, *8*, 468.

[37]　Glomb, T.; Szymankiewicz, K.; Swiatek, P. Anticancer activity of derivatives of 1,3,4-oxadiazoles. *Molecule*, **2018**, *23*, 3361.
[http://dx.doi.org/10.3390/molecules23123361]

[38]　Akhtar, J.; Khan, A.A.; Ali, Z.; Haider, R.; Shahar Yar, M. Structure-activity relationship (SAR) study and design strategies of nitrogen-containing heterocyclic moieties for their anticancer activities. *Eur. J. Med. Chem.*, **2017**, *125*, 143-189.

[http://dx.doi.org/10.1016/j.ejmech.2016.09.023] [PMID: 27662031]

[39] Jaroch, K.; Karolak, M.; Górski, P.; Jaroch, A.; Krajewski, A.; Ilnicka, A.; Sloderbach, A.; Stefański, T.; Sobiak, S. Combretastatins: *In vitro* structure-activity relationship, mode of action and current clinical status. *Pharmacol. Rep.,* **2016**, *68*(6), 1266-1275.
[http://dx.doi.org/10.1016/j.pharep.2016.08.007] [PMID: 27686966]

[40] Kamal, A.; Srikanth, P.S.; Vishnuvardhan, M.V.; Kumar, G.B.; Suresh Babu, K.; Hussaini, S.M.; Kapure, J.S.; Alarifi, A. Combretastatin linked 1,3,4-oxadiazole conjugates as a Potent Tubulin Polymerization inhibitors. *Bioorg. Chem.,* **2016**, *65*, 126-136.
[http://dx.doi.org/10.1016/j.bioorg.2016.02.007] [PMID: 26943479]

[41] Sun, J.; Ren, S.Z.; Lu, X.Y.; Li, J.J.; Shen, F.Q.; Xu, C.; Zhu, H.L. Discovery of a series of 1,3,4-oxadiazole-2(3H)-thione derivatives containing piperazine skeleton as potential FAK inhibitors. *Bioorg. Med. Chem.,* **2017**, *25*(9), 2593-2600.
[http://dx.doi.org/10.1016/j.bmc.2017.03.038] [PMID: 28363444]

[42] Altıntop, M.D.; Sever, B.; Akalın Çiftçi, G.; Turan-Zitouni, G.; Kaplancıklı, Z.A.; Özdemir, A. Design, synthesis, in vitro and in silico evaluation of a new series of oxadiazole-based anticancer agents as potential Akt and FAK inhibitors. *Eur. J. Med. Chem.,* **2018**, *155*, 905-924.
[http://dx.doi.org/10.1016/j.ejmech.2018.06.049] [PMID: 29966916]

[43] Ehrsam, D.; Porta, F.; Mori, M.; Schwabedissen, H.E.M.Z.; Dalla Via, L.; Garcia-Argaez, A.N.; Basile, L.; Meneghetti, F.; Villa, S.; Gelain, A. Unravelling the Antiproliferative Activity of 1,2,5-oxadiazole Derivatives. *Anticancer Res.,* **2019**, *39*(7), 3453-3461.
[http://dx.doi.org/10.21873/anticanres.13491] [PMID: 31262869]

[44] Han, X.; Yu, Y.L.; Ma, D.; Zhang, Z.Y.; Liu, X.H. Synthesis, telomerase inhibitory and anticancer activity of new 2-phenyl-4H-chromone derivatives containing 1,3,4-oxadiazole moiety. *J. Enzyme Inhib. Med. Chem.,* **2021**, *36*(1), 344-360.
[http://dx.doi.org/10.1080/14756366.2020.1864630] [PMID: 33356666]

[45] Srinivas, M.; Satyaveni, S.; Ram, B. Design, synthesis, and biological evaluation of 1,2,4-oxadiazol--isoxazole linked quinazoline derivatives as anticancer agents. *Russ. J. Gen. Chem.,* **2019**, *89*, 2492-2497.
[http://dx.doi.org/10.1134/S1070363219120260]

[46] Alderawy, M.Q.A.; Alrubaie, L.A.R.; Sheri, F.H. Synthesis, characterization of ibuprofen *N*-acy--1,3,4-oxadiazole derivatives and anticancer activity against MCF-7 cell line. *Sys Rev Pharm,* **2020**, *11*(4), 681-689.

[47] Hamdy, R.; Elseginy, S.A.; Ziedan, N.I.; El-Sadek, M.; Lashin, E.; Jones, A.T.; Westwell, A.D. Design, synthesis and evaluation of new bioactive oxadiazole derivatives as anticancer agents targeting Bcl-2. *Int. J. Mol. Sci.,* **2020**, *21*(23), 8980.
[http://dx.doi.org/10.3390/ijms21238980] [PMID: 33256166]

[48] Pragathi, Y.J.; Veronica, D.; Rao, M.V.B.; Raju, R.R. Design, synthesis, and anticancer activity of 1,3,4-oxadiazole incorporated 5-(pyrimidin-5-yl)benzo[d]oxazole derivatives. *Russ. J. Gen. Chem.,* **2020**, *90*, 2371-2375.
[http://dx.doi.org/10.1134/S1070363220120221]

[49] Shahzadi, I.; Zahoor, A.F.; Rasul, A.; Rasool, N.; Raza, J.; Fasal, S.; Parveen, B.; Kamal, S.; Rehman, M.; Zahid, F.M. Synthesis, anticancer, and computational studies of 1, 3,4-oxadiazole-purine derivatives. *J. Heterocycl. Chem.,* **2020**, *57*(7), 2782-2794.
[http://dx.doi.org/10.1002/jhet.3987]

[50] Bhatt, P.; Sen, A.; Jha, A. Design and ultrasound assisted synthesis of novel 1,3,4-oxadiazole drugs for anti-cancer activity. *ChemistrySelect,* **2020**, *5*, 3347-3354.
[http://dx.doi.org/10.1002/slct.201904412]

[51] Shamsi, F.; Hasan,, P.; Queen, A. Synthesis and SAR studies of novel 1,2,4-oxadiazole-sulfonamide based compounds as potential anticancer agents for colorectal cancer therapy. *Bioorg Chem,* **2020**, *98*,

103754.
[http://dx.doi.org/10.1515/tjb-2016-0240]

[52]　Polothi, R.; Raolji, G.S.B.; Kuchibhotla, V.S.; Sheelam, K.; Tuniki, B.; Thodupunuri, P. Synthesis and biological evaluation of 1,2,4-oxadiazole linked 1,3,4-oxadiazole derivatives as tubulin binding agents. *Synth. Commun.,* **2019**, *49*(13), 1603-1612.
[http://dx.doi.org/10.1080/00397911.2018.1535076]

[53]　Zhu, J.; Mo, J.; Lin, H.Z.; Chen, Y.; Sun, H.P. The recent progress of isoxazole in medicinal chemistry. *Bioorg. Med. Chem.,* **2018**, *26*(12), 3065-3075.
[http://dx.doi.org/10.1016/j.bmc.2018.05.013] [PMID: 29853341]

[54]　Hoter, A.; El-Sabban, M.E.; Naim, H.Y. The HSP90 Family: Structure, Regulation, Function, and Implications in Health and Disease. *Int. J. Mol. Sci.,* **2018**, *19*(9), 2560.
[http://dx.doi.org/10.3390/ijms19092560] [PMID: 30158430]

[55]　Zhang, C.; Wang, X.; Liu, H.; Zhang, M.; Geng, M.; Sun, L.; Shen, A.; Zhang, A. Design, synthesis and pharmacological evaluation of 4,5-diarylisoxazols bearing amino acid residues within the 3-amido motif as potent heat shock protein 90 (Hsp90) inhibitors. *Eur. J. Med. Chem.,* **2017**, *125*, 315-326.
[http://dx.doi.org/10.1016/j.ejmech.2016.09.043] [PMID: 27688186]

[56]　Zhang, M.C.; Gu, S.H.; Liu, G.P.; Li, C.C.; Xu, H.M.; Wu, Z.X.; Ye, B.P.; Lu, Y.Y.; Huang, D.C.; Wang, Z.X.; Jiang, F. Facile synthesis and cytotoxicity of phenazine-chromene hybrid molecules derived from phenazine natural product. *Comb. Chem. High Throughput Screen.,* **2019**, *22*(1), 35-40.
[http://dx.doi.org/10.2174/1386207322666190307125015] [PMID: 30848195]

[57]　Dinesh, V.C.; Hareeshbabu, E.; Krishnakumar, H. Synthesis of hybrid molecules of isoxazole derivatives in search of new anticancer drugs. *IJARIIT,* **2019**, *5*, 1348-1355.

[58]　Arunkumar, T.; Ratnakaram, V.N.; Navuluri, S.; Kishore, K. Novel hybrid molecules of isoxazole chalcone derivatives: synthesis and study of *in vitro* cytotoxic activities. *Lett. Drug Des. Discov.,* **2018**, *15*(6), 576-582.
[http://dx.doi.org/10.2174/1570180814666170914121740]

[59]　Çalışkan, B.; Sinoplu, E.; İbiş, K.; Akhan Güzelcan, E.; Çetin Atalay, R.; Banoglu, E. Synthesis and cellular bioactivities of novel isoxazole derivatives incorporating an arylpiperazine moiety as anticancer agents. *J. Enzyme Inhib. Med. Chem.,* **2018**, *33*(1), 1352-1361.
[http://dx.doi.org/10.1080/14756366.2018.1504041] [PMID: 30251900]

[60]　Shaik, A.; Bhandare, R.R.; Palleapati, K.; Nissankararao, S.; Kancharlapalli, V.; Shaik, S. Antimicrobial, Antioxidant, and Anticancer Activities of Some Novel Isoxazole Ring Containing Chalcone and Dihydropyrazole Derivatives. *Molecules,* **2020**, *25*(5), 1047.
[http://dx.doi.org/10.3390/molecules25051047] [PMID: 32110945]

[61]　Shahinshavali, S.; Sreenivasulu, R.; Guttikonda, V.R. Synthesis and anticancer activity of amide derivatives of 1,2-isoxazole combined 1,2,4-thiadiazole. *Russ. J. Gen. Chem.,* **2019**, *89*, 324-329.
[http://dx.doi.org/10.1134/S1070363219020257]

[62]　Rao, B.V.D.; Sreenivasulub, R.; Rao, M.V.B. Design, synthesis, and evaluation of isoxazole-thiadiazole linked carbazole hybrids as anticancer agents. *Russ. J. Gen. Chem.,* **2019**, *89*, 2115-2120.
[http://dx.doi.org/10.1134/S1070363219100207]

[63]　Wang, G.; Liu, W.; Huang, Y.; Li, Y.; Peng, J. Design, synthesis and biological evaluation of isoxazole-napthalene derivatives as anti-tubulin agents. *Arab. J. Chem.,* **2020**, *13*(6), 5765-5775.
[http://dx.doi.org/10.1016/j.arabjc.2020.04.014]

[64]　Kumari, P.; Mishra, V.S.; Narayana, C.; Khanna, A.; Chakrabarty, A.; Sagar, R. Design and efficient synthesis of pyrazoline and isoxazole bridged indole C-glycoside hybrids as potential anticancer agents. *Sci. Rep.,* **2020**, *10*(1), 6660.
[http://dx.doi.org/10.1038/s41598-020-63377-x] [PMID: 32313038]

# SUBJECT INDEX

## A

Abelson kinase 121
Aberrant DNA methylation 13
Ability 5, 7, 15, 66, 125, 134, 187, 189, 249
 antiproliferative 187, 189
 antitumor 189
Abl 105, 122
 kinase inhibitors 105
 mutated gene 122
Abl kinase enzyme 122, 123
 for cancer therapy 122
Acetylation, histone 130, 234
Acid 7, 18, 20, 23, 26, 27, 28, 58, 59, 67, 68,
  73, 74, 75, 76, 77, 80, 131, 132, 133,
  136, 211, 233, 234
 angelic 58, 59
 asiatic 74, 76
 betulinic 74, 76, 80
 boswellic 73
 carnosic 67
 carsonic 58
 conjugated hydroxamic 131
 corosolic 75
 deoxyribose nucleic (DNA) 7, 18, 20, 23,
  26, 27, 28, 67, 132, 133, 136, 233, 234
 dihydrobetulinic 80
 echinocystic 74
 glutamic 80
 glycyrrhetinic 77
 hydrazoic 211
 isovaleric 58, 59
 lucidenic 76
 marrubiinic 80
 marrubinic 80
 maslinic 77
 pachymic 73
 pomolic 75
 pseudolaric 68
 senecioic 58, 59
 tiglic 58, 59
 ursolic 73, 74

Acidification 212
Acids 66, 107, 145, 168, 205, 206, 233
 aromatic 66
 carboxylic 107, 205, 206
 nucleic 145, 168, 233
Actaea recemosa 74
Action-oriented tetrazole derivatives 215
Activate AMPK 75
Activation 10, 15, 20, 59, 61, 64, 65, 71, 73,
  76, 77, 117
 caspase cascade 10
 of apoptosis 59, 117
Activity 75, 120, 121, 135, 144, 145, 146,
  182, 208, 216, 219, 220, 233, 238, 240,
  242, 244, 248, 249, 250, 252, 253
 anti-breast 135
 antimitotic 182
 anti-tubulin 244
 chemoprotective 135
 diabetic 233
 mutagenesis 216
 proteasome 75
 therapeutic 250
Adipose tissues 19, 140
Agents 1, 16, 22, 28, 106, 111, 117, 116, 119,
  133,135, 169, 185, 192
 active chemo-preventive 135
 anticervical cancer 192
 anti-EGFR 117, 119
 antimitotic 111, 116, 185
 anti-mitotic 22, 111
 carcinogenic 16
 novel anticancer 169
 promising anti-neoplastic 28
Akt 8, 67
 and extracellular receptor kinase
 pathways 8
 mTOR pathway 67
 phosphorylation 8
AKT signalling pathway 69
ALDH 167, 197, 180
 inhibition 167, 197

mediated inhibitory activity 16
  pathway 61
*Nigella sativa* 77
Non-receptor tyrosine kinase (NRTKs) 117,
  121
Nucleus 107, 110, 135
  heterocyclic pyrazole 135

# O

Oncogenes 13, 61
Osteosarcoma 8
Ovarian 12, 16, 26, 153, 248
  cancer 12, 16, 26, 248
  carcinoma therapy 153
Oxygen 173, 232, 233

# P

Pancreatic cancer cells 16
Pathways 15, 59, 71, 124
  paraptosis 15
  signaling 71
  therapeutic signaling 124
  ubiquitin-proteasome 59
PERK pathway 15
Pharmacological properties, multifunctional
  70
Pharmacophores 20, 64, 68, 72, 74, 127, 138,
  169, 132, 178, 215, 218, 223
  synthesise multifunctional 169
Phosphorylation 68, 74, 127, 138
  activating transcription-3 72
  inhibiting 20
Phytoestrogen 18
Poison(s) 23, 132
  cytotoxicity 132
  mitosis 23
PP2A inhibition 61
Pro-apoptotic proteins 10, 64
Processes 2, 9, 18, 64, 67, 68, 72, 106, 124,
  137, 220
  cytokinesis 137
  fermentation 106

intrinsic 9
metabolic 124
signalling 68
Production 16, 57, 117, 118, 127, 132
  reactive oxygen species 16
Progression 8, 13, 16, 28, 117, 122
  free survival time 28
  reduced angiogenesis 8
Proliferation 13, 16, 17, 18, 61, 64, 65, 68, 72,
  79, 140, 148
  inhibiting 64
Proliferator-activated receptor gamma 79
Propylenediamine 220
Prostate cancer 6, 12, 22, 31, 32, 60, 61, 65,
  79, 121, 139, 168
  metastatic castration-resistant 22
  progression 31
Prostate carcinoma 12, 26, 31
  cells 12
Prostatic intraepithelial neoplasia 31
Protease 76
Proteasomes 71
Protein arginine 220, 223, 214, 223
  deiminases (PADs) 220, 223
  methyltransferases 214, 218
Protein kinase enzyme 27, 117
Protein kinases 64, 68, 69, 75
  mitogen-activated 68
Protein(s) 7, 10, 11, 12, 61, 64, 67, 68, 76,
  111, 127, 140, 142, 143, 167, 170, 238,
  250
  anti-apoptotic 64
  apoptotic 68
  disease-creating 167
  enzymatic 238
  phosphatase 61
Proteomic analysis 79
Pyridine nucleus 113
Pyrimidine 120
  moieties 120
  nucleus 120

www.ingramcontent.com/pod-product-compliance
Lightning Source LLC
Chambersburg PA
CBHW050816220326
41598CB00006B/231